The Nuts and
Bolts of
Paced ECG Interpretation

Commissioning Editor: Thomas V. Hartman
Development Editor: Kate Newell
Production Editor: Cathryn Gates

The Nuts and Bolts of Paced ECG Interpretation

Tom Kenny

St Jude Medical
Austin, Texas
USA

⊗WILEY-BLACKWELL

A John Wiley & Sons, Ltd., Publication

This edition first published 2009, © 2009 by St. Jude Medical

Blackwell Publishing was acquired by John Wiley & Sons in February 2007. Blackwell's publishing program has been merged with Wiley's global Scientific, Technical and Medical business to form Wiley-Blackwell.

Registered office: John Wiley & Sons Ltd, The Atrium, Southern Gate, Chichester, West Sussex, PO19 8SQ, UK

Editorial offices: 9600 Garsington Road, Oxford, OX4 2DQ, UK
      The Atrium, Southern Gate, Chichester, West Sussex, PO19 8SQ, UK
      111 River Street, Hoboken, NJ 07030-5774, USA

For details of our global editorial offices, for customer services and for information about how to apply for permission to reuse the copyright material in this book please see our website at www.wiley.com/wiley-blackwell

Library of Congress Cataloging-in-Publication Data

Kenny, Tom, 1954-
  The nuts and bolts of paced ECG interpretation / Tom Kenny.
    p. ; cm.
  ISBN 978-1-4051-8404-5
  1. Electrocardiography. 2. Cardiac pacing. I. Title.
  [DNLM: 1. Electrocardiography--methods. 2. Cardiac Pacing, Artificial. WG 140 K365n 2009]
  RC683.5.E5K46 2009
  616.1'207547--dc22

                                         2008055897

ISBN: 9781405184045

A catalogue record for this book is available from the British Library.

Set in 9.5/12 pt Minion by Sparks, Oxford – www.sparkspublishing.com

1   2009

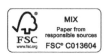

Contents

Preface

It seems that every time I start to talk about cardiac pacing and how devices work and how clinicians can better care for the device patients they see, it always comes back to the paced ECG. As much as we like to talk about advanced device features or describe the wonders of downloadable diagnostic reports, I am increasingly convinced that the key to really understanding device behavior is contained in the paced ECGs.

And yet paced ECGs are surprisingly intimidating, even to clinicians who navigate around non-paced ECGs all day long. Pacemakers can behave in unusual and unexpected ways and even when they are behaving themselves appropriately, they can leave a mysterious paced ECG behind for clinicians to deal with.

I wrote this book to supplement the first book in *The Nuts and Bolts* series, *The Nuts and Bolts of Cardiac Pacing*. That book, recently revised and updated, contains a lot of good and useful information about how pacemakers work, but it does not take the time to delve thoroughly into the mysteries of the paced ECGs.

Rather than tack this onto the pacing book, I decided to make it a stand-alone volume. Much of the material in this book applies to ICDs with pacing function as well as pacemakers. And because it is its own volume, it can be as thorough as I wanted it to be.

While some clinicians may cringe at seeing a paced ECG, I always like to see them. I like them because most of the time, they tell me that a person is getting improved quality of life and possibly better functional capacity because of a tiny implanted device. I also like them because they can sometimes be a bit of a puzzle. Yet by knowing the basics, keeping it as simple as possible (when in doubt, look at the most obvious solutions), and evaluating everything in a steady, systematic way, most clinicians can learn to interpret tracings accurately.

Early in my career, I was given a great piece of advice with respect to paced ECGs. I was told, "You see only what you look for, you recognize only what you know!" I heard it from one of my first mentors, Dr. Michael Chizner, but the original quotation comes from W. Proctor Harvey, MD, a pioneer of cardiology and professor of medicine at Georgetown University in Washington, D.C. I suspect that many young device specialists struggling to interpret a paced ECG heard that same bit of advice.

It is my privilege, as author of this book, to hand down this sage bit of advice. Don't let the simplicity of the saying deceive you. It's a powerful insight that will help you very well as you master the art and science of paced ECGs. "You see only what you look for, you recognize only what you know!"

By the way, paced ECGs (or any tracing) can be surprisingly controversial. That's one reason they call it *ECG interpretation*! I have frequently observed formal and informal sessions where respected, knowledgeable, expert colleagues have vigorously disagreed with each other about what a paced ECG might actually mean. The truth is, sometimes we do not know for sure what is going on from an ECG (particularly just one short section of a tracing and viewed apart from the patient). As we developed the workbook section of this book, I saw many ECGs that my colleagues might interpret differently than I do. In the event that you disagree with my interpretations, that's not entirely unexpected! For my part, I tried to provide evidence for my conclusions so that you can at least follow my thinking. In a few instances, my interpretation is based on "the most likely" interpretation, which, as we all know, may not always be the true one.

I must thank my very wonderful editor at Blackwell, Gina Almond, for her patience and willingness to share my passion for this admittedly unusual subject, and to Kate Newell at Blackwell who does the magic of putting these books together. This is the first time Kate and I have worked together, and it has been a pleasure. As usual, thanks to my creative team who helps translate my ideas into book form. I am indebted to Jo Ann LeQuang (who helps guide the project from my first phone call when I announce, "hey, I've got an idea" through the final printing) and Belinda Kinkade (who is one of the few professional artists in the world who can now read paced ECGs). I would also like to thank all of my colleagues at St. Jude Medical who have been overwhelmingly supportive of these books and who are always glad to hear about how useful these volumes have been in your own practice.

As always, I am indebted to my family for their patience as they provided encouragement for me and "another book." Much of the material for this book has been taken from work done here at St. Jude Medical and I thank my many colleagues for their support and suggestions to make this the best possible book.

Tom Kenny
May, 2009
Austin, Texas

Before We Start …

I wanted to start out this book at ground zero! Whether you are an old hand at ECG interpretation or brand new to the clinical world, ECG interpretation is a challenging practice that can keep you studying – and learning – for an entire career! Paced ECGs are even more of a challenge since the electrical representation of what's going on in the heart reflects not only intrinsic activity (which can be difficult enough to interpret at times) but also device activity. Device activity changes intrinsic activity and intrinsic activity changes device activity. It can be exciting to see how devices can restore a heart rhythm, but it does not make interpreting paced tracings any easier.

Your job in evaluating a paced ECG is to determine not only what's going on but to offer a clinical assessment as to the value of what's going on. Is it helping? Could the device be programmed more appropriately? Is the patient benefiting from the therapy as well as he might? Is the device not "seeing" all that it should see?

The fundamental rule in paced ECG interpretation is this: **you see only what you look for, you recognize only what you know.**

A secondary rule is that you need to approach any paced ECG systematically. Over the years, I have developed my own system and I am going to inflict that on my readers in this book. But the actual system itself is not as important as the fact that you take a careful, point-by-point approach to looking at any ECG. Don't skip over things or look at any ECG haphazardly. Too much is at stake for you to approach a paced tracing casually. It can be very tempting to home in on some unusual aspect of a tracing and miss the big picture. That's why you can't beat the system when it comes to paced ECGs.

Many of the seemingly simple ECGs you encounter in the clinical setting can turn out to be very challenging, and sometimes an odd-looking ECG is quite clear-cut. Because looks can be deceiving, the systematic approach is invaluable. It will help you uncover troublespots in ECGs that look – at a glance – to be quite normal and it will give you confidence to interpret unusual tracings.

The first portion of this book is going to train you to recognize some of the key landmarks on paced rhythm strips. We'll go over pacing spikes, paced events, timing cycles, fusion and pseudofusion, and how to determine pacing rates. This entire first section of the book is my attempt to show you the many things that you are going to need to be able to find and distinguish on a paced ECG.

You'll learn with visual examples. These first chapters are roughly arranged in order of difficulty, but it is my experience as a teacher that those rankings are subjective. If you find a topic particularly challenging, stay with it until you learn the basics.

And with paced ECGs, it always comes back to the basics! It's all about pacing spikes, sensing, capture, and timing cycles. Just keep those four principles in mind. From there, we'll build up to rates and special features. It's a matter of building from the ground up – because you can't really begin to understand hysteresis behavior until you understand the basics. So please do not rush through the first part of this book, and do not hesitate to revisit it periodically as a refresher.

You'll also see examples of pacemaker features in action that can complicate the paced ECG. For instance, it's not unusual in paced patients to see a paced rhythm at a rate above or below the programmed base rate! Oversensing and undersensing are not uncommon on paced rhythm strips. Fusion and pseudofusion have puzzled many clinicians! And if the patient has high-rate intrinsic atrial activity, the pacemaker can demonstrate what we call "upper-rate behavior" or mode switching, all of which show up on the ECG.

The Nuts and Bolts of Paced ECG Interpretation, 1st edition. By Tom Kenny.
Published 2009 by Blackwell Publishing, ISBN: 978-1-4501-8404-5.

Once you know what to look for, you can evaluate most paced ECGs without much trouble, **because you are going to recognize what you know**.

The second part of the book is my favorite. I've found about 100 paced ECGs that I have collected over the years. Most of them are not particularly unusual ECGs. In fact, I'd venture to say that if you worked full-time at a pacing clinic, you'd run into the things illustrated in these strips routinely over the course of a year. I saved these particular strips because they illustrate the very things that clinicians ought to look for (and that means these are the things clinicians must know!). They're assembled in a workbook format so you can try your hand at evaluating the paced ECG yourself and then read through my systematic analysis on the next pages.

I divided the workbook into sections, rather subjectively classified as easy, moderate, and tough. Then at the very end, I offer a section I called "scramble," which takes strips of all difficulty levels and offers them in random order. That's actually the way they will be handed to you if you work in a clinic! You just never know what you will see next.

One last caution. For the purposes of this book, we had an artist re-draw all of our ECGs. We did this mainly for the sake of allowing you to focus on the principles of paced ECG interpretation rather than the vagaries of real-world ECG equipment. In practice, you'll see strips at different speeds, in different sizes, and you'll see stuff that can be grainy or blurry. In the real world, you'll see device artifacts and ECGs that seem to want to fly off the page. Don't be put off by the fact that the paced ECGs in this book look a little bit too polished or too "perfect." We did this so you can focus on the basic principles and then apply them to your real-world clinical practice.

Finally, I want to say that I called this book *The Nuts and Bolts of Paced ECG Interpretation* because "interpretation" is all you can do with an ECG. The clues or evidence that appears on a tracing has to be put together with other factors in order to arrive at a "likely explanation" for what appears on the tracing. Tracings don't lie, but they aren't always outspoken with the truth, either. I fully expect that you or other colleagues may occasionally disagree with my interpretation or at least consider a possible ECG interpretation that I dismiss. My interpretation is just that – my interpretation. But it's based on many years of clinical and industry experience. Over that time, primarily as an educator, I gained a keen appreciation of what seems to trip clinicians up when confronting a paced ECG. Many of these strips were selected with that in mind.

An ECG is just one piece of the puzzle in the care of a pacemaker patient and most ECGs can only tell us about how the patient and device interacted over a few moments of time. Patient symptoms, history, and a routine physical exam are all important in the care of a pacemaker patient. Thus, this book is a bit lopsided in that you will get my interpretations based solely on a strip – something I would not do in the clinic if the patient was available!

And remember: **you see only what you look for, you recognize only what you know!**

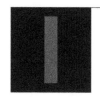

PART I
Timing Cycles and Troubleshooting Review

SECTION 1

Calculating Rates and Intervals

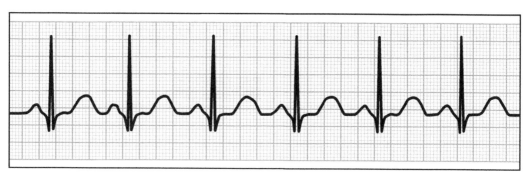

Figure 1.1

Few clinicians can escape their training without having to learn to read a basic ECG. The illustration above is a textbook-type ECG, a perfect example of an ECG that you would probably never see in real-life clinical practice. That's fine, since you should learn from textbooks and then apply your knowledge to the messier ECGs you'll come up with in the clinic.

A surface ECG is a graphic representation of electrical energy. The electricity that generates this tracing is obtained from the surface of the skin of the patient. It's amazing that the heart (about the size of a clenched fist) can generate enough electricity so that it can be picked up on the skin.

The smallest rounded bumps on the ECG are the P-waves, which graphically depict the atrial depolarization. This is followed closely by the largest waveform on the ECG, a pointed wave that goes both below and above the baseline. Called the QRS complex (also sometimes nicknamed an R-wave), this sharp, pointed waveform depicts the depolarization of the ventricles. It's much larger on the tracing because the ventricles are much larger than the atria and produce more electricity as they squeeze together to pump out blood. After a short pause is another rounded waveform known as the T-wave.

The T-wave represents the ventricular repolarization, that is, the time period where the ventricles go back to baseline, in other words, from depolarization to repolarization.

Standard ECG paper has a grid on it that can help you "eyeball" timing. The gridwork is made up of many tiny blocks that are 1 mm square. Each of these tiny boxes is 40 ms duration. Heavier lines are used to make larger squares of five boxes tall and five boxes wide. Each larger square has a duration of 200 ms. Five of these larger squares (200 × 5) equals 1000 ms or 1 sec.

By counting out the grids, you can get a fast approximation of the duration of a particular cardiac cycle or timing cycle. This is going to become increasingly important as we get into paced ECGs. With the heart, timing is everything!

Test your knowledge

1 Looking at this non-paced ECG, would you say that this patient has a regular or an irregular rhythm?
2 Using just this tracing, approximate how long (in ms) the duration is from one P-wave to the next P-wave.

The Nuts and Bolts of Paced ECG Interpretation, 1st edition. By Tom Kenny.
Published 2009 by Blackwell Publishing, ISBN: 978-1-4501-8404-5.

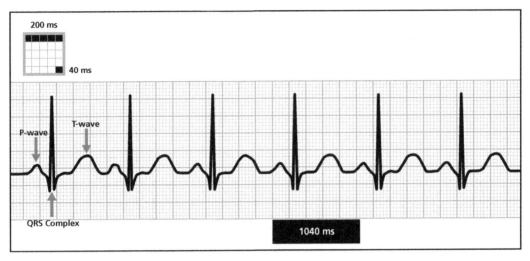

Figure 1.2

This rhythm is regular. Once your eye gets trained to reading ECGs, it is easy to look at a rhythm and appreciate something that is regular or irregular. What makes this rhythm regular, however, is not that the QRS amplitudes are the same or the T-waves have the same morphology (shape). (Those things matter, but for different reasons that we'll get into later on.) The regularity of this rhythm refers to its even timing. Notice that the complexes all have the same duration. It doesn't matter whether you measure from P-wave to P-wave, R-wave to R-wave, or T-wave to T-wave, you'll see the same results. In fact, if you go to the very last complex on the strip, and then added some blank grid paper, you would know enough to draw in where the next P-wave and QRS complex would fall.

In this tracing, we can see that the distance between one P-wave and the next consecutive P-wave is about 1040 ms. That's based on 4 big squares (4 × 200 = 800) plus 6 little boxes (6 × 40 = 240). You could also measure QRS to QRS or any other complexes. The trick is to measure from the one waveform to the next consecutive waveform *of that type*.

When clinicians talk about heart rate, we generally use terms like "70 beats per minute" or "82 bpm" or we might say a patient's heart rate is 120/min. In fact, pacemakers almost always program rate in terms of pulses per minute (ppm) even though this information is not obvious on the ECG. While we humans tend to prefer beats per minute as a way to express rate, pacemakers (and ECG machines) use durations or intervals. That is, this strip does tell us the rate in the form of an interval value (1040 ms). But what rate is that?

Clinicians who work with pacemakers have to be able to convert intervals to rates and vice versa. There are conversion tables that do this and many pacemaker programmers will assist you as well. However, it can also be done with some basic arithmetic or a simple calculator. If one cardiac cycle (i.e., one beat) took 1040 ms, how many beats would occur in a minute? First, we know that 1 minute = 60 seconds or 60,000 ms (60 × 1000). By dividing 1040 (the interval duration) into 60,000 ms (1 minute), you arrive at the rate (57.69 beats a minute, which you would probably state as 58 bpm).

The formula works backward, too. For instance, if you know that a patient's heart rate is right around 80 bpm, you could expect to see a cardiac cycle interval duration on the ECG of about 750 ms (80 divided by 60,000). That's three big boxes on the ECG paper and almost four little boxes (3 × 200 = 600 and 4 × 40 = 160).

The nuts and bolts of rates and intervals

- A regular rhythm refers to the timing of the events on the ECG (not necessarily the consistency of waveform shapes).
- Grid paper on an ECG can help you rapidly approximate intervals. Each tiny box is worth 40 ms, the heavier-lined squares count as 200 ms.
- When calculating the interval of a cardiac cycle, measure from one type of event (P-wave or QRS complex or T-wave) to the next consecutive such event.
- Devices tend to "think" in intervals, people tend to think in rates, but they are really just two different ways of expressing the same thing. Convert rate to interval by dividing 60,000 by the rate; convert interval to rate by dividing 60,000 by the interval. For example, 60 ppm converts to a pacing interval of 1000 ms.

Pacing Spikes

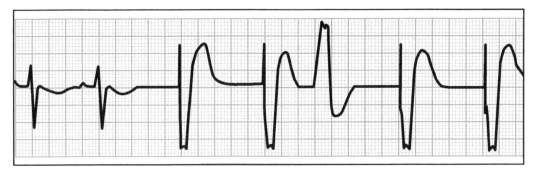

Figure 2.1

This is a paced ECG. You can immediately see it starts to look quite different than a non-paced ECG! The large vertical lines on the strip are pacemaker "spikes," sometimes called pacing artifacts. This is an electrical signal left on the ECG from the pacemaker output pulse. The output pulse leaves a straight line rather than a more filled out space because a pacemaker output pulse has a very short duration. On average, pacemaker output pulses are about 0.4 ms (that's less than one thousandth of one second)! That sort of ultra-short but strong energy will just make a line on the tracing rather than a curved or even pointed shape.

These output pulses are quite large. A pacing expert might look at this tracing and tell you the pacemaker was "unipolar." You'll also encounter pacemaker spikes that are much shorter (bipolar systems). There can be other reasons for prominent pacing spikes or less visible ones. For instance, the gain control on the ECG monitor may affect the size of the pacing artifact. As a rule of thumb, unipolar pacing involves larger, more visible spikes compared to bipolar pacing. However, new ECG equipment can help adjust the spikes so that unipolar and bipolar spikes appear equivalent.

Unipolar and bipolar are pacing terms that are actually a little bit misleading. They refer to the electrical circuit formed when the pacemaker emits an output pulse. All electricity travels in a circuit, and all circuits have two poles (an anode or positive pole and a cathode or negative pole). A unipolar pacemaker has a lead that forms its electrical circuit using the electrode on the lead itself and the pacemaker can. A bipolar system has a lead with two electrodes that forms a circuit. Thus, the terms "unipolar" and "bipolar" really refer to *how many poles are in use on the lead*. A unipolar pacemaker has electricity that travels over a wider area than a bipolar pacemaker. As a result, you can expect unipolar pacemakers to show larger pacing spikes than bipolar pacemakers.

The first two QRS complexes on this strip are non-paced. The pacemaker spike appears before the QRS complex in the rest of the complexes. Note that the pacing spike changes the morphology or shape of the QRS complex. This occurs to varying degrees by patient and by the lead observed, but a clinician can often "see" the difference between a paced ventricular depolarization and an intrinsic ventricular depolarization.

There is also an odd-looking event in the middle of the strip. It's an upward deflection with notches.

Test your knowledge

1 Can you see atrial activity on this rhythm strip? Is there atrial pacing going on?

The Nuts and Bolts of Paced ECG Interpretation, 1st edition. By Tom Kenny.
Published 2009 by Blackwell Publishing, ISBN: 978-1-4501-8404-5.

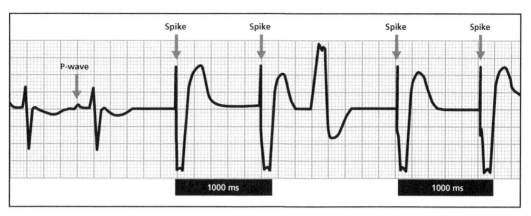

Figure 2.2

2 How many pacing spikes do you see on this strip? Which chamber of the heart is being paced?

3 Using the grid, approximately how long is the interval between the last pacemaker spike and the one before it?

4 Is that the same as the interval between the first pacemaker spike and the one immediately following it? What rate would this be?

5 What is that odd-looking event in the middle of the strip?

Atrial activity does show up on this ECG but it is not consistent. An imperfect atrial rhythm is nothing unusual, since patients with pacemakers have serious cardiac rhythm problems! The P-wave indicated in the illustration marks an intrinsic atrial depolarization, that is, there is no pacemaker spike to show that a pacemaker output pulse was in any way associated with that atrial event.

There are four pacemaker spikes on this strip. They are large spikes and they show up in association with ventricular events. You can also see that the paced ventricular beats look noticeably different than the intrinsic ventricular events that appear at the beginning of this strip. If you get ECGs with lots of paced and non-paced ventricular activity, it is often possible to use morphology alone to distinguish paced from intrinsic beats.

Looking at the first ventricular spike and the one immediately following it and the last ventricular spike and the one immediately preceding it, the grid work gives us an approximate interval duration of 1000 ms (5 large squares × 200 ms). Converting 1000 ms to a

rate is the easiest of all of the interval values: 1000 ms equals 60 beats per minute. The intervals between the two sets of pacing spikes we measured are the same, which shows a nice, consistent pacing rate. (In the clinic, you should check this against how the device was programmed. For this particular patient, expect to see a ventricular pacing rate of 60 ppm.)

In the middle of this strip, there is an odd-looking upward deflection. It looks a lot like a paced ventricular event, but it has a different morphology (shape) and there is a noticeable absence of pacemaker spike. Since this depolarization is not paced, it has to be intrinsic. It appears that about 600 ms (3 large squares × 200 ms) after the previous ventricular output pulse, the ventricles contracted on their own. This is a premature ventricular contraction or PVC. They are not uncommon to see in clinical practice, and they show up on paced ECGs just like non-paced ECGs.

The question with the PVC is this: what does the pacemaker do with it? All pacemakers do only two things: they sense and they pace. We see evidence of ventricular pacing in this strip. Here, with the PVC, we also have good evidence of ventricular sensing. If you try to calculate the interval from the previous pacemaker spike to the PVC, you'll see that it is much shorter than 1000 ms. That's because this was a PVC, that is, it occurred much earlier in the cardiac timing cycle. However, once the PVC occurred, the pacemaker should have "sensed" it and used it to reset the pacemaker timing. That is, the distance between the PVC and the next ventricular output pulse should be 1000 ms.

If you measure from the initial upward deflection of the PVC to the next pacemaker spike, you will get five large squares or 1000 ms. This means the pacemaker sensed the PVC, counted it as an intrinsic ventricular event (which it was) and then timed its next pacemaker output to occur 1000 ms later. That is good evidence of appropriate ventricular sensing.

When a pacemaker senses intrinsic cardiac activity that occurs in certain time periods (called "alert periods"), the pacemaker counts the event and uses it as a "landmark" on which to base future timing. In this case, the intrinsic ventricular event (premature ventricular contraction or PVC) caused the pacemaker to withhold a pacemaker output until 1000 ms after the PVC. Had the PVC not occurred, the next pacemaker spike would have occurred much earlier, that is, 1000 ms after the previous spike. The ability of the pacemaker to withhold pacing when events are sensed is known as "inhibition." Here, a PVC occurred which inhibited the ventricular output until the appropriate interval timing could be restored.

The nuts and bolts of pacing spikes

- Pacemaker output pulses appear on the ECG as spikes, vertical lines. They can be large or small, depending on the pacemaker system and ECG equipment but will be consistent within the strip.
- Unipolar devices tend to leave larger spikes on the ECG than bipolar systems. Both unipolar and bipolar devices provide excellent pacing reliability. The difference is the size of the electrical "antenna." A unipolar device delivers an output pulse that makes a larger circuit through the body than a bipolar device.
- Unipolar and bipolar in pacing are actually misnomers. All electrical circuits have two poles! A unipolar device has one pole *on the lead*, a bipolar device has two poles *on the lead*.
- When pacing at the programmed base rate, you should see spikes appear at precisely timed and consistent intervals. However, if intrinsic events occur between paced events, it can reset the timing.
- Pacemakers can only do two things: sense and pace. One evidence for pacing is the tell-tale spike. You cannot "see" sensing as obviously, but you can measure it. When an intrinsic event resets timing, that is good evidence that it has been seen or sensed by the pacemaker.
- Inhibition occurs when a pacemaker withholds ("inhibits") an output pulse because of intrinsic cardiac activity.
- Paced QRS complexes tend to have a different morphology than intrinsic QRS complexes. Paced ventricular beats tend to be wider and might have a notch. This is not always the case, but is common.
- Pacing at the right-ventricular (RV) apex typically causes a wider QRS complex and a QRS morphology that resembles left bundle-branch block (LBBB). Most patients with conventional pacemakers are paced from the RV apex.
- Seeing a pacemaker spike followed by a wider notched QRS complex is good evidence of ventricular capture.

SECTION 3

The Basics of Capture and Sensing

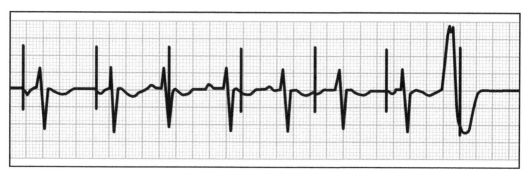

Figure 3.1

This paced ECG shows atrial and ventricular activity, but notice where the pacing spikes fall. This is an ECG from a device pacing the atrium. In the very first complex, there is an atrial spike, an atrial event, and an intrinsic ventricular event. It happens again in the second complex. But now look at the third complex.

In this particular complex, the pacing spike falls right in the middle of the ventricular complex. The QRS complex is not paced; it has the same morphology as the intrinsic QRS complexes that preceded it. What's going on? *The spike occurs on the atrial channel* and although it occurs at the same time as the ventricular event, it is unrelated to the intrinsic ventricular event.

The next pacing spike occurs after an intrinsic ventricular event. Then there is another "displaced" spike. In terms of what is going on in the heart, the spikes seem to just occur at random. But take a closer look! It isn't random at all. Measure the distance between the spikes. You can eyeball it or get out the calipers. You'll be able to count out 840 ms between spikes (4 large squares and 1 small box or 4 × 200 = 800 + 40 = 840 ms) which converts to about 71 beats a minute.

This pacing behavior is not random at all; the atrial spikes appear at precise intervals. However, they are not synchronized or working with the intrinsic activity.

This strip is an example of what we would call an asynchronous pacing mode. It's AOO pacing. The device paces the atrium but it does not sense; in fact, is has no regard for intrinsic activity.

In clinical practice, you won't see asynchronous pacing very much, but it can be used for testing, backup pacing, and may be used in certain unusual situations. You should be aware of what asynchronous pacing looks like, though! In this strip, it is appropriate since the device is programmed to AOO pacing, and this is clearly AOO pacing. In most instances, however, clinicians would want to avoid this kind of pacing.

By the way, "appropriate" is a favorite word for pacing experts because it refers to what the device "ought to do." Since this pacemaker was programmed to AOO pacing, the above strip is absolutely appropriate. However, if the pacemaker was programmed to AAI pacing and this strip appeared, there would be a problem. That's why, as a clinician, it is always useful (even if not always possible) to know the pacing mode and other programmed settings.

By the way, appropriate means the expected behavior of the device as programmed. Sometimes a

The Nuts and Bolts of Paced ECG Interpretation, 1st edition. By Tom Kenny.
Published 2009 by Blackwell Publishing, ISBN: 978-1-4501-8404-5.

pacemaker performs appropriately, but it is not necessarily the optimal pacing therapy for the patient. This strip might be a good example of pacing that is appropriate, but not optimal!

Test your knowledge

1 Would you say that there is atrial capture going on in this strip? If so, where?

2 Would you say that there is atrial sensing going on in this strip? If so, where?

3 How would you explain the last complex in this strip?

4 Is there any ventricular pacing going on in this strip?

5 If somebody were to ask you to "prove" this strip showed asynchronous pacing, how would you prove it?

Atrial capture occurs when there is an atrial pacing spike that causes an immediate atrial depolarization, which would show up on the strip as an atrial event (P-wave). The first, second, and next-to-last complex all show an atrial pacing spike and an immediate atrial depolarization. But was it capture? It is what a pacing specialist might call "apparent capture." That is, it looks like capture but it is hard to know for certain.

The reason that it is "apparent capture" rather than "definitely capture" is that the strip shows other intrinsic atrial activity for this patient. The atria are beating on their own, although not regularly and not every complex. So it is possible that a pacing spike just happened to occur precisely at the moment the atria depolarized. From this tracing by itself, it is just not possible to be sure there was true capture.

Atrial sensing means that the pacemaker would "see" intrinsic atrial activity and then adjust pacing behavior. That is not happening. For instance, the fourth pacing spike falls relatively quickly after an intrinsic atrial event. Had the pacemaker "seen" that intrinsic atrial event, it would have inhibited the atrial output.

You can also get a clue that there is no sensing going on by the fact that although the patient's rhythm is a bit erratic, the pacing spikes appear with military precision every 840 ms. When a pacemaker is sensing, you will only see such exact pacing spikes when the patient has a very stable rhythm. (By the way, since this is AOO or asynchronous atrial pacing, you also know from the mode that there is no sensing. This is covered in the next "In Depth" section.)

The last complex in this strip looks a bit strange. The event is a PVC. However, the device delivers an atrial output pulse at the same time. On the ECG, they appear together, but the PVC is an intrinsic ventricular event while the spike occurs on the atrial channel.

If you were to just have one or two complexes of this tracing, it might be hard to say if the pacing spikes were atrial or ventricular. That's because the ECG captures all electrical activity in both chambers and reports it in one tracing. You can't readily see whether the spike is coming from an electrode

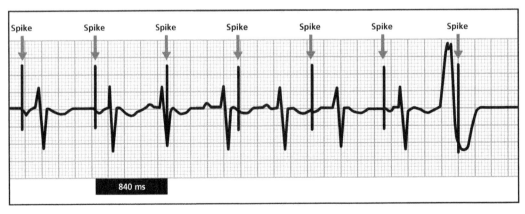

Figure 3.2

in the atrium or the ventricle! But if you look at the larger picture of several complexes, you can see that there is apparent atrial capture in three of the complexes and no examples of apparent or even possible ventricular capture in the rest of the strip.

But the real clincher that shows this is an AOO and not a VOO system is the third complex. If a ventricular output pulse actually occurred in the middle of a ventricular intrinsic beat, it would very likely distort the QRS morphology. The distortion may not be dramatic, but the QRS would show some electrical impact. Since that isn't going on here, the evidence strongly suggests that the spike is atrial.

If you knew the patient had an atrial pacemaker but you did not know the mode and suspected asynchronous pacing, you could demonstrate AOO mode by measuring the distance between pacing spikes. Since asynchronous pacemakers do not sense, there is nothing to change the timing cycles. Pacing spikes appear at regular intervals with no deviation, even if the patient's rhythm is unstable. Further evidence is the fact that intrinsic atrial events do not seem to impact the timing of atrial pacing. If the device could sense atrial activity (and was not sensing inappropriately), the fourth pacing spike would have been greatly delayed. This is almost "textbook" atrial asynchronous pacing!

The nuts and bolts of capture and sensing

- Capture is strongly suggested when a pacing spike is followed immediately by a depolarization.
- When pacing spikes occur at exact intervals with no variation in timing, even when the patient's own rhythm is somewhat unstable, this means the pacing is asynchronous. Asynchronous means pacing occurs without sensing.
- Asynchronous pacing will pace without regard to what is going on in the patient's native rhythm. That means you may see pacemaker spikes falling in unusual places!
- If you look at isolated events on an ECG, it is not always possible to determine if a pacemaker spike was atrial or ventricular in origin; you need to consider all the evidence presented in the strip.
- It is not common to see asynchronous pacing in the average pacemaker patient, but asynchronous pacing may be used for testing situations, backup pacing, or other special circumstances.

Section 4

In Depth: Modes

Whenever you see paced ECGs, it is always a good idea to get as much information as possible about how the pacemaker is programmed. One of the most basic and useful bits of information to know is the pacing mode. Mode refers to how the pacemaker is set up to pace and sense cardiac activity.

Single-chamber modes have pacing function only in one chamber, typically the ventricle. Atrial single-chamber pacemakers do exist, but are not as common to see in clinical practice as ventricular single-chamber pacemakers. **Dual-chamber pacemakers** pace in both chambers. In many practices today, dual-chamber pacemakers are the most typical device you will encounter. Dual-chamber pacing is a bit more complex than single-chamber pacing and will be covered in more detail in later chapters.

The pacemaker code in common use provides three or four letters that are shorthand for how the device functions. The first letter shows where the device paces, the second letter shows where the device senses, and the third letter shows what it does if it senses an event. If the device offers rate response (covered in a later chapter), the fourth letter will be an R. If there is no fourth letter, you should assume the device is not rate responsive.

A VVI pacemaker paces in the ventricle (V), senses in the ventricle (V) and when it senses in the ventricle, its response is to inhibit (I) or withhold an output pulse.

An AAI device is the same thing, but in the atrium.

VVT pacing refers to a device that paces in the ventricle (V), senses in the ventricle (V), but when it senses something in the ventricle, its response will be to track (T) or pace in response. Tracking means that an output pulse is required of the device. AAT is the atrial counterpart to VVT mode.

For dual-chamber devices, the most common annotation is DDD or DDDR. A DDDR device paces in both chambers (D or dual), sensed in both cham-

bers (D) and when it senses something may either inhibit or track (D for dual response) and it has rate response (R).

The "either inhibit or track" response conveyed by the third D in DDD is a bit tricky. If the pacemaker senses an intrinsic atrial event, it will inhibit an atrial output pulse; likewise, if it senses an intrinsic ventricular event, it will inhibit a ventricular output pulse. However, if the DDDR pacemaker senses an atrial event, it will force a ventricular output if an intrinsic ventricular event does not occur at the proper time ("tracking"). The purpose of atrial tracking is to allow the pacemaker to provide 1:1 AV synchrony (one atrial event matched to one ventricular event), even if the patient's intrinsic atrial rate goes above the programmed pacing rate. Thus, a DDD pacemaker that senses an atrial event will withhold the next atrial output pulse (inhibition) but may pace the ventricle in response (tracking).

All of these types of pacing could be called "synchronous" pacing. An older term for synchronous pacing was "demand pacing" (the pacemaker paced when the patient's heart required or demanded it). **Synchronous pacing** means that the pacemaker senses cardiac activity and attempts to fill in the missing beats only if necessary. Synchronous pacing (VVI, VVIR, AAI, AAIR, VVT, AAT, DDD, DDDR, DDI, DDIR, etc.) might be thought of as pacing that tries to sync up or time itself to work with the patient's intrinsic activity. Synchronous pacing always involves both pacing and sensing.

Asynchronous pacing is pacing without sensing. When you see asynchronous pacing, there will be regular pacing spikes but they may fall in strange places with regard to the patient's own rhythm. There is no attempt to sync pacing activity to the patient's intrinsic cardiac activity. As a general rule, asynchronous pacing is not beneficial for most patients and is rarely, if ever, used. Asynchronous modes are available for testing purposes and special

The Nuts and Bolts of Paced ECG Interpretation, 1st edition. By Tom Kenny.
Published 2009 by Blackwell Publishing, ISBN: 978-1-4501-8404-5.

Mode	What it does	What to expect on the ECG
VOO	Asynchronous ventricular pacing	Regular ventricular pacing spikes without any regard to intrinsic activity
VVI	Paces and senses the ventricle	Ventricular capture (with widened QRS morphologies), ventricular inhibition when a ventricular depolarization occurs on its own
VVT	Paces the ventricle at regular intervals or when an intrinsic ventricular event occurs	Ventricular capture (with widened QRS morphologies) at regular intervals – this happens when there is no intrinsic ventricular depolarization. If intrinsic ventricular depolarizations occur, you'll see a somewhat different QRS morphology with a spike in it. These may occur at more irregular intervals (matching the patient's intrinsic ventricular rate)
AOO	Asynchronous atrial pacing	Regular atrial pacing spikes without any regard to intrinsic activity; it may not be immediately clear if the spikes are atrial or ventricular unless you can see several complexes
AAI	Paces and senses the atrium	Apparent atrial capture and atrial inhibition when an intrinsic atrial event occurs
AAT	Paces the atrium at regular intervals or when an intrinsic atrial event occurs	Apparent atrial capture at regular intervals – this happens when there is no intrinsic atrial depolarization. If intrinsic atrial activity occurs, you'll see atrial events with a spike. These may occur at more irregular intervals (matching the patient's intrinsic atrial rate)
DOO	Paces and senses both atrium and ventricle but does not sense	Two spikes per complex, with atrial and ventricular spikes occurring at exact intervals with no relation to the patient's own rhythm
DDI	Paces and senses both atrium and ventricle but will inhibit pacing when an intrinsic depolarization occurs	This is a fairly complex ECG which should show atrial capture or sensed atrial activity and ventricular capture or sensed ventricular beats. If the patient has intrinsic atrial activity above the programmed base rate, the ventricles will not be paced to keep up with the native atrial rate.
DDD	Paces and senses both atrium and ventricle but will inhibit pacing when an intrinsic depolarization occurs in one chamber; if it senses an atrial event, it will require the ventricle to depolarize, either by pacing it or sensing an intrinsic event within a certain timing cycle	This paced ECG is both complex and quite common in clinical practice. It will usually show pacing activity going on in both atrium and ventricle. You will often see paced atrial events and paced ventricular events. If sensed events appear, you should see how they were "taken into account" by the pacemaker; in other words, the device inhibits a ventricular spike if there was a native ventricular event. One unique feature of a DDD-paced ECG is that in the presence of rapid intrinsic atrial activity, you may see rapid ventricular pacing, even at rates above the base rate! This is atrial tracking – and we'll cover it more in depth in later sections

circumstances. They are AOO, VOO, and DOO plus their rate-responsive counterparts, AOOR, VOOR, DOOR.

How do you find out the mode? If you have access to a pacemaker programmer and can download programmed settings, the pacemaker's mode will be prominently displayed in most diagnostic and general reports. If the patient carries a pacemaker ID card or other information from his or her doctor, the pacemaker mode may be stated. Pacemaker ID cards state the highest mode to which the pacemaker can be programmed, and this is usually (but not necessarily) how the device is programmed. (A DDDR pacemaker can be programmed to pace as a DDD or DDI or even a VVIR or VVI device! How-

ever, a VVI device cannot be programmed "up" to DDD since it only has one lead.)

If you cannot figure out the mode but know the manufacturer, you can call the Technical Services hotline of the manufacturer and ask about the mode for that particular model of pacemaker. Otherwise, the clinician has to "deduce" the mode by looking at clues on the ECG. Believe it or not, with some practice, most clinicians get fairly adept at recognizing classic pacemaker behavior. By far the most common pacing modes are VVI and VVIR for single-chamber devices and DDD and DDDR for dual-chamber devices.

Modes are programmable, which means that physicians are free to program what they deem the most appropriate mode for a patient. While this is not common practice, it is not unusual for a mode to be changed in response to a clinical situation. For instance, a patient with a DDD device may be repro- grammed to VVI pacing if he has atrial fibrillation. Thus, even if you think you know the mode of the device, you should still look carefully at the paced ECG.

The nuts and bolts of modes in depth

- Most of the time, pacemakers you see in clinical practice will be VVI, VVIR or DDD, DDDR systems. It is rare to see the other modes.
- If you know the name or model number of the device, you can get the mode by going online or calling the manufacturer's Tech Services department. Modes stated are the highest modes available, which is usually what is programmed. However, modes can be changed. You will sometimes encounter patients with a pacemaker that has been programmed to a different mode (i.e., a DDD device set to DDI or VVI).
- Asynchronous pacing is not common but it is usually easy to identify: you'll see pacing spikes at exact intervals without any regard to intrinsic events.
- Synchronous pacing is much more common and it tries to synchronize pacing events with the patient's own cardiac activity. As a result, the pacing spikes can be anything but at exact intervals!
- Inhibition occurs when the device senses an intrinsic event and, in response, withholds (or "inhibits") a pacing spike.
- Tracking means that when the device senses

an intrinsic event, it requires the device to pace. Tracking may occur in a single-chamber pacemaker (VVT or AAT) but those modes are fairly unusual to see in clinical practice. Tracking is most commonly observed in dual-chamber pacemakers (DDD and DDDR). In such cases, when an atrial event is sensed, the device is then "required" to deliver a ventricular output pulse if no intrinsic ventricular depolarization occurs within the proper timing window.
- The pacemaker code is a common shorthand used to describe how devices function. It is used across all manufacturers and in all countries.
- You may sometimes see SSI or SSIR as a pacemaker code. This is actually a manufacturer's designation (not part of the official pacemaker code) but is widely understood. The S means "single." An SSI pacemaker is a single-chamber system which can be implanted in the ventricle (where it would then be known as a VVI pacemaker) or in the atrium (where it would become an AAI pacemaker). Until it is implanted, it may be called an SSI device.

SECTION 5

Ventricular Sensing

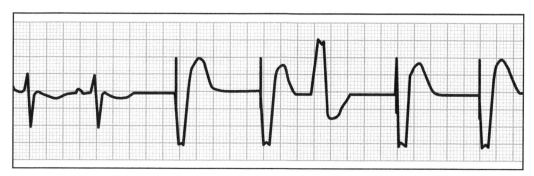

Figure 5.1

With the exception of unusual mode programming, most pacemakers are set up so that they "fill in the blanks" or "put in the beat that is missing" in the patient's own intrinsic cardiac rhythm. That means they listen to the heart (sense) and pace when the heart does not beat within a programmable time limit. If the heart does beat within that timing cycle on its own, the pacemaker withholds or inhibits the pacemaker spike.

Let's come back to this example of VVI pacing. When intrinsic ventricular activity occurs, the pacemaker goes on standby, that is, it inhibits the output pulse. When the patient's heart does not respond in the right timing, the pacemaker delivers an output pulse.

In clinical practice, it is very common to see sensed and paced events occur together. This can be perfectly appropriate pacing behavior in that it indicates that the patient's heart rate is sufficiently fast some of the time, but not all of the time.

Notice the premature ventricular contraction (PVC) about midway on the tracing. When it occurred, it was sensed. If you take calipers and measure the distance spike to spike, you'll see that the timing from the premature ventricular event to the next ventricular pacing spike is exactly the same as the timing from spike to spike. This shows how the

pacemaker "adds" ventricular events where they might have been missing naturally, synchronizing them to intrinsic activity.

Inhibition is also proof that the pacemaker is sensing.

Test your knowledge

1 Counting the very first ventricular complex on the strip, how many sensed ventricular events are there on this strip?
2 How many paced ventricular events are there on the strip?
3 At what rate (pulses per minute) is this pacemaker pacing?
4 Based on this strip, would you say this VVI pacemaker was sensing properly?

There are three sensed ventricular events on this strip. The premature ventricular contraction (PVC) in the middle of the strip may be an unusual ventricular event, but it counts as a sensed ventricular event the same as a more "normal" ventricular contraction. Notice the QRS morphology of the different types of ventricular events:

- The pointy, narrow sensed "normal" intrinsic ventricular depolarization

The Nuts and Bolts of Paced ECG Interpretation, 1st edition. By Tom Kenny.
Published 2009 by Blackwell Publishing, ISBN: 978-1-4501-8404-5.

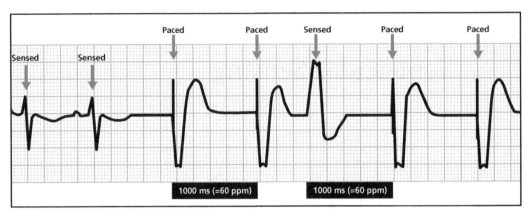

Figure 5.2

- The wider, notched, paced ventricular depolarization (which follows the pattern of left bundle-branch block or LBBB)
- The wider, notched non-paced premature ventricular contraction (PVC)

There are four paced ventricular events on this strip, evidenced by the large ventricular pacing spike immediately preceding the ventricular depolarization.

If you measure the distance between two ventricular pacing spikes (with no intervening sensed events), it measures 1000 ms, which converts to a rate of 60 ppm. The VP-VP interval is also known as the ventricular pacing interval and is sometimes called the "automatic interval." This is a VVI pacemaker pacing at 60 ppm. Notice that the premature ventricular event resets the interval timer so that the timing from the premature ventricular contraction to the next paced ventricular event is also 1000 ms (or 60 ppm).

This strip shows capture (a pacing spike that causes a depolarization) and sensing (an intrinsic event that inhibits the pacemaker from delivering an output pulse).

Sensing appears to be appropriate in that *every intrinsic ventricular event has caused the pacemaker to respond by inhibiting the output pulse and resetting the time cycle*. If the sensed ventricular events had not inhibited the ventricular output pulses, there would be pacing spikes at inappropriate places. The fact that the 1000 ms (60 ppm) timing marches through the strip indicates sensing is appropriate.

The nuts and bolts of ventricular sensing

- Pacemakers are designed to "fill in the missing beats" in a patient's own rhythm. This means they stay on standby when the patient's heart beats on its own, but they pace when a natural beat does not occur within the proper timing interval.
- You can check sensing by noticing if the device resets its timing in the presence of intrinsic events.
- For most commonly used modes, an intrinsic event will inhibit the pacemaker's output.
- As far as the pacemaker is concerned, a premature ventricular contraction is a sensed ventricular event.

SECTION 6

Pacing Intervals

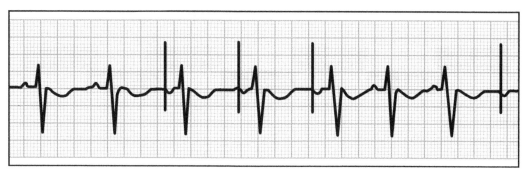

Figure 6.1

This pacing strip shows atrial pacing and sensing. The patient's atrial rate is not always fast, but he appears to have good AV conduction in that every atrial event (sensed or paced) conducts across the AV node and down to the ventricle.

This pacemaker could be an AAI device or it might even be a DDD pacemaker. A dual-chamber pacemaker sometimes functions like an AAI device when the patient has good AV conduction and the ventricles beat in response to the atrial depolarization, regardless of whether it is sensed or paced.

The pacing interval or automatic interval is a timing cycle in pacing that is defined as the time between two consecutive paced events in the same chamber without an intervening sensed event. To find the pacing intervals in this strip, you would measure from one paced atrial event to the next paced atrial event. (As there is only atrial pacing, we're going to have to measure the atrial pacing interval.)

When you measure off pacing intervals with calipers, you should find that in non-rate-responsive devices, the timing between one paced event and the next paced event is exactly the rate interval. A pacemaker set to pace at 60 ppm should have pacing intervals of 1000 ms.

However, when sensed events occur, they will deviate from this strict timing. The time from two sensed atrial events can be anything less than 1000 ms (once the 1000 ms timer times out, the device paces). The time from one paced atrial event to the next sensed atrial event can be anything less than 1000 ms (again, once the timing cycle times out, the pacemaker spike is delivered).

The time from one sensed atrial event to a paced atrial event is going to be 1000 ms. Why? It's because the pacemaker waited for the patient's own heart to beat and when the timing cycle expired (at exactly 1000 ms), the pacemaker paced.

Test your knowledge

1 How many sensed atrial events do you count on this strip?
2 How many sensed ventricular events are there on the strip?
3 Using calipers or another system, mark off the pacing intervals.
4 Are all of the pacing intervals the same length? Is that a problem?

This strip shows four sensed atrial events (atrial contractions with no associated pacing spike) and

The Nuts and Bolts of Paced ECG Interpretation, 1st edition. By Tom Kenny.
Published 2009 by Blackwell Publishing, ISBN: 978-1-4501-8404-5.

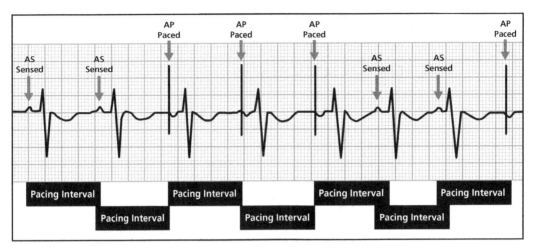

Figure 6.2

four paced atrial events (atrial contractions with a pacing spike … counting the last event that nearly runs off the page). Note that the pacing interval can also be called the "automatic interval."

There is no ventricular pacing going on; every ventricular event is sensed (seven total). The pacing mode shown on this strip is AAI mode. While AAI is not a common mode, there are a couple of reasons why this might happen. First, the pacemaker could be an AAI device. With no ventricular pacing lead, an AAI device will only ever exhibit atrial sensing and pacing and never offer ventricular sensing and pacing.

But AAI-type pacing can occur in DDD devices. In fact, *this is more likely* in that DDD devices are more commonly seen in clinical practice than AAI devices. Here's how this happens in a DDD pacemaker: the pacemaker finds that the atrium does not always beat in the proper timing, so it "fills in" with atrial pacing. However, AV conduction is good so every time the atrium depolarizes (whether on its own or thanks to a pacemaker spike), the ventricles depolarize. A DDD device would then withhold (inhibit) ventricular pacing.

Since this strip shows only atrial pacing, the pacing intervals run from atrial event to atrial event. You can see that using the notations AP (for atrial paced event) and AS (for atrial sensed event) the pacing intervals include

- AS-AS
- AP-AP
- AS-AP
- AP-AS

When the pacing intervals are AP-AP or AS-AP, the timing will match the programmed rate. In this case, those pacing intervals are about 840 ms (about 70 ppm). Unless the device has rate response or other special features that can affect the rate, the rate should remain very consistent in these kinds of pacing intervals.

However, in AS-AS or AP-AS intervals, the concluding sensed event means that the timing cycle did not expire, so the interval will be shorter than the programmed interval (i.e. < 840 ms). The first two sensed atrial events occurred very close to the pacing interval; in fact, unless you really get in with calipers, it's hard to tell that this interval is just a hair shorter than 840 ms. However, the last two sensed atrial events are good examples of an AS-AS pacing interval that is obviously shorter than the programmed pacing rate.

Every atrial event "resets" the pacing or escape interval. You'll notice from the bars below the ECG that sometimes a pacing interval is "cut off" before it can naturally expire by the presence of a sensed event. This is not a problem; it is the expected behavior of the device.

The nuts and bolts of pacing intervals

- The pacing interval is the time between two consecutive paced events in the same chamber without an intervening event. Another name for the pacing interval is automatic interval.
- If the device is not programmed with rate response or other features that can affect rate timing, the pacing interval between two consecutive paced events in the same chamber should be consistent and equivalent to the pacing rate. For instance, a device programmed to 60 ppm should have pacing intervals between paced events of 1000 ms.
- The interval from a sensed event to a paced event is called the "escape interval." The escape interval should match the programmed rate interval.
- Intervals that terminate in a sensed event will be shorter than the programmed rate interval.
- The presence of pacing intervals of varying length on a rhythm strip is not abnormal and is actually quite typical, particularly when the patient has a mixture of paced and sensed events.
- Other causes of rate variation will be addressed later but include such special features as rate hysteresis, rate response, and AF Suppression™ pacing.

7

SECTION 7

Loss of Capture

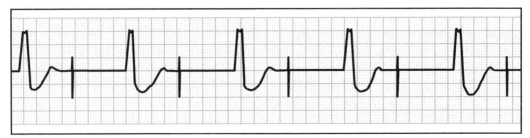

Figure 7.1

This rhythm strip comes from a patient with a VVI pacemaker. You can see large ventricular pacing spikes "marching through" the strip. But these spikes appear disconnected from any cardiac activity. The ventricles are beating on their own. Although these ventricular complexes are wide and notched, they are not captured ventricular events. This is an idio-ventricular rhythm with a slow, wide QRS from a point of origin in the ventricle. In other words, this is a ventricular escape rhythm.

If the pacemaker were capturing the ventricles, the ventricular spikes would be immediately fol-lowed by a ventricular depolarization. The distance between spike and ventricular depolarization alone demonstrates clearly that capture is not occurring.

Loss of capture can occur for several reasons; it can be consistent (as in this example) or inter-mittent. One common reason for loss of capture is insufficient energy, that is, the output pulse is too weak to capture the heart. A capture threshold test is performed at implant and should be performed at every follow-up. However, the patient's capture threshold is not constant and can change with many factors, including drug therapy and disease progres-sion. Capture thresholds can also change if pacing lead impedance changes. For that reason, the pace-maker that captured reliably one day may lose cap-ture in the future; that is why frequent pacemaker follow-up is so important.

This strip shows that the pacemaker is not captur-ing the heart and the cause should be investigated quickly. After all, capture is one of the main things that a pacemaker has to do in order to provide the patient with pacing therapy!

Test your knowledge

1 It is clear that this pacemaker is not capturing. But is it sensing?

A pacemaker senses when it "sees" an intrinsic event and allows that event to reset timing. If we look at the pacing intervals on this strip, we end up with two main types of intervals. The first is from a ventricu-lar paced event (VP) to a ventricular sensed event (VS) and the other is from a ventricular sensed event (VS) to a ventricular paced event (VP). If you use calipers and look at the VS-VP pacing intervals, they are consistent in duration. The VS-VP intervals are all 840 ms (about 70 ppm).

That means that the pacemaker "saw" the VS and used it to reset the timing. When the ventricles did not depolarize on their own within the 840 ms tim-ing cycle, the pacemaker responded with a ventricu-lar pacing spike. That is good evidence that those intrinsic ventricular events were sensed.

Notice the timing cycles that end with a VS. They are all shorter than the 840 ms timing cycle. This is

The Nuts and Bolts of Paced ECG Interpretation, 1st edition. By Tom Kenny.
Published 2009 by Blackwell Publishing, ISBN: 978-1-4501-8404-5.

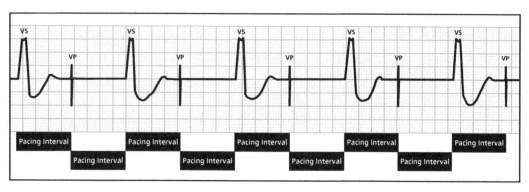

Figure 7.2

also further evidence (though not conclusive in and of itself) that the pacemaker was sensing in that the VS event "inhibited" the output pulse and reset the interval timing.

This strip is a good example of a pacemaker that is not capturing at all but appears to be sensing appropriately.

The nuts and bolts of loss of capture

- Capture is vitally important to a pacing system; capture is really what pacing is all about! Therefore, it's always crucial to check appropriate capture.
- Loss of capture is often the result of insufficient energy in the pacing spike. This is governed by the output parameters (pulse width and pulse amplitude).
- To increase the output pulse energy, you need to increase the "output parameters." Output parameters are pulse amplitude (in volts) and pulse width or pulse duration (in milliseconds). As a general rule, it is usually more efficient and more common to increase pulse amplitude.
- Loss of capture can occur even in a patient who had good capture previously. Capture can be lost if the patient's capture threshold changes or if pacing lead impedance changes.
- Capture thresholds in a patient are not fixed values. They change for many reasons and are affected by many factors. Two of the main factors that can change a patient's capture threshold are drug therapy and disease progression.
- Good evidence for capture on a paced ECG is a pacing spike followed immediately by a depolarization.
- In the case of ventricular depolarizations, paced morphology is different than sensed morphology. Specifically, most paced

ventricular beats create a wider, more notched waveform than a sensed ventricular beat. (While paced ventricular events almost always have a different morphology than sensed ventricular events, a "wider notched" QRS is just one common form of that distinct morphology. It is possible for paced ventricular events to appear narrower or without the notch.)
- A capture threshold test should be performed at every follow-up session to provide the capture threshold value. This is the smallest amount of energy required to consistently capture the heart.
- When programming output parameters, always use the capture threshold and a safety margin (for example, 2 to 3 times the threshold voltage). Thus, a patient with a capture threshold of 1 V at 0.4 ms should be programmed to output settings of 3 V at 0.4 ms.
- Capture problems can also be caused by problems with the leads. This is rare and occurs more often in the acute phase than in chronic systems.
- Capture problems need not be constant. Some patients will experience only intermittent capture problems (which are harder to identify but must also be addressed).
- To evaluate sensing, you need to figure out if the pacemaker is "seeing" intrinsic events. This involves determining if the intrinsic events have inhibited outputs and/or reset timing cycles.

Oversensing

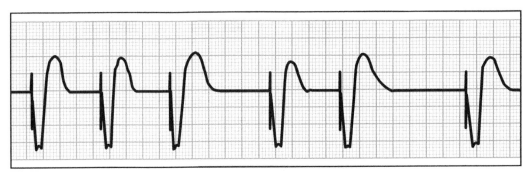

Figure 8.1

This tracing comes from a VVI pacemaker. There are clear pacing spikes followed immediately by ventricular depolarizations. The wider, notched ventricular waveform morphology suggests that these output spikes are indeed capturing the ventricle. In fact, from this strip, it is pretty clear that the pacemaker is capturing appropriately.

There are no intrinsic ventricular events in this strip. So why are the pacing spikes at uneven intervals? There are a few examples of pacing intervals (VP to VP) of 840 ms (which is equivalent to 70 ppm), but there are also two instances in this strip of pacing intervals that are much longer.

Since there are no intrinsic ventricular events on this strip, it is not clear if they would have inhibited ventricular pacing.

Test your knowledge

1 Can sensing be evaluated on this strip at all?
2 Why are there big gaps between paced ventricular events in some places and not in others?

One way to evaluate proper sensing is to look for evidence that an intrinsic event was "seen" by the pacemaker. Since this strip (like many you'll run

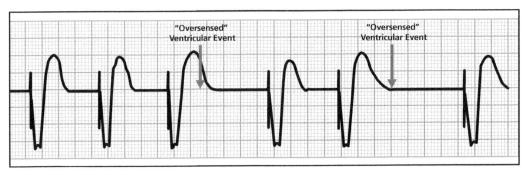

Figure 8.2

The Nuts and Bolts of Paced ECG Interpretation, 1st edition. By Tom Kenny.
Published 2009 by Blackwell Publishing, ISBN: 978-1-4501-8404-5.

into at the clinic) does not show any intrinsic ventricular activity, it cannot be determined if a sensed ventricular event would have inhibited pacing.

However, something is throwing off the pacemaker timing. The first three complexes are paced at 840 ms pacing intervals (70 ppm). That same timing is shown again in the middle of the strip. But something has extended two of the pacing intervals.

This is a classic example of "oversensing." The pacemaker in this case has "seen" what it believes to be intrinsic ventricular activity that is simply not there! Oversensing is typically the result of sensitivity settings that are too sensitive. The pacemaker may be picking up muscle noise or other extraneous signals and mistakenly thinking that they represent ventricular depolarizations.

You should always suspect oversensing when you see "under-pacing." In this case, there is a sensing problem, namely the device is so sensitive it is seeing signals that simply do not correspond to cardiac activity! The sensitivity settings should be adjusted.

The nuts and bolts of oversensing

- One type of evidence for appropriate sensing is a sensed event that inhibits the pacemaker output pulse. In real life, rhythm strips do not always offer that kind of evidence!
- When sensed events reset the timing, that provides another form of evidence of appropriate sensing. In fact, even when you don't see intrinsic events, the timing on the paced ECG can still provide important clues about sensing.
- Oversensing occurs when the pacemaker is so sensitive, it thinks it "sees" cardiac events that are not there. Oversensing is caused by sensitivity settings that are too high.
- Sensitivity is programmable; it is programmed in millivolts (mV).
- To make a pacemaker less sensitive, increase the mV value. Conversely, to make a device more sensitive, decrease the mV value.
- Oversensing leads to under-pacing! When you see pauses or gaps in the rhythm strip where you expected to see paced events … investigate possible oversensing!

SECTION 9

In Depth: Sensing

If you are new to pacing and cardiac rhythm management devices, it can be a bit of a hurdle to make sense out of sensing. The concept of sensing is simple: the pacemaker has to be able to "see" or sense intrinsic cardiac activity. When a pacemaker senses intrinsic events appropriately, it knows when to inhibit pacemaker outputs (and remain on standby) and when to pace the heart. Appropriate sensing assures that the pacemaker does not pace unnecessarily, but it also makes sure that the pacemaker does not remain on standby when pacing is required.

A pacemaker senses electrical activity in the heart through electrodes on the pacing lead. This sounds easier than it really is. On the one hand, the pacemaker has to be sensitive enough that it picks up even very small cardiac signals. Many patients have intrinsic electrical signals that are fairly low amplitude. If the pacemaker isn't sensitive enough, it can easily overlook those signals.

On the other hand, if you make the pacemaker too sensitive, then it may start picking up extraneous signals. Believe it or not there is a lot of electrical noise in the body. Muscle noise, for instance, can be picked up by an overly sensitive pacemaker – which then counts it as an intrinsic cardiac event!

The two main problems that clinicians encounter with sensitivity will be:

- Oversensing (the device senses signals that do not represent intrinsic cardiac events)
- Undersensing (the device misses signals that do represent intrinsic cardiac events)

When you look at the rhythm strips, you'll see that:

- Oversensing leads to under-pacing (look for pauses)
- Undersensing leads to over-pacing (visible as "too many spikes")

In order to correct the problem, you need to adjust the sensitivity setting. Pacemakers allow you to program the sensitivity (in millivolts or mV) so that sensitivity can be adjusted for each individual patient. However, programming sensitivity settings can seem counterintuitive, because increasing the mV setting decreases sensitivity, while decreasing the mV setting increases sensitivity.

To understand this better, you have to visualize how the device "sees" signals. Setting sensitivity is like creating a wall that blocks out signals. You build the wall to a certain height defined in mV. If you build a wall that is 5 mV tall, the only signals that the device can "see" are those that are taller than 5 mV. On the other hand, if you build a wall that is just 1 mV tall, the device can see any signal taller than 1 mV.

Thus, if you set sensitivity to 5 mV, the pacemaker is fairly insensitive. It takes a pretty large signal to

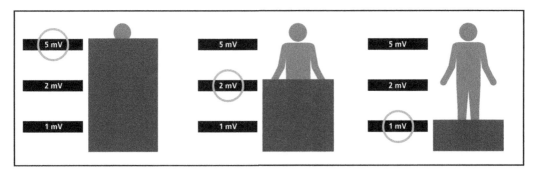

Figure 9.1

The Nuts and Bolts of Paced ECG Interpretation, 1st edition. By Tom Kenny.
Published 2009 by Blackwell Publishing, ISBN: 978-1-4501-8404-5.

get the device's attention. On the other hand, setting the sensitivity to 2 mV makes it more sensitive; a lot more signals have the potential to be seen by the pacemaker.

Before programming sensitivity settings, it is a good idea to do a sensing threshold test. This is a semi-automatic and/or automatic test by the pacemaker and programmer which determines the sensing threshold by finding the point at which sensing is lost. The sensing threshold can change with time, disease progression, drugs, and many other things, so it should be checked at every follow-up, even if the rhythm strip reveals appropriate sensing.

The normal safety margin for sensitivity is 2:1. If a patient has a 2 mV sensing threshold in the ventricle, sensitivity should be 1 mV. Many programmers will automatically recommend a good sensitivity setting value after you run the sensing threshold test.

When adjusting sensitivity, go slowly. Big changes in the mV settings may solve one problem, but they'll cause new problems! For most cases, undersensing or oversensing can be corrected with small adjustments.

The nuts and bolts of sensing in depth

- Sensing is governed by the programmable sensitivity setting, which can be adjusted in millivolt (mV) value. Increasing the mV setting decreases sensitivity and vice versa.
- A pacemaker that is too sensitive will lead to oversensing (seeing intrinsic cardiac events that are not there) and under-pacing (not pacing when required).
- When you see pauses in the paced ECG, suspect oversensing. When you see too may spikes on a paced ECG, suspect undersensing.
- A pacemaker that is not sensitive enough will lead to undersensing (not seeing intrinsic cardiac events) and over-pacing (pacing even though an intrinsic event had just occurred).
- Check sensing threshold and capture threshold at every follow-up. These thresholds are vitally important to pacing system operation and they are not static values. They can change over time, with disease progression, with drug interaction, and even during the course of the day.
- Sensing problems are one of the most common reasons for pacemaker troubleshooting. Always be vigilant about sensing disorders.
- While sensing problems on an ECG mean you should definitely conduct a sensing threshold test and adjust sensitivity settings, just because sensing looks normal on the ECG is no reason not to run a sensing threshold test during a check-up.
- Sensing problems can be constant or intermittent.

SECTION 10

QRS Morphologies

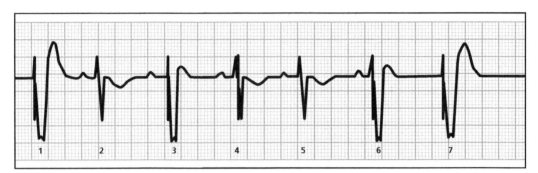

Figure 10.1

This tracing shows some intrinsic atrial activity, some intrinsic ventricular activity, and some ventricular pacing. It is quite normal to see different QRS waveform morphologies for sensed and paced events. But look closely at this strip and you'll see *four different morphologies*! The first and last complexes have one morphology. The second and fifth beats have another QRS morphology. The third and sixth beats look alike in terms of QRS shape. And the fourth beat looks unique.

Clearly, the second and fifth ventricular beats are sensed events. There is no pacing spike and the QRS waveform has a narrow, pointed look.

The first, third, sixth and seventh beat all are paced; you can see the widened QRS and the characteristic notch. But why are the first and last beats "wider" than the other two? The answer is a phenomenon called "fusion." Fusion occurs when the pacemaker spike is delivered at precisely the moment the heart was going to beat on its own. When a pacemaker output and a natural contraction occur at once, the result is a "fused beat." The pacemaker output actually contributes to the contraction; that's why you'll see the widened, notched look. However, the heart was going to beat intrinsically anyway. In this case, the fused beats look sort of like a cross between a

paced and sensed beat – narrower than a paced beat, wider than a sensed beat.

The first and last complexes are paced ventricular events, the third and sixth beats are "fused" ventricular beats. A fused beat is not unusual; they turn up a lot on paced ECGs. A fused beat counts as capture; after all, the pacemaker output "helps" the heart to depolarize. Fused beats are not harmful, and they are not noticeable to the patient. However, they are wasteful in that a pacemaker output pulse was delivered when one was probably not necessary.

But what about the strange-looking fourth beat? There is a pacemaker spike but the QRS complex looks intrinsic. This phenomenon is called "pseudofusion" in that it might look like fusion, but it really is not. Pseudofusion occurs when the pacemaker spike collides with an intrinsic depolarization. The output pulse has no effect on the heart, which depolarized on its own (and that's why the beat looks intrinsic). The pulse was wasted energy; it did not help the depolarization.

Pseudofusion does not confirm capture (nor does it refute it). It is simply a case of "bad timing" where the pacemaker delivered energy as the heart was depolarizing on its own. Pseudofusion is not dangerous to the patient, is not uncommon on ECGs,

The Nuts and Bolts of Paced ECG Interpretation, 1st edition. By Tom Kenny.
Published 2009 by Blackwell Publishing, ISBN: 978-1-4501-8404-5.

but when it is frequent, it can be a good reason to reprogram pacemaker timing cycles.

Test your knowledge

1 Would you say from this strip that the device is sensing appropriately?
2 Is there proper capture?
3 Why is there no atrial event preceding the last QRS complex on this strip?
4 What is the functional mode of this pacemaker?

Using calipers, find the pacing interval from paced ventricular event to paced ventricular event (using the last two complexes). If you apply that interval to the other complexes, you can see from the first event (paced) to the next event (sensed), the duration is less than the pacing interval. Going from that sensed ventricular event, the pacing interval exactly lands on the pacing spike in the next complex. This means the pacemaker "saw" the sensed ventricular event and used it to reset the timing. If you look at the pseudofusion complex, it is clear that the next sensed event occurs before the pacing interval times out and it inhibits the ventricular output and resets timing. These are all examples of proper sensing.

The first and last complexes definitely indicate proper capture: a ventricular pacemaker spike causes a ventricular depolarization. Although the third and

sixth depolarizations are fused, they also confirm capture. Fused beats indicate capture. The fourth depolarization (pseudofusion) does not confirm capture; neither do the two sensed events on the strip. However sensed events and pseudofusion do not disprove capture, either! They merely indicate that the heart depolarized on its own. Thus, from this segment of the ECG, you can see appropriate capture. There is no time when the pacemaker should have captured the heart that it failed to do so.

This patient appears to have intrinsic atrial activity, although the distance of the atrial event to the ventricular event is a bit variable. However, the atria do not depolarize before the last ventricular event on this strip. This indicates the patient has some sort of atrial arrhythmia, although you would need more than just these few complexes to better understand that rhythm disorder.

This pacemaker is pacing in the ventricle, and the absence of any pacing spikes in the atria – even when there is a missing atrial beat – indicates that there is no pacing in the atrium. The pacemaker's response to sensed events is inhibition. This means the device is a VVI system. This does not necessarily mean the pacemaker is VVI; it means the functional mode (the way the device is currently performing) is VVI. It may be a dual-chamber device programmed to VVI or a VVIR device with rate response turned off or otherwise inactive. However, it is functionally VVI.

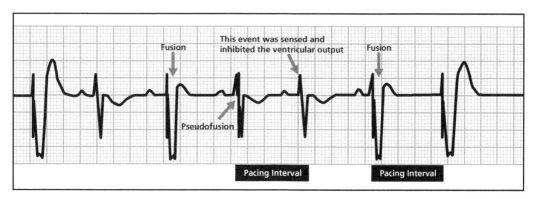

Figure 10.2

The nuts and bolts of QRS morphologies

- Fusion occurs when a pacemaker output pulse and an intrinsic depolarization occur simultaneously; the pacemaker contributes to the heartbeat but it does not totally cause it, since the heart is naturally trying to depolarize on its own.
- Fused beats look like a cross between a truly paced event and a sensed depolarization.
- Fusion confirms capture!
- Although fusion is not necessarily desirable, it is not uncommon to see on paced ECGs and is not harmful to the patient.
- Pseudofusion occurs when a pacemaker spike falls on top of a cardiac depolarization. In this case, the pacemaker output pulse has no effect on the cardiac depolarization. A pseudofusion ventricular event looks like an intrinsic ventricular event with a pacemaker spike.
- Pseudofusion neither confirms nor refutes capture.

SECTION 11

Fusion and Pseudofusion

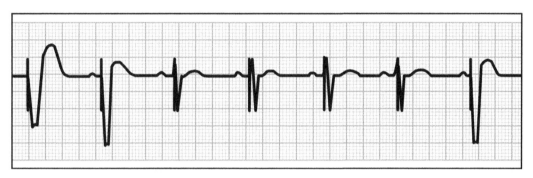

Figure 11.1

This VVI tracing shows examples of fusion, pseudo-fusion, and pacing. The paced complex (first one) and the fused beats confirm proper capture. The pseudofusion beats neither confirm nor refute capture. Using just this much of the ECG, most pacemaker specialists would say the device appears to be capturing the heart appropriately.

What is unclear from this strip is sensing. In order to evaluate sensing, you need intrinsic activity to appear on the strip. In this case, there is intrinsic activity in the form of pseudofusion. But since the pacemaker paced into these intrinsic events, the pacemaker counted them as paced events and used them to reset device timing. In other words, sensing cannot be assessed!

There may be other clinical scenarios that prevent you from evaluating appropriate sensing. Some patients have such slow underlying rhythms (or no underlying rhythm) that the device paces 100% of the time. Such patients may be called pacemaker-dependent in that they rely on the pacemaker to keep their heart beating. There are actually degrees of pacemaker dependence and lots of opinions on the subject. It may not be prudent to subject a pacemaker-dependent patient to sensing tests that involve withholding pacing even for

very short periods of time. However, most pacemaker patients are not device dependent. The "typical pacemaker patient" has enough underlying rhythm that the device is on standby at least some of the time.

To evaluate sensing, the clinician needs to inhibit pacing long enough for intrinsic events to break through and then to see if those intrinsic events are sensed. For the non-dependent patient, this may be done by temporarily changing pacing parameter settings to the point that the patient's own rhythm starts to prevail.

However, there are many clinical situations where you simply cannot "force" intrinsic events to occur. Thus, there will be times when you cannot evaluate proper sensing function.

In this particular patient, the first step would be to run more ECG to see if evidence of sensing might be found. If there was none, the chart should be checked and, if the patient had a strong enough underlying rhythm, the pacing rate could be reduced for a brief period to allow intrinsic activity to occur. A sensing test could be conducted using the programmer's automatic sequence or the clinician could look at the strip and see if sensed events inhibited pacing output pulses.

The Nuts and Bolts of Paced ECG Interpretation, 1st edition. By Tom Kenny.
Published 2009 by Blackwell Publishing, ISBN: 978-1-4501-8404-5.

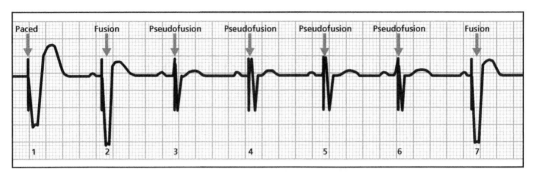

Figure 11.2

Test your knowledge

1 Locate the fused beat(s) on this strip.
2 Locate the captured beat(s) on this strip.
3 Locate the pseudofusion beat(s) on this strip.
4 Locate the sensed event(s) on this strip.

The first beat is a normal paced beat and demonstrates capture. The ventricular spike causes a wider, notched QRS complex indicating energy from the pacemaker depolarized the ventricles.

The second and seventh beats on this complex are fused beats. The pacemaker spike contributes but does not totally cause the ventricular contraction. Fused beats confirm capture.

Since both the first and second beats show a pacing spike followed immediately by a depolarization, how do we know to classify one as a paced event (capture) and the other as a fused event? The morphology of the two events is clearly different, which means the events are different. A spike followed immediately by a depolarization can be one of three things: true capture (paced event), fusion, or pseudofusion. Both the first and second events show a widened, notched QRS characteristic of capture: this means the events are paced or fused (pseudofu-

sion is an intrinsic event with a spike on top, so the QRS morphology is not going to show evidence of capture). The two reasons to label the first event a paced event and the second event a fused event are:
• The first event looks "more paced," that is, wider and with a more prominent notch, than the second
• The spike is closer to the depolarization on the second event (a fused event is a timing problem in which the spike gets "too close" to an intrinsic event)

The third, fourth, fifth and sixth beats of this complex show pseudofusion. The pacemaker spike and the intrinsic ventricular contraction collide. The ventricular spike does nothing to contribute to the contraction; that's why it looks intrinsic. Pseudofusion does not confirm capture, but it does not disprove it, either. If you were to remove the spike, the morphology of pseudofusion resembles the morphology of an intrinsic event.

Although this strip shows four intrinsic contractions, there is no way to use this strip to confirm proper sensing function. That's because the pacemaker output spike caused the device to "see" these events as paced events; it does not see the intrinsic contraction or use it to reset timing.

The nuts and bolts of fusion and pseudofusion

- To confirm capture, you have to force the device to pace and see if pacing spikes cause immediate depolarizations.
- To confirm sensing, you have to force intrinsic events to occur and see if the pacemaker can "see" them and whether or not they inhibit the pacemaker output.
- Sensing is sometimes difficult (and even impossible) to confirm if you cannot force intrinsic events to occur. This can happen when the patient's own heart rate is extremely low, the underlying rhythm is weak, or the patient becomes symptomatic without pacing at lower rates.
- Pacemaker-dependent patients have virtually no reliable underlying rhythm. There are degrees of pacemaker dependence; it is not a black-and-white diagnosis.
- It is a good idea to flag or sticker charts of extremely pacemaker-dependent patients so that clinicians know that their pacing rates should never be reduced, even for testing purposes.
- While pacemaker dependency is not easy to define, it is an easy concept to understand. Warning signs that suggest pacemaker dependency: the patient is paced 100% of the time, has a very severe arrhythmia, or has an underlying rhythm of 30 beats a minute or below.
- Most pacemaker patients are not dependent on their devices, in that the device may be inhibited some of the time and the patient can endure brief periods of non-pacing without symptoms.
- When comparing paced events to fused events, paced events will look "more paced" in terms of waveform morphology. Fused events will have a spike that occurs in closer proximity to the depolarization than a true paced event; this may be discernible on the ECG (if you know enough to look for it).

In Depth: Single-Chamber Timing Cycles

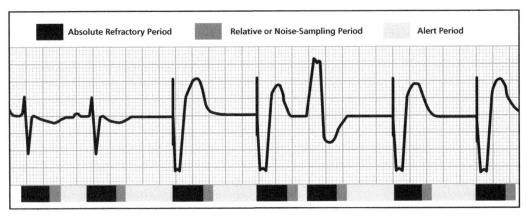

Figure 12.1

Timing cycles refer to the internal "clocks" within the pacemaker that govern how the device functions. Many pacemaker timing cycles are programmable, which gives the clinician great control over how the device paces. Most timing cycles start because of a specific type of event and then count down until either something specific happens to terminate them or they expire. Sometimes the expiration of a timing cycle will trigger something or launch a new timing cycle.

For instance, the **pacing interval** is an example of a timing cycle. A paced event launches that timing cycle, and the cycle starts to count down. If an intrinsic event occurs before it expires, it inhibits the output and resets the timer. If no intrinsic event occurs before the pacing interval expires, a pacing output spike is delivered.

There are also timing cycles on the sensing circuits that govern how the device performs. Whenever a paced or sensed event occurs, the device launches a timing cycle known as the **absolute refractory period** followed immediately by another

(shorter) timing cycle called the **relative refractory period** or **noise-sampling period**. Sometimes these two cycles are combined and called the "**refractory period**." In simplest terms, the device does not sense during the refractory period.

That is actually a bit oversimplified. During the absolute refractory period, the device is literally "blind" to all incoming signals. It does not see, count, or record any electrical signals at all. During the relative refractory period, the device can see signals, but it will not respond to them. Intrinsic events can be counted during the relative refractory period but no matter what the device senses during the relative refractory period, it will not affect its behavior.

The pacemaker will not pace during any portion of the refractory period (absolute or relative).

When the refractory period expires, the device goes into an alert phase. During the **alert period**, the device senses intrinsic cardiac events. In fact, it is on the lookout for intrinsic events. An intrinsic event that occurs in the alert period will be sensed and the pacemaker will respond to them.

The Nuts and Bolts of Paced ECG Interpretation, 1st edition. By Tom Kenny.
Published 2009 by Blackwell Publishing, ISBN: 978-1-4501-8404-5.

The nuts and bolts of single-chamber timing cycles in depth

- Timing cycles are vitally important to pacemaker operation.
- Single-chamber timing cycles at their most basic include a refractory period and an alert period.
- The refractory period is likely to be programmable but the alert period is not. However, other parameter settings (such as rate) affect the alert period.
- During the alert period, the device tries to sense intrinsic events and respond to them.
- During the refractory period, the device will not respond to intrinsic events.
- The refractory period is actually subdivided into an absolute refractory period and a relative refractory period, which may or may not be independently programmable. During the absolute refractory period, the device is blind to intrinsic signals. During the relative refractory period, it can see (and can even count) intrinsic events but it will not respond to them.

SECTION 13

Intermittent Oversensing

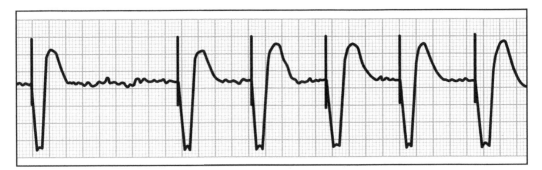

Figure 13.1

This tracing shows VVI pacing with apparent ventricular capture. There are ventricular pacing spikes immediately preceding what appear to be ventricular paced beats. All of the QRS morphologies look similar, indicating capture and no fusion.

This patient seems to have a lot of intrinsic atrial activity going on, as evidenced by the multiple atrial waves preceding each QRS complex. This would be typical of a pacemaker patient with atrial fibrillation or at least atrial tachycardia. Many pacemaker patients have atrial tachyarrhythmias. While there are different ways to approach pacing a patient with atrial tachyarrhythmias, one way is to simply ignore the atrial activity and pace the ventricle. This may be an example of that approach since the device is functioning as a VVI system.

Look at the pacing interval. If you measure the interval from paced event to paced event in the middle of the strip, you get a consistent value that marches through the strip. *Except there is a beat missing!* The span between the first and second pacing spikes is very long. In fact, it's nearly twice as long as the others.

This is an example of "oversensing." Somewhere between the first and second spikes, the pacemaker thought it saw an intrinsic ventricular event and inhibited the pacemaker output pulse.

Test your knowledge

1 Using the pacing interval, indicate the spot on the strip where the pacemaker oversensed.
2 How would you suggest correcting this kind of problem?
3 Why did oversensing occur only in one place on this strip?

This is functional VVI pacing with a consistent pacing interval. If you mark them out, you can see the point (circled) where the device inappropriately "sensed" a ventricular event. While this inhibition indicates that the device is indeed trying to sense, the sensing is not appropriate because the pacemaker is too sensitive. It's seeing things that are not there! What appears to be atrial activity might actually be noise on the ventricular channel leading to ventricular oversensing.

The clinician should run a sensing threshold test and then reprogram the sensitivity setting (in mV). The device should be made somewhat less sensitive, which means increasing the millivolt setting. Most programmers offer a semi-automatic or automatic way of evaluating sensing.

Although the pacemaker oversensed one ventricular beat (and thus missed a beat), the rest of the

The Nuts and Bolts of Paced ECG Interpretation, 1st edition. By Tom Kenny.
Published 2009 by Blackwell Publishing, ISBN: 978-1-4501-8404-5.

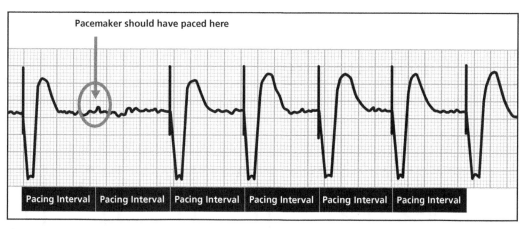

Figure 13.2

pacing looks appropriate. Many sensing problems in pacemakers are intermittent. It may be that the slightly larger than normal atrial wave on the tracing was so large that the device inappropriately perceived its signal as ventricular in origin. There may have been muscle noise or some other electrical signal in the body that caused the system to oversense here but not in other cases.

Because sensing problems can be intermittent, it is always good clinical practice to evaluate sensing thresholds (if possible) at every check-up.

The nuts and bolts of intermittent oversensing

- Sensing problems can be intermittent; in fact, they usually are. This is why clinicians need to be on the lookout for them and to check sensing and sensitivity at every check-up (if possible).
- Oversensing leads to under-pacing. When you see a "skipped" beat that really ought to be there, you should first suspect oversensing since it is a likely culprit.
- Likewise, when you see "extra" beats, you should suspect undersensing.
- A good way to check on sensing is to measure out pacing intervals.

SECTION 14

Undersensing

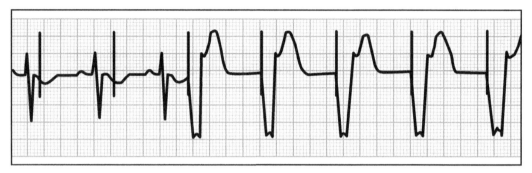

Figure 14.1

This tracing comes from a VVI pacemaker. The complexes in the middle of the strip show what appears to be normal ventricular capture. The ventricular pacing spike is followed immediately by a wider, notched QRS complex.

The first three ventricular complexes in this strip are intrinsic events. They are narrower and not preceded by a ventricular pacing spike.

The "problem" in this strip is that there are two ventricular pacing spikes that appear on this strip "unconnected" to any other events. They also appear in unexpected places. The first intrinsic event is followed quickly by a ventricular pacing spike. The second intrinsic event is also followed by a ventricular pacing spike.

The third intrinsic event is followed by a ventricular pacing spike that captures the ventricle.

Test your knowledge

1 Map out the pacing intervals for this strip. What does this tell you?
2 Would you say that there is a sensing problem on this strip? Why?
3 Would you say that there is a capture problem on this strip? Why?

4 How would you troubleshoot this sort of situation?

If you use calipers to measure out a nice clean pacing interval from two clearly captured paced events in the middle of the strip, you can see that the pacing intervals show the points at which pacing spikes were delivered. But should they have occurred there?

If the device was a VOO system, that is, if it did not sense, this would be appropriate. However, we know that this is a VVI device and should be sensing. The first intrinsic event in this strip should have been sensed. As a sensed ventricular event, it would have reset the pacing interval. Likewise, the second intrinsic ventricular event should have inhibited the ventricular output pulse and reset the pacing interval. Even the third intrinsic ventricular event should have inhibited the ventricular output pulse and reset the timing interval.

This indicates a sensing problem. The device is not sensing intrinsic events that it ought to see. This is "undersensing" and it causes too much pacing.

The output pulse can capture the ventricle when it occurs in the right timing. But why do the first two spikes fail to capture the heart? They occur

The Nuts and Bolts of Paced ECG Interpretation, 1st edition. By Tom Kenny.
Published 2009 by Blackwell Publishing, ISBN: 978-1-4501-8404-5.

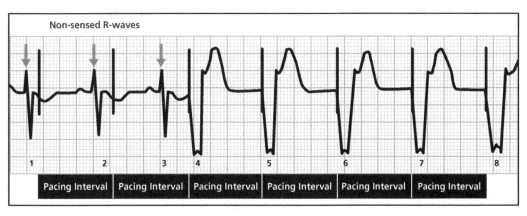

Non-sensed R-waves

Figure 14.2

right after a ventricular depolarization during the heart's physiological refractory period. This means that no electrical pulse, not even a very large one, would be capable of causing a cardiac depolarization. Thus, these spikes would *never be capable of causing a ventricular depolarization*. They are not evidence of non-capture, but rather of undersensing. This is sometimes called "functional non-capture."

The fourth through eighth complexes on this strip show good capture. The first three complexes are intrinsic and the two stray pacemaker spikes neither confirm nor disprove capture. Thus, it appears that capture is normal.

The best way to troubleshoot this sort of strip is to run a sensing threshold test and adjust the sensitivity. It is very likely the device should be made more sensitive (decrease the mV setting).

The nuts and bolts of undersensing

- If a pacemaker spike falls during the heart's physiological refractory period, it cannot cause a cardiac depolarization. This does not prove or disprove the ability of the pulse to capture the heart; it just shows the pulse occurred at the wrong time.
- Undersensing can cause too much pacing; it may look like there are too many spikes on the strip or

  it can cause the strip to look like asynchronous pacing.
- Undersensing can be dangerous in that it may cause asynchronous pacing; some patients do not tolerate asynchronous pacing well and pacing onto a T-wave may induce a tachyarrhythmia.
- Sensing problems should be addressed first and foremost by evaluating the device's sensitivity.

SECTION 15

Hysteresis Intervals

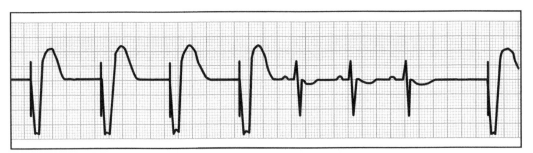

Figure 15.1

This strip comes from a VVI pacemaker that has been programmed to pace at 60 ppm, which translates to a pacing interval of 1000 ms (60 divided by 60,000 = 1000). If you look at the first two pacing spikes, you can see just from the tracing that there are five big blocks on the grid paper between spikes (5 × 200 ms = 1000 ms which converts back to 60 ppm). If you get out your calipers, you'll see that the next few paced beats are textbook perfect: the spikes appear in the right places and produce nice, wide, notched QRS complexes.

In the middle of the strip, an intrinsic ventricular event occurs. The timing from the previous pacing spike to the next intrinsic event is less than 1000 ms. That's why the intrinsic event can break through and inhibit the pacemaker output. The timing between the next intrinsic events is less than the pacing interval of 1000 ms.

But look at the last two complexes. The time between the last intrinsic ventricular event and the next paced ventricular event is quite long! It's approximately 1200 ms! If the pacing interval is 1000 ms, why didn't the spike appear sooner? Everything else on this strip makes it seem like the pacemaker is capturing and sensing appropriately. What is going on?

Test your knowledge

1 Would you say that there is appropriate capture in this strip?
2 Is sensing appropriate?
3 How would you attempt to figure out what is going on in the last complex? What kind of information would you like?
4 Why is the last interval on this strip longer than the programmed pacing interval?

This strip shows good evidence of capture. Notice the pacing spikes all result in an immediate ventricular depolarization with a different and distinct QRS morphology consistent with a paced ventricular event. There is evidence of appropriate sensing. The intrinsic ventricular depolarizations in the middle of the strip inhibited the ventricular pacing output. Every pacing interval but the last one is consistent with the programmed pacing rate of 60 ppm or 1000 ms.

Rate variations (even in relatively simple strips like this one) do turn up in paced ECGs more often than you would think! Whenever you're confronted with a rate variation, the best source of information is to look at how the device is programmed. This

The Nuts and Bolts of Paced ECG Interpretation, 1st edition. By Tom Kenny.
Published 2009 by Blackwell Publishing, ISBN: 978-1-4501-8404-5.

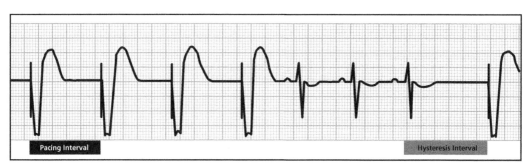

Pacing Interval

Hysteresis Interval

Figure 15.2

information may not always be available, but when it is, it can tip you off to programmed settings that can influence rate behavior.

In this case, the VVI pacemaker had hysteresis programmed on. Hysteresis automatically extends the pacing interval to a "hysteresis rate interval" periodically. This means that every so many minutes, the device will pace at a longer pacing interval than the programmed rate. This slower rate is intended to encourage intrinsic cardiac activity to break through and inhibit pacing.

If you evaluate a pacemaker that has hysteresis, expect to find occasionally longer-than-normal intervals. Likewise, if you don't know how a device is programmed but see something like an occasional longer interval, hysteresis should be the first thing you think of.

The nuts and bolts of hysteresis intervals

- Hysteresis is a programmable feature in pacemakers that periodically extends the pacing interval in an effort to extend the alert period to look for intrinsic cardiac activity. If an intrinsic event is found, the pacemaker will keep the extended pacing interval in place.
- The goal of hysteresis is to encourage intrinsic cardiac activity and, in that way, to reduce pacing.
- Hysteresis is a fairly common feature in most pacemakers and ICDs today; it is not unusual to see hysteresis appear on paced ECGs.
- Hysteresis works best in patients whose native cardiac rate is close to the pacing rate.

16

SECTION 16

In Depth: Hysteresis

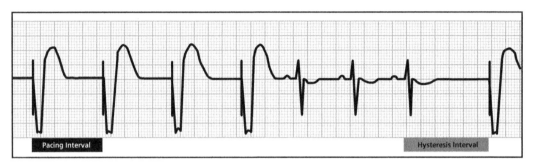

Pacing Interval   Hysteresis Interval

Figure 16.1

Hysteresis is a commonly used feature in most pacemakers on the market today. The goal of hysteresis is to encourage the patient's intrinsic cardiac activity to inhibit the pacemaker. The thought behind this is that unpaced cardiac activity is always beneficial, providing the patient still gets adequate rate support. Besides that, any time the pacemaker does not have to pace, there is less drain on the device battery.

Hysteresis works best in patients who have an intrinsic rate near the programmed base rate. For instance, let's say a pacemaker is programmed to 60 ppm. This means that unless the patient's own heart beats more rapidly than 60 ppm, the pacemaker is going to pace. Even if the patient's heart could beat 59 beats a minute on its own, the pacemaker would still take over and pace.

The idea with hysteresis is to impose a sort of "secondary" or interim rate known as the hysteresis rate. The *hysteresis rate is always lower than the programmed rate* but it is not vastly lower. If a pacemaker was programmed to pace at 60 ppm, a typical hysteresis rate would be 50 bpm.

Hysteresis works by extending the escape interval to the slower hysteresis interval at periodic intervals. These periodic intervals are programmable, usually in minutes. A typical set-up for hysteresis might be

50 bpm hysteresis rate for one interval every five minutes. Every five minutes, the pacemaker would impose the hysteresis interval and "search" or look for intrinsic activity. If no intrinsic events occurred, the device would deliver a pacing spike and pacing would resume at the programmed rate.

On the other hand, if an intrinsic event did occur during the hysteresis interval, the hysteresis interval would remain in effect. Different manufacturers offer different ways for hysteresis to work, but generally the hysteresis interval remains in effect until it is clear that there is no more intrinsic activity. At that point, the device goes back to the programmed pacing rate until it is time for the search to begin again.

To really understand hysteresis on the ECG, you have to understand the different kinds of intervals that appear on a paced ECG. Two paced events in the same chamber without an intervening sensed event at the base rate is sometimes called the **automatic interval** (it's what happens automatically when the heart needs rate support) or **pacing interval**. The **escape interval** occurs when a sensed event occurs followed by a paced event. The sensed event launches an alert period but it times out before another intrinsic event occurs; as a result, the pacemaker is forced to pace (and "escape" out of the intrinsic

The Nuts and Bolts of Paced ECG Interpretation, 1st edition. By Tom Kenny.
Published 2009 by Blackwell Publishing, ISBN: 978-1-4501-8404-5.

rhythm). The best evidence of hysteresis in a device is the appearance of pacing intervals or escape intervals at a rate below the programmed base rate.

Because hysteresis is a fairly common feature and because it usually imposes a search interval every few minutes, it is not unusual to see an occasional extended pacing interval on a rhythm strip! This is one of the main (but certainly not the only) causes of rate variations on a paced ECG.

The nuts and bolts of hysteresis in depth

- Hysteresis extends the pacing interval at periodic intervals to look for intrinsic cardiac activity, with the goal that intrinsic activity at rates near the base rate will inhibit pacing.
- Hysteresis is one of the main reasons for seemingly confusing "rate variations" you'll encounter on paced ECGs. If possible, check device settings when looking at a paced ECG.
- The best evidence for hysteresis will be pacing intervals at rates below the base rate.
- Hysteresis requires the programming of a hysteresis rate, which is slightly lower than the pacing rate, and a search interval, usually programmed in minutes.
- Hysteresis works well in patients who have an underlying rhythm (even if intermittent) that is in the vicinity of the programmed pacing rate.
- It is generally not recommended that there be a big gap between the hysteresis rate and the pacing rate; if you program a pacing rate of 80 ppm, the hysteresis rate should be 70 ppm or possibly 65 ppm. A bigger differential than that can result in uncomfortable "rate bumps" for the patient.

- The idea behind hysteresis is that it is generally beneficial for the intrinsic rate to inhibit the pacemaker if the patient still gets adequate rate support.
- Other reasons hysteresis is programmed include reducing battery drain, encouraging intrinsic activity (even if intermittently) while protecting the patient from sharp rate drops.
- If a patient has a very slow underlying rhythm, it can make sense for hysteresis to be programmed off. However, in clinical situations you may see such patients with hysteresis programmed on. In such cases, hysteresis will never go into effect (that is, you'll never see runs of extended-interval intrinsic activity) but you may see periodic extended search intervals on the rhythm strip.
- If a patient has an underlying rhythm that can support him or is fairly close to the paced rate (even if it is not consistent), hysteresis may be of great benefit. However, in clinical situations, you may see such patients with hysteresis programmed off. In such cases, programming hysteresis on is probably a good idea.

17

SECTION 17

Rate Response

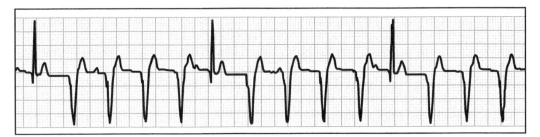

Figure 17.1

This strip comes from a single-chamber ventricular pacemaker. The wider downward ventricular complexes are paced events (you can see a little notch where a small bipolar pacing spike appears), while the three narrow upward ventricular events are sensed ventricular events. Although it is not typical for paced and sensed events to have opposite deflections, it is something that may be seen in the clinic from time to time. This has to do with the angles of the signals, however, not the fact that one is paced or sensed.

The pacing interval is a general term given between any two cardiac events in the same chamber, but it often is useful to look at it in terms of the duration between two consecutive paced events in the same chamber (this is the automatic interval). Those intervals that start with a sensed event but end with a paced event can be called an escape interval.

Paced intervals should match the programmed pacing interval (calculated from the programmed pacing rate). Escape intervals should also match the programmed pacing interval. Only when an interval ends with a sensed event will the interval duration be different than the programmed interval; in fact, *when an interval ends with a sensed event, the interval should be shorter than the programmed pacing interval* since the sensed event interrupted it and inhibited the output.

This strip contains automatic intervals (paced event to paced event) and escape intervals (sensed event to paced event).

Test your knowledge

1 What is unusual about the pacing rate?
2 How would you explain the rate?

You can measure the pacing rate by looking at the distance between ventricular pacing spikes. The first two spikes on the strip cover two big boxes and four little boxes on the grid (200 × 2 = 400 plus 4 × 20 = 80 results in 480 ms). That converts to 125 ppm, which might not be ominous if the heart were beating on its own – but this is a paced rate! It is highly unlikely that the pacemaker would be programmed to a pacing rate of 125 ppm.

The pacemaker appears to be capturing normally (pacing spikes result in ventricular depolarizations) and sensing appropriately (sensed ventricular events inhibit the output) and escape intervals look like they match the pacing intervals (480 ms or 125 ppm). But why so fast?

If you had access to information about the device, you would have seen that the pacemaker is VVIR. Rate response (the R in VVIR) means that the pacemaker will speed up the rate according to sensor

The Nuts and Bolts of Paced ECG Interpretation, 1st edition. By Tom Kenny.
Published 2009 by Blackwell Publishing, ISBN: 978-1-4501-8404-5.

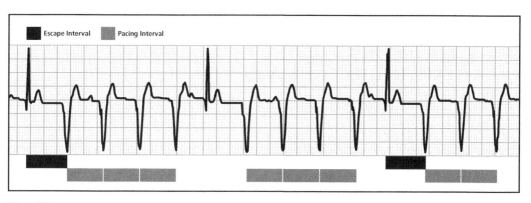

Figure 17.2

input. Unfortunately, the ECG does not tell us that the rate at this moment is sensor driven, but it is the most likely explanation for a rapid paced rate in a VVIR device.

Rate response may cause some unusual-looking things to appear on the paced ECG. You may see pacing at rates above the programmed base rates or rate variations (even from beat to beat) or both. In this case, the rate remained relatively stable at 125 ppm, it is just rapid. The idea behind rate response is that pacing at 125 ppm allows the patient enough cardiac output to meet the metabolic demands of his activity level at that moment.

The nuts and bolts of rate response

- Rate response may cause the paced ECG to show pacing at rates above the pacing rate. This can be consistent or intermittent. If the device is rate responsive and under sensor control, these rate variations are quite likely to be appropriate.
- Rate response is also called rate modulation and rate adaptation. It is indicated by an R in the fourth position of the mode code (VVIR, DDDR). Rate response is governed by a sensor and the rate-responsive rate is sometimes called the sensor rate or the sensor-driven rate. These terms all mean the same thing.
- The goal of rate response is to pace more rapidly when the patient is active (as indicated by the sensor) so that the patient's heart can provide sufficient cardiac output to meet his or her metabolic demand at that moment.
- Expect to see a lot of rate-responsive pacing

in the clinic; this feature is very common and frequently programmed on.
- Some devices allow rate response to be programmed to a PASSIVE setting so that the clinician can download diagnostics and assess how rate response might have performed had the sensor truly been in control. A device with the sensor set to PASSIVE will not actually pace in a rate-responsive manner. It allows for diagnostic information only.
- When the sensor does not show sufficient activity to invoke a faster pacing rate, the pacemaker will behave like a non-rate-responsive device. Just because you're looking at a paced ECG strip from a rate-responsive pacemaker does not mean that you will observe faster-than-base-rate pacing.

SECTION 18

Annotated ECGs

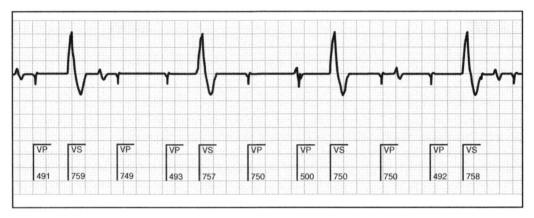

Figure 18.1

This strip comes from a VVIR pacemaker programmed to a base rate of 70 ppm (about 857 ms). The marks at the bottom are annotations, which many programmers automatically place on ECGs produced through the device programmer. Although every pacemaker company annotates a bit differently than the others, most annotations are intuitive and easy to follow. In this case VP stands for a ventricular paced event and VS stands for a ventricular sensed event. The numbers indicate the milliseconds that elapse between the vertical line just to the left and the next vertical line to the right.

When looking at annotations, it is crucial to realize that *annotations are the device's interpretations of what is going on*. Annotations may not match what is going on in the ECG but they always tell you what the pacemaker "thinks" is going on! When annotations do not match the strip, it is cause to adjust the pacemaker. (When the ECG and the annotations disagree, the ECG is presumed correct.)

This strip shows four intrinsic ventricular events (VS), which are the largest events on the tracing. There are also some pacing spikes on the strip (right

above the VP annotations) but these are very small spikes characteristic of bipolar pacing.

If you just looked at the annotations, you would see pacing intervals 750 ms (80 ppm) and escape intervals (VS-VP) at 750 ms. This would be consistent with a VVIR device with a pacing rate of 80 ppm.

However, the tracing shows a different story!

Test your knowledge

1 Is there capture?
2 Is there sensing?
3 Knowing the device is VVIR with a pacing rate of 70 ppm, is sensor drive active?
4 How would you troubleshoot this situation?

There is no capture on this strip, although the pacemaker "thinks" that there is capture (VP). Notice that the small pacemaker spikes do not cause a ventricular depolarization. The only ventricular events on this strip are the four intrinsic ones marked VS on the annotation. Annotations can be great time savers, but you should always compare them against the ECG!

The Nuts and Bolts of Paced ECG Interpretation, 1st edition. By Tom Kenny.
Published 2009 by Blackwell Publishing, ISBN: 978-1-4501-8404-5.

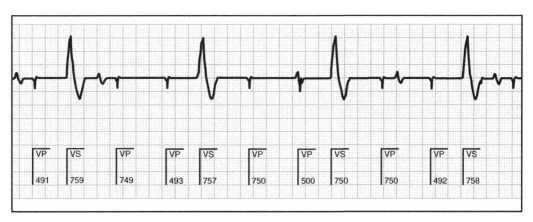

Figure 18.2

The pacemaker appears to be sensing normally. When an intrinsic event (VS) appears on the strip, it inhibits the output pulse. If you check the pacing intervals (VP-VP), you see they are 750 ms. If you look at the escape intervals (VS-VP) you see they are also 750 ms. This indicates that the pacemaker truly sees ventricular events and uses them to reset the timing. By comparing the VS annotation to the actual intrinsic ventricular event on the strip, you can tell that the pacemaker is seeing what is actually happening as far as intrinsic activity is concerned.

However, 750 ms correlates to 80 ppm, which is faster than the programmed base rate. Since the device is rate responsive, the most likely explanation for the higher-than-base-rate pacing is that the sensor is driving the rate.

The problem on this strip is a clear loss of capture. In fact, there is not even one captured ventricular event on the whole strip! The most likely cause of loss of capture is that the output pulse is not "big" enough to capture the ventricle. The best course of action is to conduct a pacing threshold test (which may be automatic or semi-automatic on the programmer) and reprogram the output parameters (pulse amplitude and pulse width) to greater settings.

The nuts and bolts of annotated ECGs

- Annotations are letter codes, symbols, and numbers that the programmer automatically puts on paced ECGs and intracardiac electrograms to help aid clinicians in evaluating a tracing.
- The real value of annotations is that they show you exactly what the pacemaker "thinks."
- Always check to see if annotations match what is going on in the rhythm strip! Never use annotations without double-checking with the tracing. If the tracing disagrees with the annotations, assume the tracing is right.
- Just because annotations show VP or ventricular paced events, do not assume that there is capture. The pacemaker only annotates pacing spikes, not resultant depolarizations.
- Interval durations on the rhythm strip are valuable to help you see pacing intervals and escape intervals. The interval duration measures what has elapsed between the two vertical lines that enclose it.
- You may sometimes encounter events on the strip that do not appear in the annotations. This tells you the pacemaker did not "see" those events.
- You may sometimes see annotations that do not correspond to anything on the strip or do not match the type of event on the strip. This tells you the pacemaker counted these events inappropriately.

- Capture problems are very serious and should be resolved whenever encountered. The best method is to run a pacing threshold test (also called a capture threshold test) and to reprogram the pulse amplitude and/or pulse width accordingly (increase them).
- The most likely cause of capture problems is an insufficient output. However, loss of capture may also be caused by lead problems.
- Capture thresholds are not static; they change not only over time, but even over the course of the day! Many things can affect them, including drugs and disease progression. For these reasons, it is important to check capture thresholds at every follow-up. Capture problems can occur suddenly, even in a patient who never had such problems previously.
- Capture problems may also be intermittent. That is another good reason to always review pacing threshold values and output settings at every follow-up.
- It is not unusual for clinicians to have to adjust the output settings (pulse amplitude and pulse width) on a device many times over its life. This kind of fine-tuning is not indicative of any problem with the device or the patient. In fact, it's actually indicative of good pacemaker patient management!

SECTION 19

AV Synchrony

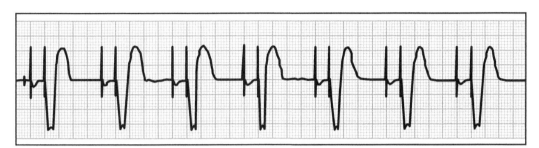

Figure 19.1

This is a textbook perfect ECG from a dual-chamber (DDD pacemaker). In fact, this ECG shows a lot of what's right with great DDD pacing.

First, notice that there is atrial pacing going on. You see big atrial pacing spikes followed each time by an atrial depolarization, suggesting appropriate atrial capture. Each atrial paced event is followed by a ventricular pacing spike and a resulting depolarization with the widened, notched morphology characteristic of a paced ventricular event.

This strip exhibits 1:1 AV synchrony which means that there is one atrial beat for every ventricular beat. One-to-one AV synchrony is highly desirable in paced patients because it closely mimics the behavior of the healthy heart. With 1:1 AV synchrony, the patient is more likely to derive the benefits of the atrial contribution to ventricular filling, which could result in better hemodynamics. Anecdotally, many patients seem to prefer dual-chamber pacing and report feeling better when 1:1 AV synchrony can be achieved.

Dual-chamber pacing is a bit more complicated than just atrial pacing on top of ventricular pacing. The atrial channel interacts with the ventricular channel and vice versa, creating some new (and sometimes challenging) timing cycles to contend with. For now, let's stick with the basics.

Test your knowledge

1 Is there appropriate atrial and ventricular capture?

2 Is there appropriate atrial and ventricular sensing?

3 What is the pacing rate, measured from atrial event to atrial event?

4 What is the pacing rate, measured from ventricular event to ventricular event?

5 How long is the delay between atrial pacing spike and ventricular pacing spike? Is it consistent?

On any dual-chamber strip, you have to evaluate appropriate capture and sensing twice: once for the atrium and once for the ventricle. In terms of capture, there is clearly atrial capture; every spike is followed by a P-wave or atrial contraction. On the ventricular channel, every spike is followed by a QRS complex that looks like a typical "paced QRS."

You cannot evaluate sensing from this strip, simply because the only thing the device is doing here is pacing. Intrinsic (sensed) events must be present in order to evaluate sensing. If this patient were in the clinic, you might be able to force intrinsic activity to appear on the strip by making temporary adjustments to the pacemaker's settings. This is only

The Nuts and Bolts of Paced ECG Interpretation, 1st edition. By Tom Kenny.
Published 2009 by Blackwell Publishing, ISBN: 978-1-4501-8404-5.

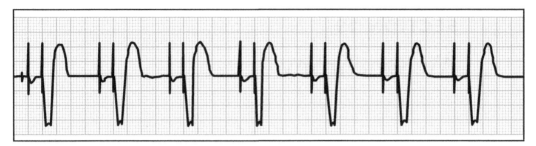

Figure 19.2

advisable in patients who can tolerate brief periods of no pacing, that is, patients with a relatively strong underlying rhythm. In some cases, it may literally be impossible for the clinician to evaluate appropriate sensing.

The pacing interval is the time between two consecutive paced events *in the same chamber*. In this case, the atrial pacing intervals are all 1000 ms (five big boxes) which translates to a pacing rate of 60 ppm. You can also measure the ventricular pacing intervals; again, you arrive at 1000 ms (60 ppm). This rate consistently marches through the strip.

If you were to find out that this patient had a DDD pacemaker set to a pacing rate of 60 ppm, you would literally have to concede this is a picture-perfect strip! Of course, we drew this strip … this kind of perfect ECG is something you don't often see in actual practice.

Notice that there is a pause between the atrial paced event and the ventricular paced event. It measures 200 ms and it's consistent across the strip. This is a timing cycle in dual-chamber systems known as the paced AV delay. The paced AV delay mimics the pause in the cardiac cycle between atrial depolarization and ventricular depolarization. This is a very important timing cycle in proper dual-chamber function. Think of the AV delay interval as the "electrical PR interval"!

The nuts and bolts of AV synchrony

- For dual-chamber pacemakers, base-rate pacing means pacing at the programmed pacing rate in a single channel (atrial or ventricular).
- Dual-chamber pacing allows for pacing and sensing in both the atrium and the ventricle. However, it's a bit more complicated than just two single-chamber pacemakers working independently. The atrial and ventricular channels actually interact.
- One way that atrial and ventricular channels interact has to do with the "AV delay." This is a timing cycle between an atrial event and the next paced ventricular event. The purpose of the AV delay is to impose a pause (similar to the physiologic pause that occurs in the healthy unpaced heart) between atrial contraction and ventricular contraction.

- Think of the AV delay as an electrical PR interval.
- When evaluating a dual-chamber strip, you still look for appropriate capture and appropriate sensing, but you do it twice: once for the atrium and once for the ventricle.
- The atrial and ventricular channels in dual-chamber pacing are independent in that they involve separate leads, separate electrodes, and separate portions of the heart. As such, it is possible to have appropriate capture in one chamber but a loss of capture in the other. The same applies to sensing.
- When calculating pacing rate from a dual-chamber paced rhythm strip, measure atrial pacing intervals or ventricular pacing intervals. (This will get a bit more involved later on, but this is a good basic principle.)

SECTION 20

Atrial Tracking

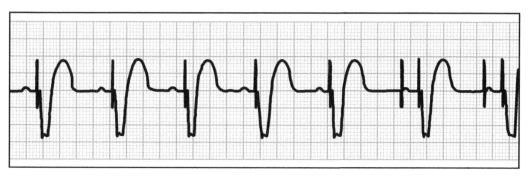

Figure 20.1

If you were presented with this ECG and no information on the patient or pacemaker, you should be able to conclude that this comes from a dual-chamber pacemaker. The reason is that you're seeing both ventricular pacing spikes and atrial pacing spikes, although they are not showing up in every single complex. However, the presence of atrial and ventricular pacing means dual-chamber pacing.

There are no sensed ventricular events on the strips but there are five sensed atrial events. The presence of intrinsic atrial events without spikes around them indicates appropriate sensing. The presence of atrial spikes (the last two complexes) with a resulting immediate atrial depolarization suggests appropriate atrial capture.

Another way to determine atrial capture in a dual-chamber system is to look for consistent AP-VS intervals. The theory is that in a patient with intact AV conduction, an atrial depolarization (if it truly occurred) would be able to elicit a ventricular response (depolarization). If that atrial event were paced, the AP-VS interval would be consistently timed. This is a moot point for this strip, since there are no AP-VS intervals, but it is another good way to assess atrial capture in a dual-chamber strip.

This particular patient has some good intrinsic atrial activity, but it is not reliable. Note that when-

ever any atrial activity occurs (sensed or paced), the ventricle requires pacing. This suggests that the patient has some degree of heart block, in other words, the atrial depolarization has difficulty conducting across the AV node and down to the ventricles.

Test your knowledge

1 Does this strip show 1:1 AV synchrony? Why or why not?
2 What is the ventricular pacing interval? What rate does that translate to?
3 Is the ventricular pacing interval consistent?

One-to-one AV synchrony means there is one atrial event for each and every ventricular event. It does not matter if those events are sensed or paced. In this case, there is one atrial contraction for every ventricular contraction although some of the atrial events are intrinsic and some are paced. Thus, this patient is deriving the benefits of 1:1 AV synchrony.

The ventricular pacing interval would be measured from one ventricular spike to the next ventricular spike. If you look at the first ventricular pacing interval on the strip, it amounts to about 880 ms, which converts to a rate of about 68 ppm (880 into 60,000 = 68.18). The second pacing interval is

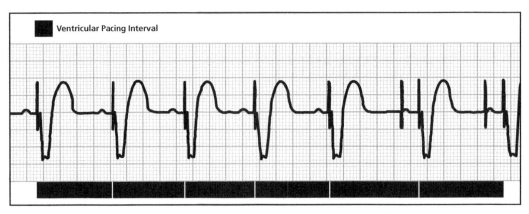

Ventricular Pacing Interval

Figure 20.2

a bit shorter. But the third pacing interval is much shorter. (You can see this very clearly if you have calipers and try to "march" through the intervals.) The third interval is about 840 ms (71 ppm). Now look at the next-to-last ventricular pacing interval. It's 1000 ms (60 ppm)!

Why is the ventricular rate interval bouncing around like that? This illustrates an important point about dual-chamber timing. The ventricular spike is timed to work with the preceding atrial event. In the case of sensed atrial events, the pacemaker senses the intrinsic atrial depolarization, imposes the AV delay, and then paces the ventricle. If the patient has a consistent intrinsic atrial rate, you'll see relatively consistent ventricular pacing intervals (which are shown at the beginning of this strip). However, if the intrinsic atrial rate becomes too slow, atrial pacing occurs and the ventricle will time itself against the paced atrial event.

In a strip with consistent atrial and ventricular pacing, you may actually see consistent pacing intervals. In a strip like this with some sensed and some paced events, you are unlikely to see rock-stable intervals. The ventricular spike is going to take its timing cue from the preceding atrial event.

The nuts and bolts of atrial tracking

- When a dual-chamber pacemaker paces both chambers of the heart consistently, it is possible to see stable pacing intervals on the rhythm strip. If there are sensed events on the strip, pacing intervals may show some variation. In fact, you should expect it.
- A dual-chamber pacemaker times events based on the activity in the preceding chamber. For instance, an atrial event (sensed or paced) launches a timing cycle (the AV delay) and

the next ventricular pacing spike will be synchronized to that atrial event.
- Likewise, a ventricular event launches a timing cycle (refractory period) which will only allow an atrial event to be sensed or paced after a specific time period.
- As a result, intrinsic atrial or ventricular activity on a dual-chamber paced ECG will likely cause you to see variations in the pacing rate.

SECTION 21

AV Conduction

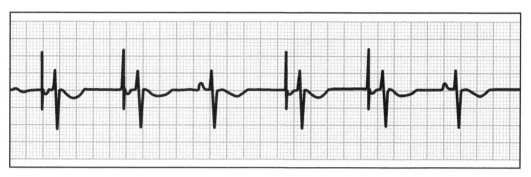

Figure 21.1

A quick look at the ECG reveals some atrial pacing spikes (plus some intrinsic atrial events) and sensed ventricular events. If you did not know anything about the pacemaker, you would not be able to determine whether this patient had an AAI pacemaker (or possibly AAIR) or a DDD (DDDR) device. This particular strip is from a dual-chamber (DDD) device that at this moment happens to be functioning in AAI mode. In truth, single-chamber atrial pacemakers are quite rare so if you see this kind of strip, it is much more likely a dual-chamber device functioning as AAI than a single-chamber atrial pacemaker.

This strip has four atrial pacing spikes and it appears by the atrial depolarization immediately after the spike that there is atrial capture. There are two sensed atrial events on the strip and the inhibition of an atrial pacing spike around these intrinsic events suggests appropriate atrial sensing.

This strip shows only intrinsic ventricular events. Since there are no ventricular pacing spikes delivered nearby, ventricular sensing appears to be appropriate. You cannot assess ventricular capture from this strip since there is no pacing going on at all. Ventricular capture may or may not be appropriate.

This patient appears to have intrinsic AV conduction in that once the atria depolarize, the electricity conducts reliably out over the AV node and down into the ventricles. Thus, this patient does not seem to suffer from AV block, but does have unreliable atrial activity.

Test your knowledge

1 Does this patient have 1:1 AV synchrony? Why or why not?
2 Is there a pacing interval that can be measured? If so, where is it and what is its duration?

One-to-one AV synchrony occurs when the patient has one atrial event for each ventricular event, regardless of whether the events are sensed or paced. In this case, the patient always has one atrial event followed by one ventricular event. Thus, this patient has 1:1 AV synchrony.

There are two pacing (or "automatic") intervals (paced event to next consecutive paced event in the same chamber) that can be measured on this strip. They are both 1000 ms, which converts to a rate of 60 ppm. There is also one atrial escape interval that

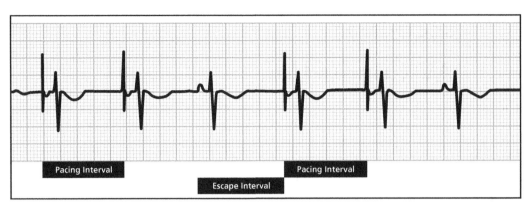

Figure 21.2

can be measured (atrial sensed event to next consecutive atrial paced event) and it is 1000 ms, the same rate as the atrial pacing interval.

The time between the atrial event and the sensed ventricular event varies; this is because we're seeing intrinsic events, which can be erratic in a pacemaker patient.

The nuts and bolts of AV conduction

- When the patient has intact AV conduction, an atrial event (paced or sensed) will likely conduct reliably out over the AV node and down into the ventricles. This will depolarize the ventricles and result in a sensed ventricular event.
- For patients without intact conduction (e.g. heart block, also called AV block), you should expect to see a lot of ventricular pacing, even if there is intrinsic atrial activity.
- One-to-one AV synchrony can occur with paced or sensed events or a mixture of both. The important thing is that every atrial event is followed by a ventricular event.
- Paced atrial events may or may not look the same as sensed atrial events. One common way that paced and sensed atrial events may vary in morphology is by deflection (one is positive or above the line and the other is negative or below the line).

SECTION 22

States of Dual-Chamber Pacing

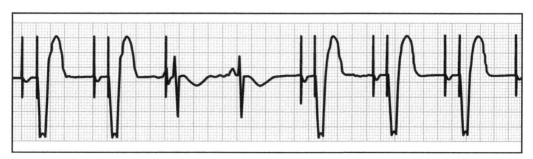

Figure 22.1

This is a dual-chamber ECG. The first two complexes are the AP-VP pacing state; this state occurs again at the end of the strip. In the middle of the strip is an AS-VS pacing state. Preceding that there appears to be an AP-VS pacing state. Thus, this strip shows pacing and sensing in both chambers.

There are only four states in dual-chamber pacing: AP-VP, AP-VS, AS-VS, and AS-VP. This strip exhibits three of those states. In most patients, one or two pacing states tend to dominate pacing behavior. It is unusual to see three states so closely together.

To evaluate this strip, we first need to confirm capture in both chambers. Atrial capture is present in the first two complexes and in the last four complexes. Notice the morphology of the paced atrial beat, which looks altogether different from the morphology of the one sensed atrial beat in the middle of the strip. But now look at the third atrial event. There is an atrial pacing spike, but the resulting atrial beat looks strange. It does not look like a paced atrial beat, nor does it look like a sensed atrial beat.

Ventricular capture is present in the first two and the last three complexes. Notice the morphology is different than that of the two sensed ventricular events in the middle of the strip. All of this suggests appropriate ventricular capture.

Is sensing appropriate? The one sensed atrial event in the middle of the strip inhibits an atrial output pulse, so that suggests appropriate atrial sensing. Likewise, the two sensed ventricular events in the middle of the strip inhibit ventricular pacing spikes. This again suggests appropriate ventricular sensing.

The base rate can be measured from atrial paced event to atrial paced event. It is consistent and measures 1000 ms or 60 ppm.

The paced AV delay on this strip (distance from paced atrial event to paced ventricular event) is consistent at 200 ms.

Test your knowledge

1 What do you think the third atrial event is?
2 What would you do to troubleshoot this third atrial event?
3 What is the value of the sensed AV delay?
4 What, if any, determinations might be made about this patient's underlying rhythm?

The third atrial event in this strip is atrial fusion. Fused atrial beats are sometimes harder to identify than their ventricular counterparts, simply because the atrial waveform morphology is much smaller and differences between captured and fused atrial beats can be more subtle than such differences in ventricular beats. However, in this example, this third atrial beat resembles neither a paced atrial

The Nuts and Bolts of Paced ECG Interpretation, 1st edition. By Tom Kenny.
Published 2009 by Blackwell Publishing, ISBN: 978-1-4501-8404-5.

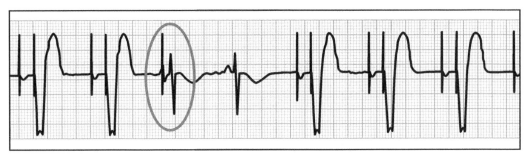

Figure 22.2

event nor a sensed atrial event. The atrial spike occurs simultaneously with the native atrial contraction, causing a sort of hybrid event that is neither truly paced nor truly intrinsic. The spike contributes to the beat and like any fused beat, this event confirms capture.

Fused beats are not necessarily problematic, so there is no urgency to address this, unless the patient is experiencing long runs of fused beats. If you were to try to address fusion, you should bear in mind that it is a timing problem, not a capture problem. Fusion occurs because the patient's intrinsic rhythm is very close to and competing with the programmed base rate. To deal with fusion, either program hysteresis on or lower the base rate slightly or both.

The paced AV delay on this strip is 200 ms. To measure a sensed AV delay you need to find an AS-VP pacing state (sensed atrial event followed by a ventricular paced event). There is none on this strip, so you cannot measure the sensed AV delay.

Sometimes a paced ECG reveals a lot about a patient's underlying rhythm. In this case, the patient's rhythm is erratic. There is a nearly textbook-perfect cardiac complex in the middle of the strip, but most of the time, the atria do not beat reliably on their own. There appears to be some degree of conduction (two complexes show an atrial event conducting over the AV node to the ventricles, causing an intrinsic ventricular depolarization), but it is not reliable, either. Like most pacemaker patients, this patient has intermittent rhythm problems. The patient has sick sinus syndrome and some degree of AV block. Despite these problems, with the pacemaker, this patient is still getting 1:1 AV synchrony!

The nuts and bolts of states of dual-chamber pacing

- The four states of DDD pacing are AS-VS, AS-VP, AP-VS, and AP-VP. Those are the only complexes possible on a paced dual-chamber ECG.
- Most patients tend to have one or two "favorite" states of DDD pacing. Patients who experience a lot of AS-VS and AP-VS activity demonstrate intact AV conduction but intermittent sinus node function. Patients who have mostly AS-VP or AP-VP activity have slow AV conduction.
- If possible, try to measure sensed and paced AV delays on a paced dual-chamber ECG. Not all strips will show them.

- Fusion and pseudofusion both mean that the patient's intrinsic rate is competing with the programmed base rate. Fusion and pseudofusion are timing issues. If they occur frequently, adjust the base rate so that it does not give the patient's native rate so much competition! This can be accomplished by programming hysteresis on or lowering the base rate slightly or both.
- Fusion and pseudofusion will sometimes occur no matter how well the pacemaker is programmed. Occasional fusion and pseudofusion events are no cause for alarm.

SECTION 23

Maximum Tracking Rate

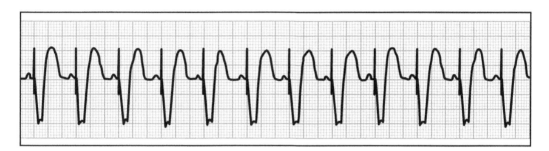

Figure 23.1

This ECG comes from a patient with a DDD pacemaker (no rate response) programmed to pace at 60 ppm (equivalent to a 1000 ms interval). A pacing rookie might be tempted to think that this could actually be a ventricular pacemaker (after all, there's no atrial pacing going on) that just happens to be set at a high rate. However, most experienced pacemaker clinicians would think this is far more likely to be a dual-chamber device.

Notice the intrinsic atrial activity. This patient has a pretty rapid natural atrial rate. If you measure the distance of one P-wave to the next consecutive P-wave, you can see that the intrinsic atrial rate is about 600 ms (100 bpm). Every intrinsic atrial depolarization is followed by a paced ventricular event (AS-VP pacing).

That's not likely to be an accident! This patient has maintained 1:1 AV synchrony, despite the fact that his atrial rate is faster than the programmed pacing rate. This is a good example of atrial tracking. The pacemaker will try (within limits) to match each intrinsic atrial event to a paced ventricular event, even if it means pacing the ventricle at rates above the programmed base rate. However, there is a speed limit. It's called the **maximum tracking rate** (or Max Track, for short, sometimes also called just MTR) and it defines the highest rate at which the

pacemaker will pace the ventricle in response to intrinsic atrial activity.

Test your knowledge

1 What is the ventricular pacing interval?
2 Does the intrinsic atrial rate match the ventricular pacing interval?
3 Looking at this DDD paced strip, what do you know about the Max Track setting in this particular case?
4 Why is the sensed AV delay so short?
5 Would you troubleshoot this situation and, if so, how?

This particular strip shows a very consistent high intrinsic atrial rate of about 100 bpm (600 ms). In clinical practice, you may also see high-rate intrinsic atrial activity at more irregular rates. Using calipers from one ventricular pacing spike to the next, the ventricular pacing interval in this example turns out to be 600 ms as well. The intrinsic atrial rate and the paced ventricular rate are identical, which is one of the characteristics of atrial tracking.

The purpose of atrial tracking in DDD devices is to provide for 1:1 AV synchrony, even in cases where the patient may experience high intrinsic atrial

The Nuts and Bolts of Paced ECG Interpretation, 1st edition. By Tom Kenny.
Published 2009 by Blackwell Publishing, ISBN: 978-1-4501-8404-5.

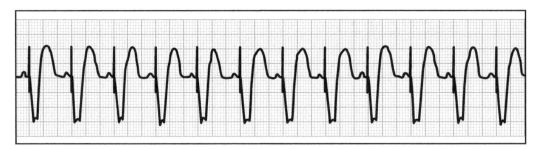

Figure 23.2

rates. This patient may be susceptible to atrial tachy-arrhythmias at the lower end of the tachyarrhythmia spectrum (intrinsic atrial rates of 80, 90, 100 bpm). This patient might also have been doing something strenuous, and the increased atrial rate could be a natural sinus tachycardia in response to exertion. High intrinsic atrial rates can also occur during fever. Whatever the cause, the purpose of atrial tracking is to maintain the benefits of 1:1 AV synchrony, even when the intrinsic atrial rate goes up.

Like anything else in pacing, moderation is the key! Atrial tracking would be extremely dangerous if the patient experienced atrial fibrillation and the pacemaker tried to pace the ventricle at rates of 200 ppm or higher! For that reason, it is important to program the Max Track setting to a ventricular pac-ing rate that the patient can tolerate. To find out the Max Track setting for this particular patient, you would need to check the programmed parameter settings shown on the programmer. Since the de-vice is tracking the atrium at a rate of 100 ppm, one

thing we know for sure is that the Max Track is set to a value over 100 ppm! (A typical setting that works for most patients is around 120 ppm.)

The sensed AV delay is very short on this ECG. In fact, you may have trouble using your calipers to measure it! That is because many pacemakers have algorithms that automatically shorten the sensed AV delay as the intrinsic atrial rate goes up. In the healthy non-paced heart, the pause between atrial and ventricular contractions naturally shortens as the heart rate increases. Pacemakers are designed to mimic this very behavior!

Far from troubleshooting this scenario, what you are seeing here is expected behavior of the device. The patient is getting 1:1 AV synchrony at a rate he can presumably tolerate well. If you saw this ECG and the patient complained of having a racing heart, being out of breath, or other symptoms that would lead you to think he cannot tolerate 100 ppm ven-tricular pacing, you would be well advised to repro-gram the Max Track value to a lower setting.

The nuts and bolts of maximum tracking rate

- Atrial tracking occurs when the pacemaker paces the ventricle to keep up with an intrinsic atrial rate that is higher than the programmed base rate but lower than the programmed maximum tracking rate.
- Atrial tracking is a good thing (up to a point) because it maintains 1:1 AV synchrony.
- Atrial tracking only occurs in DDD and DDDR devices. A DDI device does not track the atrium (the third D in DDD stands for "dual" meaning it inhibits and/or tracks in response to sensed activity; the I in DDI stands for "inhibited" meaning it will *only inhibit* in response to sensed activity and not track intrinsic atrial events).
- The maximum tracking rate (MTR) or Max Track is a programmable value that defines how fast the ventricle will be paced in order to keep up with a higher-than-base-rate intrinsic atrial rate. Think of it as a speed limit on atrial tracking. It should be set to the highest paced ventricular rate the patient can tolerate well.
- Expect to see sensed AV delays shorten automatically as the intrinsic atrial rate increases; this is common in most recent devices and mimics the behavior of the healthy heart.

SECTION 24

Pacemaker Multiblock

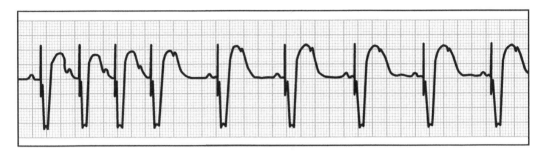

Figure 24.1

This very unusual-looking strip is actually a typical example of one type of **upper rate behavior** in a dual-chamber pacemaker. Upper rate behavior is a general term for how a DDD pacemaker responds when the patient's intrinsic atrial rate goes above the programmed maximum tracking rate or MTR. (This is not unusual!)

In this case, the patient's intrinsic atrial rate is high but remains fairly stable. Yet notice how the device paces the ventricle. At first the pacemaker paces the ventricle fairly rapidly – in fact, at the beginning of the strip, there is 1:1 atrial tracking. Then the paced ventricular rate slows down. When it slows down, the patient loses 1:1 AV synchrony! You can notice two atrial sensed events for every one paced ventricular event (look for atrial events on the T-wave, which indicate the atria depolarized during ventricular repolarization). However, every ventricular paced event was immediately preceded by a sensed atrial event, so there is some degree of AV synchrony and a discernible pattern.

This type of behavior is called **2:1 multiblock**. It's a form of what is collectively called **pacemaker multiblock**. The 2:1 reference means that this patient experiences two sensed atrial events for every one paced ventricular event (by the same token, 3:1 multiblock would mean three sensed atrial events for every one paced ventricular event).

Test your knowledge

1 What would make the paced ventricular rate suddenly slow down?

2 Why does the pacemaker not "see" all of the atrial events on this strip?

3 How do you think the patient would respond to being paced in this way?

4 Would you troubleshoot this situation and, if so, how?

Not only can a pacing expert explain how multiblock occurs, he or she can actually predict the rate when it will happen! To do this, you have to understand some dual-chamber timing cycles. The sensed AV delay is already a familiar concept: it's the programmable amount of time between a sensed atrial event and the following paced ventricular event. The PVARP (which stands for post-ventricular atrial refractory period) is a timing cycle that starts with any ventricular event and simply times out. During PVARP, the atrial channel will not respond to any signals. Atrial events that occur during PVARP will not provoke a device response. (PVARP is designed to help prevent retrograde P-waves from possibly triggering a pacemaker-mediated tachycardia.)

If you look at the timing cycles on the ECG, you can see that at first, the atrial signals fell in the alert

The Nuts and Bolts of Paced ECG Interpretation, 1st edition. By Tom Kenny.
Published 2009 by Blackwell Publishing, ISBN: 978-1-4501-8404-5.

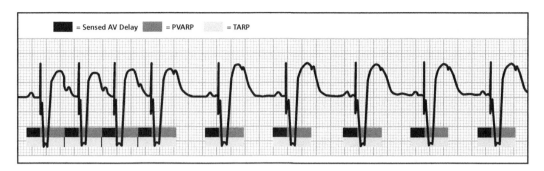

Figure 24.2

period but eventually, atrial signals started to occur during PVARP. Any atrial signal that occurs during PVARP will simply not cause a device response. The pacemaker is not "seeing" any intrinsic atrial events that occur during PVARP.

You can predict the rate at which 2:1 multiblock will occur. This is useful information for device programming and can be crucial if your patient does not tolerate 2:1 multiblock well. To calculate when 2:1 multiblock is going to occur, you need to understand TARP.

TARP (which stands for total atrial refractory period) is the name given to the sensed AV delay plus the PVARP. TARP is not a programmable setting on the programmer screen (but the sensed AV delay is and so is PVARP, so TARP is indirectly programmable) but it is a useful way of talking about dual-chamber timing. In this particular example, the sensed AV delay is set to 200 ms, the PVARP is

240 ms and so the TARP would be 440 ms (200 + 240).

If you divide TARP into 60,000, you will get the intrinsic atrial rate which will force the device to go into 2:1 multiblock. In this example, 440 divided into 60,000 equals 136 bpm. As soon as the intrinsic atrial rate hits 136 bpm, 2:1 multiblock will occur.

Patients have varying responses to multiblock. Some may not notice it, but to others, the abrupt rate transition can be disturbing or unsettling. Two-to-one multiblock cuts the pacing rate in half in one beat, so this patient went from 136 ppm ventricular pacing to 68 ppm ventricular pacing in about one second! For this reason, many clinicians will try to use other programming options to avoid multiblock with its abrupt rate transitions. However, when multiblock occurs, as in this strip, it is appropriate and expected DDD device behavior. The device is doing exactly what it is supposed to do.

The nuts and bolts of pacemaker multiblock

- Two-to-one multiblock means that the patient experiences two intrinsic atrial events for every one paced ventricular event. Multiblock pacing can occur in other patterns (3:1 multiblock, for example).
- Multiblock involves an abrupt rate slowdown which some patients find unpleasant or uncomfortable. However, multiblock is not a device "problem." It's the expected and appropriate behavior of DDD or DDDR systems in certain situations.
- Multiblock occurs when some intrinsic atrial events fall in the PVARP and are not counted. Sensed atrial events in the alert period will be "seen" and responded to, but atrial events in the PVARP will not cause a device response.
- PVARP is a programmable timing cycle. It starts with any ventricular event (sensed or paced) and times out. A typical setting for PVARP is 250 ms.
- Clinicians often find it useful to talk about TARP or the total atrial refractory period. TARP is not directly programmable. It refers to the total period of time that the atrial channel is unresponsive to incoming signals. It starts with the AV delay (sensed or paced) and runs through the PVARP. To calculate the TARP, just add the AV delay and the PVARP.
- Although you can't program the TARP, you can program the AV delay and the PVARP. Thus, you can indirectly control how long the TARP is.
- The length of TARP determines when 2:1 multiblock will occur. To find the intrinsic atrial rate that will result in 2:1 multiblock, divide TARP into 60,000.
- Multiblock is expected device behavior. It is not a device error or a programming problem!

SECTION 25

Pacemaker Wenckebach

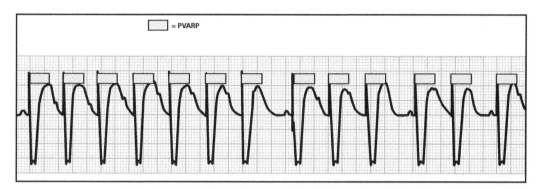

Figure 25.1

If you are familiar with non-paced ECGs, this paced DDD strip may remind you a bit of Wenckebach behavior, which occurs naturally when the PR interval gradually lengthens until an atrial beat is dropped. This strip is a good example of so-called **"pacemaker Wenckebach."** This is another case of the pacemaker mimicking what the non-paced heart will do in the presence of intrinsic high-rate atrial activity.

The ventricular pacing spikes on this strip show a lot of pacing at about 500 ms (120 ppm), which happens to be the Max Track rate for this particular device. Every ventricular event launches the PVARP timing cycle, which is shown here as a box to give you a clearer picture of the timing cycles. Intrinsic atrial events that occur *during the PVARP* are not counted by the device, but intrinsic atrial events *outside the PVARP* are sensed.

This pacemaker is trying to do two things. First, it is trying to maintain 1:1 AV synchrony even in the presence of high intrinsic atrial activity. Second, it is observing the 120 ppm (500 ms) "speed limit" on ventricular pacing imposed by the maximum tracking rate. The result is that the programmed sensed AV delay value of 150 ms cannot consistently be maintained (to keep the 150 ms interval, the pace-

maker would have to pace the ventricle above the Max Track rate – and it will not do that).

In about the middle of the strip, a sensed atrial event falls in the PVARP and is not counted. The next sensed atrial event occurs in the alert period, is sensed, and the ventricular pacing resumes.

Pacemaker Wenckebach is the expected and appropriate behavior of a DDD device when high-rate intrinsic atrial activity occurs.

Test your knowledge

1 Which of the atrial events on this strip were sensed? Which were not?
2 Look at the long complex in the middle of the strip. Why did the ventricular rate not come in at 120 ppm? What was the pacemaker waiting for?
3 If you knew this pacemaker was set to a sensed AV delay of 150 ms and a PVARP of 250 ms, at what rate would 2:1 multiblock occur? Is that faster or slower than this strip?

All but one atrial event on this strip was sensed (see downward-pointing black arrows). The only intrinsic atrial beat that fell in the PVARP occurred

---

The Nuts and Bolts of Paced ECG Interpretation, 1st edition. By Tom Kenny.
Published 2009 by Blackwell Publishing, ISBN: 978-1-4501-8404-5.

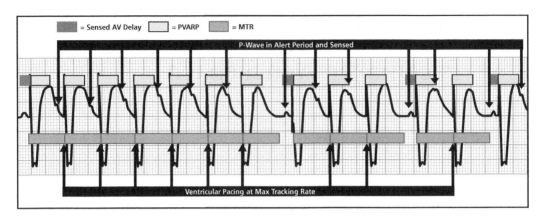

Figure 25.2

in the middle of the strip. Although the P-wave appears on the paced ECG, the pacemaker will not respond to it because it occurred during PVARP.

In the first portion of this strip, the pacemaker will not exceed the Max Track rate of 120 ppm. Although atrial events occur earlier and earlier, the pacemaker will not impose the sensed AV delay because, if it did, the paced ventricular rate would exceed the 120 ppm limit. (It may be useful for you to see how this would look by using calipers; maintaining the sensed AV delay would result in very rapid ventricular pacing.) However, in the middle of the strip, an intrinsic atrial event is not sensed. Thus, the pacemaker goes on "alert" and starts to look for an intrinsic atrial event. At this point, the pacemaker is going to do whichever of these occurs first:
- The programmed pacing interval (1000 ms or 60 ppm) times out
- An intrinsic atrial event occurs.

Well before the 1000 ms pacing interval can expire, an intrinsic atrial event occurs in the alert period. This launches the sensed AV delay timing cycle (150 ms) and after that, the device delivers a ventricular output pulse. The next intrinsic atrial event occurs so soon afterward, that if the pacemaker were to pace after the 150 ms sensed AV delay, the ven-

tricular paced rate would exceed the programmed Max Track limit of 120 ppm. The pacemaker will not break the speed limit, so the device senses the atrial event and delivers a ventricular pacing output just as soon as possible (at the 120 ppm rate). The pacemaker is willing to adjust the sensed AV delay duration in order to maintain the Max Track speed limit.

In this example, the TARP equals the sensed AV delay (150) plus the PVARP setting (250), so TARP would be 400 ms. Using the formula of dividing TARP into 60,000 results in 150 bpm. Thus, 2:1 multiblock can be expected to occur in this particular device when the patient's intrinsic atrial rate hits 150 bpm.

Pacemaker Wenckebach occurs when the patient's intrinsic atrial rate exceeds the Max Track rate but has not yet reached the multiblock rate. In other words, the various stages of upper-rate behavior for this particular patient would be:
- 1:1 AV synchrony at intrinsic atrial rates below 120 bpm (Max Track rate)
- Pacemaker Wenckebach at intrinsic atrial rates of 121 bpm to 149 bpm (higher than Max Track but lower than the multiblock rate)
- 2:1 pacemaker multiblock when the intrinsic atrial rate meets or exceeds 150 bpm

The nuts and bolts of pacemaker Wenckebach

- Pacemaker Wenckebach looks a lot like physiological Wenckebach, in that you'll see a progressive lengthening of the PR interval (distance from an intrinsic atrial event to the next ventricular event) until eventually an atrial event is missed.
- During pacemaker Wenckebach, the pacemaker will pace the patient's ventricle at the Max Track rate. It will not be able to maintain the programmed sensed AV delay value because to do so would violate the Max Track rate.
- Pacemaker Wenckebach occurs because eventually an intrinsic atrial event will occur during PVARP and be missed.
- When a DDD patient has intrinsic high-rate atrial activity, he or she will have 1:1 AV synchrony up to the Max Track rate; at intrinsic atrial rates above the Max Track rate but below the multiblock rate, pacemaker Wenckebach will occur. Once the intrinsic atrial rate hits the multiblock rate (TARP divided into 60,000), 2:1 pacemaker multiblock will occur. This is sometimes called the "atrial rate continuum" for DDD pacing.
- Upper rate behaviors such as shown in this example are not problems, but are the normal and appropriate behavior of the device. If the patient does not tolerate them, steps can be taken to help avoid them. However, the device is functioning exactly as programmed.

SECTION 26

Pacemaker-Mediated Tachycardia

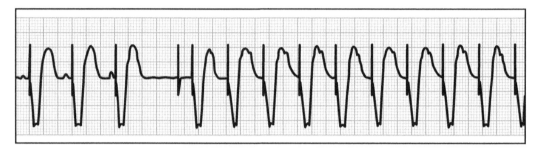

Figure 26.1

The first few complexes on this DDD pacemaker strip show AS-VP activity. The pacemaker is pacing the ventricle above the programmed base rate in an effort to preserve 1:1 AV synchrony (one atrial event for every ventricular event). These first few complexes are textbook examples of "atrial tracking" and that is the expected and appropriate behavior of a dual-chamber pacemaker in the presence of high-rate intrinsic atrial activity.

A pause follows. Notice there are suddenly no intrinsic atrial events at all. If you measure the atrial pacing spike backward to the previous intrinsic atrial event, it measures 1000 ms or 60 ppm. This atrial spike has timed itself to the previous intrinsic atrial event.

The immediately apparent problem on this strip is that the atrial spike did not capture the atrium. The loss of atrial capture results in a pacemaker-mediated tachycardia or PMT. In fact the abrupt loss of atrial capture is the most common cause of PMT.

Let's see how it happened. The atrial pacing spike is delivered; it fails to capture but the pacemaker launches a paced AV delay interval and paces the ventricle. The stage is set for this ventricular event to conduct in a retrograde manner and launch what is known as a "retrograde P-wave." The pacemaker senses the retrograde P-wave and continues to try to maintain 1:1 AV synchrony by tracking the atrium.

The pacemaker does not "realize" that it's trying to track retrograde P-waves. The result is that the retrograde P-wave drives up the ventricular pacing rate. Ventricular pacing will not go on indefinitely fast. The maximum tracking rate or MTR will eventually set a limit on how fast the ventricle can be paced in response to intrinsic atrial activity. A typical MTR programmed setting is around 120 ppm.

This cascade of events is known as a pacemaker-mediated tachycardia because it is a tachycardia (too-rapid heart rate) that is facilitated in part by the pacemaker. A PMT does not just happen out of the blue; it is usually precipitated by a triggering event, typically a loss of atrial capture. Most devices have special protective algorithms that can be set up to go into effect to break a suspected PMT.

Test your knowledge

1 What is the programmed Max Track rate of this device?

2 Why did the loss of atrial capture cause a PMT?

3 How long would this PMT likely last?

The loss of atrial capture in the middle of the strip precipitated a PMT that quickly attained and maintained at the MTR. The MTR interval is 460 ms which means the MTR was programmed to 130

The Nuts and Bolts of Paced ECG Interpretation, 1st edition. By Tom Kenny. Published 2009 by Blackwell Publishing, ISBN: 978-1-4501-8404-5.

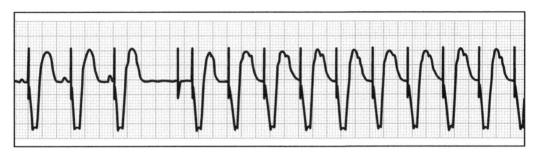

Figure 26.2

ppm. Notice that during the PMT portion of the strip, the patient is subjected to consistent ventricular pacing at a rate of 130 ppm. This rate may not be well tolerated by the patient, particularly for a prolonged period of time.

A PMT requires a trigger. Typical triggers are a premature ventricular contraction (PVC) or sudden loss of atrial capture – something that gets the rhythm out of sync! PMTs can be treacherous because neither PVCs nor a loss of atrial capture are all that unusual in a paced rhythm.

The trigger for this particular PMT was the loss of atrial capture. Had the atrial output captured the atrium, the atrium would have depolarized and then repolarized normally. It would not have been physiologically capable of depolarizing again so soon after the ventricular paced event.

A PMT requires several things in order to occur: a dual-chamber pacemaker, a patient with retrograde conduction, and a triggering event. Not all patients have retrograde conduction. If this patient did not have retrograde conduction, the intrinsic atrial event could not have gotten caught in the endless loop that perpetuates the PMT.

A PMT can last for a long period of time unless there is a special PMT algorithm to help break it. In the "olden days" of pacing, PMTs could be very troublesome. Today there are many automatic and programmable algorithms to help break a suspected PMT. But left alone, this PMT would last until the patient's intrinsic atrial rate slowed down.

Most PMT algorithms work by automatically extending the PVARP (so that the retrograde atrial events can "fall into the refractory" and thus do not get sensed, breaking the cycle). If this strip was longer, we might be able to see the PMT algorithm go into effect, and a normal paced rhythm return.

The nuts and bolts of pacemaker-mediated tachycardia

• A pacemaker-mediated tachycardia (PMT) is a ventricular tachycardia facilitated and sustained by the pacemaker! It usually occurs when a triggering event, such as loss of atrial capture, precipitates rapid tracking of the retrograde P-wave at rates typically quickly approaching and staying at the MTR.
• PMTs can be automatically detected and even corrected by pacemakers today. Many years ago,

technology had fewer ways of handling this, so PMTs posed more of a problem for dual-chamber pacing patients than today.
• Most PMT algorithms work by automatically extending the PVARP when a PMT is suspected. This prolonged PVARP will cause some atrial activity to be "fall into the PVARP" and not be sensed. This will break the PMT.

SECTION 27

Mode Switching

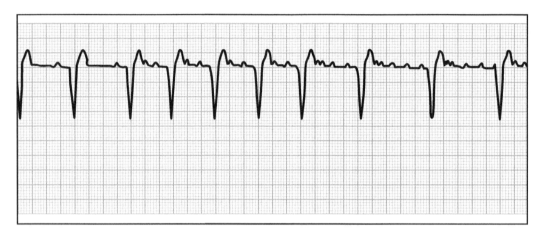

Figure 27.1

It doesn't take a lot of experience with DDD pacemakers to see that high intrinsic atrial activity, particularly atrial tachyarrhythmias, can be problematic for pacemaker patients. High-rate intrinsic atrial activity may trigger ventricular pacing at the Max Track rate, which is probably too high to be comfortable for long-term use. That was the impetus behind a dual-chamber pacemaker feature known as mode switching or automatic mode switching (AMS).

In this DDD paced strip, it is clear that the patient is experiencing high-rate atrial activity. Some of the intrinsic atrial events are "falling into" the PVARP and being missed. However, enough atrial activity is occurring that it is causing relatively rapid ventricular pacing.

Toward the end of the strip, the ventricular pacing rate slows down. There is still a lot of atrial activity, but the device seems oblivious to what's going on in the atrium. This is AMS in action. AMS essentially turns off the atrial channel. During AMS, the pacemaker will not respond to any atrial activity. It literally changes mode by turning off atrial tracking (in this example, it goes from DDD to VVI).

Actually, there are two fine points about AMS to bring up. First, during AMS episodes, the pacemaker still "sees" and counts atrial events; it just won't respond to them. That's the reason that you can still get diagnostic information on intrinsic atrial activity during an AMS episode. The pacemaker counts, it just doesn't react to atrial events. (The pacemaker needs to count intrinsic atrial events during AMS episodes to know when it's safe to turn AMS off!)

Second, although this example shows a mode switch from DDD to VVI pacing, in many devices, clinicians can program the mode change desired. For instance, it may be possible to switch from DDD to DDI instead (which turns off atrial tracking). Mode switches from DDD to VVI or DDDR to DDIR or VVIR are often possible. The programmable options will depend on the particular pacemaker.

AMS was introduced in the 1990s and quickly became a "must-have" device feature. Today, all commercially available pacemakers have AMS and it is

The Nuts and Bolts of Paced ECG Interpretation, 1st edition. By Tom Kenny.
Published 2009 by Blackwell Publishing, ISBN: 978-1-4501-8404-5.

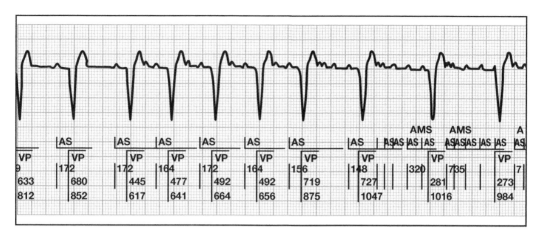

Figure 27.2

Test your knowledge

1 Which atrial events appear to be sensed?
2 If you were to draw a line on the ECG where you think AMS kicked in, where would that line be?
3 For what type of underlying rhythm(s) would you want to use AMS? For what type of patients would AMS not matter?

Early in the strip only a few of the many atrial events were sensed, as indicated by the AS (atrial sense) annotations. The other atrial events fell in the PVARP and were not sensed or annotated. Ventricular pacing tried to keep up with the sensed high-rate intrinsic atrial activity but ended up just bumping into the Max Track rate.

After a flurry of sensed rapid atrial events, the patient entered AMS (this is frequently called "AMS entry"). Although the annotations call out a rapid series of AS events, these are not events that the pacemaker will respond to. It will count them and annotate them, but they have no impact on how the

relatively uncommon to see pacemakers in clinic that do not have this feature.

device paces any more, since atrial tracking has been temporarily shut down. The device is now pacing the ventricle like a VVI system. This allows ventricular pacing to go back to the programmed base rate.

Mode switching remains in effect until the high-rate intrinsic atrial activity stops (that's why the algorithm allows the atrial events to be seen, so they can still be counted). When the atrial rate returns to normal (and there are programmable settings to determine what this rate would be and how long it must last), the device will do an "AMS exit" and restore the originally programmed mode, in this case, DDD pacing.

Mode switching is a great algorithm for pacemaker patients with known or suspected atrial tachyarrhythmias, including atrial fibrillation (AF). In fact, even patients with just short runs of high-rate intrinsic atrial activity can benefit from AMS. The algorithm is not useful in patients with no high-rate intrinsic atrial activity. However, since atrial tachyarrhythmias can develop suddenly, even in patients who had no previous history of them, the AMS algorithm is a good safety net to program on, even if it is not used by every DDD pacemaker patient.

The nuts and bolts of mode switching

- Mode switching or automatic mode switching (AMS) is a very popular, frequently used feature, that switches off atrial tracking in the presence of high-rate intrinsic atrial activity.
- Mode switching is governed by a number of programmable features which vary slightly by manufacturer. Basically, the clinician can set up the atrial cutoff rate (when the intrinsic atrial rate is high enough to mode switch), what mode the device switches to, and how long it stays in AMS before exiting. Some devices also allow the clinician to set up an interim AMS base rate, a pacing rate during AMS episodes that is slightly higher than the normal base rate (to prevent abrupt and possibly uncomfortable rate transitions).
- The AMS algorithm goes into effect when the device detects a too-high intrinsic atrial rate. It turns off atrial tracking, such as switching from DDD to DDI or DDD to VVI pacing.
- Mode switch algorithms also work for rate-responsive settings. You can switch DDDR to VVIR or DDIR.
- During an AMS episode, the pacemaker will not track any atrial events. Technically, it will still "see" and even count sensed atrial events, but it will not track them.

SECTION 28

In Depth: Upper-Rate Behavior in Dual-Chamber Pacemakers

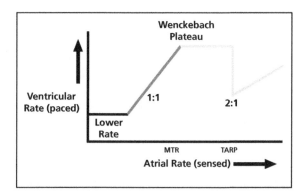

Figure 28.1

DDD and DDDR pacemakers try to maintain 1:1 AV synchrony by tracking the atrium. As long as the patient's intrinsic atrial rate behaves itself (or is too slow), this works well. But if the patient experiences intrinsic atrial activity at high rates, this poses a problem. Should the pacemaker try to pace the ventricle more rapidly to maintain 1:1 AV synchrony, or should it abandon attempts at 1:1 AV synchrony and just try to synchronize chambers as best it can? Or should it forget 1:1 AV synchrony altogether?

Those are actually the three main ways DDD(R) devices manage high-rate intrinsic atrial activity (tracking, Wenckebach/multiblock, mode switching). Upper-rate behavior in pacemakers is very important to understand because, unfortunately, atrial tachyarrhythmias are not at all uncommon.

Tracking

The maximum tracking rate or Max Track rate is the fastest rate at which the ventricle can be paced in response to atrial activity (i.e., atrial tracking). By programming the Max Track rate carefully, you can prevent the patient from experiencing unpleasant runs of rapid ventricular pacing. On the other hand, the Max Track rate will cause the pacemaker

to resort to other types of behavior to cope with the rapid intrinsic atrial rate without violating the Max Track limit.

Wenckebach/multiblock

Once the intrinsic atrial rate hits the Max Track rate, the device will have to abandon any hope of keeping up 1:1 AV synchrony. It will then use pacemaker Wenckebach (sometimes called pseudo-Wenckebach), which resembles physiologic Wenckebach behavior. The PR interval will extend progressively until an atrial event is missed because it falls into the PVARP. This allows the pacemaker to "catch its breath" and a longer-than-Max-Track ventricular interval will occur.

If the intrinsic atrial rate gets too rapid, the pacemaker may go into 2:1 multiblock where every other atrial beat is missed. The rate at which multiblock will occur may appear automatically on the programmer whenever you program the device.

If it does not appear, it is easy to calculate. The formula: TARP divided into 60,000 will equal the rate at which multiblock will occur. TARP may or may not appear on the programmer screen as an independent value; it is not programmable as such.

The Nuts and Bolts of Paced ECG Interpretation, 1st edition. By Tom Kenny.
Published 2009 by Blackwell Publishing, ISBN: 978-1-4501-8404-5.

TARP consists of the sensed AV delay value (in ms) plus the programmed PVARP value (in ms). For instance, if the sensed AV delay is set to 180 ms and the PVARP is 250 ms, the TARP is 430 and multiblock will occur at atrial rates of about 140 beats per minute. If you extend the PVARP by just 30 ms to 280 ms, TARP becomes 460 (180 + 280) and multiblock will occur at atrial rates of about 130 beats per minute. Adjusting the PVARP or the sensed AV delay setting will impact TARP and thus impact the multiblock rate.

While pacemaker Wenckebach and 2:1 multiblock are reasonable ways to approach high-rate intrinsic atrial activity, not all patients tolerate them well. In fact, many patients need a relatively low Max Track rate to feel comfortable, since ventricular pacing at a high Max Track setting can cause symptoms.

Mode switching

Since pacemaker Wenckebach and pacemaker multiblock are not always the ideal solutions to managing high-rate intrinsic atrial activity, dual-chamber pacemakers usually offer a mode switching feature which turns off atrial tracking in the presence of intrinsic atrial activity exceeding a programmable atrial cutoff rate. By carefully programming the atrial cutoff rate for a mode switch, it may be possible to pre-empt 2:1 multiblock episodes even if the atrial rate gets very high. Using the previous example, if you know the pacemaker will go into 2:1 multiblock at an atrial rate of 140 bpm, programming the atrial cutoff rate for mode switching to 130 bpm will cause the device to mode switch (turn off atrial tracking, usually resulting in VVI-type pacing) before multiblock can occur.

The nuts and bolts of dual-chamber upper rate behavior in depth

- It is not unusual for DDD(R) pacemaker patients to have occasional episodes of atrial tachyarrhythmias. The most common approach to manage this situation is to program a mode switch algorithm which allows the device to turn off atrial tracking when the intrinsic atrial rate exceeds a programmable limit (usually called an atrial cutoff rate or atrial tachycardia detection rate).
- During a mode switch episode, the pacemaker stops atrial tracking. It "sees" and counts intrinsic atrial events, but it will not try to track them by pacing the ventricle to keep pace with them.
- Mode switching got its name because it changes the mode in which the device operates. The switch is automatic and temporary; when the high-rate atrial episode is over, the device will automatically restore the previously programmed mode. Originally, the mode switch algorithm changed from DDD to VVI or DDDR to VVIR. Many devices available today allow even more latitude in selecting which mode is used for mode switch. It may be DDI, DDIR, VVI, or VVIR.
- When a mode switch goes into effect, the pacing rate will drop abruptly. Typically, the pacemaker had been pacing at the Max Track rate and will go, usually in one beat, to the programmed base rate. This may involve a change from, say, 120 ppm to 60 ppm! For that reason, some devices

- offer a programmable interim "mode switch base rate," which is the temporary pacing rate during mode switch episodes. Using the previous example, a temporary mode switch base rate of 80 ppm might be set up so that the patient would go from 120 ppm to 80 ppm and then back to 60 ppm upon mode switch exit.
- Mode switch data are contained in the device diagnostic reports which can be easily downloaded from the programmer.
- The Max Track rate is a very important parameter to program. It determines the fastest rate at which the ventricle will be paced in response to intrinsic atrial activity. It must be a ventricular pacing rate that the patient can tolerate well. It also sets the boundary at which 1:1 AV synchrony will be lost.
- Pacemaker Wenckebach will occur before 2:1 block.
- Pacemaker Wenckebach is the normal expected behavior of the device. Many patients tolerate it well. Two-to-one block may be more challenging for patients.
- All of these upper rate behaviors involve the loss of 1:1 AV synchrony and usually involve an abrupt rate drop (which some patients do not notice but others find bothersome). However, even the non-paced heart has to struggle to deal with atrial tachyarrhythmias!

SECTION 29

Troubleshooting the Paced ECG

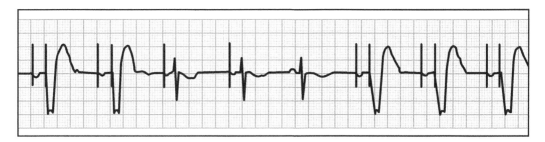

Figure 29.1

This is a dual-chamber paced strip which shows both intrinsic and paced activity in the atrium and ventricle. There is good evidence of capture and sensing in both chambers. The best way to determine the pacing rate on a strip like this is to measure the atrial automatic interval, that is, the time between two consecutive paced atrial events. That turns out to be 1000 ms, which converts to a pacing rate of 60 ppm.

It is important to measure the atrial automatic interval, if available, because dual-chamber pacemakers base their pacing rate decisions on what's going on in the atrium rather than what's going on in the ventricle.

In this example, the ventricular automatic interval is also 1000 ms and the escape interval (sensed event to next paced event in one chamber) is also 1000 ms. This presents a nice example of a stable rate.

The paced AV delay can be measured on this strip. Using calipers, it appears to be 200 ms. (Calipers are a great tool and I highly recommend getting adept with them, but they are less exact than programmer annotations.) There is no example of a sensed AV delay on this strip to measure.

Test your knowledge

1 How many of the four pacing states are evident on this strip?

2 What would you guess is this patient's underlying rhythm?

3 Would you troubleshoot or change anything based on this strip?

This strip shows three of the four DDD pacing states: AP-VP, AP-VS, and AS-VS. The one state that does not occur here is AS-VP. The type of pacing state that occurs most frequently in a patient can often provide clues as to the patient's diagnosis or underlying rhythm. In this strip, it is clear that the patient has some degree of intrinsic activity in both chambers and some conduction.

This strip is just a snapshot of this patient's paced rhythm. But if it were a good sample, more than half of the time (four complexes out of seven), the patient is subject to AP-VP pacing. This indicates sinus node dysfunction (the intrinsic atrial rate is slow) and slow conduction. However, the patient sometimes has good AV conduction because two of the seven complexes showed a paced atrial event conducting successfully over the AV node down to the ventricles. Thus the slow conduction is intermittent and not too severe.

There is even one event of the seven shown here that is a completely normal, almost textbook perfect, intrinsic complex (AS-VS). To whatever extent possible, this kind of event should be encouraged. Since some intrinsic ventricular events did manage

The Nuts and Bolts of Paced ECG Interpretation, 1st edition. By Tom Kenny.
Published 2009 by Blackwell Publishing, ISBN: 978-1-4501-8404-5.

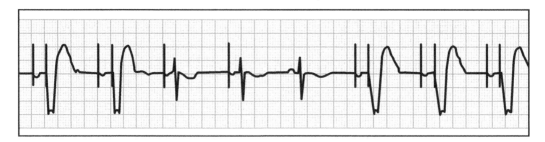

Figure 29.2

to break through on the strip (three out of seven ventricular events are sensed rather than paced), this suggests that the patient probably has a native ventricular rate that may be near the programmed base rate.

For this reason, it would probably be a good idea to program a feature like rate hysteresis for this kind of patient to encourage more intrinsic activity to prevail.

The nuts and bolts of troubleshooting the paced ECG

- When measuring rates in dual-chamber pacing strips, focus on atrial intervals since the pacemaker bases its rate decision on what is going on in the atrium rather than what is going on in the ventricle.
- There are four states in DDD pacing and knowing their relative frequency in a patient can provide clues in terms of the patient's underlying rhythm and insights for programming particular features.
- Patients with some degree of intrinsic activity at or near the base rate can benefit from programming rate hysteresis on because it allows the intrinsic rate more opportunity to prevail.

SECTION 30

More Troubleshooting the Paced ECG

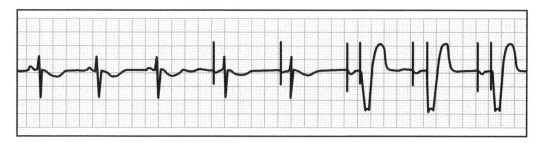

Figure 30.1

This DDD tracing shows AS-VS states at the beginning, progressing to AP-VS, and then AP-VP complexes. There appears to be good atrial capture (notice the different morphologies between paced and sensed atrial events); the same is true for the ventricle.

Atrial sensing looks appropriate. When intrinsic atrial events occur at the outset of the strip, they inhibit the atrial output pulse. Using calipers to measure the atrial pacing interval (AP-AP), it appears that the first paced atrial event times itself to the previous intrinsic atrial rate (AS-AP) at the atrial pacing interval. That means atrial sensing is functioning properly.

Ventricular sensing also appears to be appropriate, in that intrinsic ventricular events inhibit the ventricular output.

Based on this strip, it is difficult to say what the patient's real underlying rhythm is. Intrinsic events occur in both chambers and there is clearly some degree of intact AV conduction, but the atrial rate is not reliably rapid and sometimes the ventricle does not depolarize in response to an atrial depolarization. Since this strip provides us with so little data (just seven complexes, about evenly split by AS-VS, AP-VS, AP-VP) it is clear the patient requires a pacemaker, but his dominant underlying rhythm is not apparent.

What is going on in this strip?

Test your knowledge

1 Is everything really functioning appropriately in this paced ECG?
2 Why is the baseline smooth in some parts but not in others?
3 Would you troubleshoot the pacemaker parameters for this patient? If so, how?

This rhythm strip like the others in this book is a bit artificial, in that we only have a very small amount of information to work with. In the clinic, you can and should get longer strips which offer more data. But based on what we have, it appears that capture and sensing are appropriate.

Whenever you evaluate a paced ECG, rely on the tracing to do as much of the work for you as possible. On a dual-chamber rhythm strip, you need to evaluate capture in both chambers and sensing in both chambers. This strip provides that information along with showing appropriate rate and nothing unusual. Based on what we have to go on, this strip shows a pacemaker working properly.

The baseline on this strip may seem a bit wobbly to some, but that is likely a result of the ECG machine or even the way the paper was fed through the printer.

Troubleshooting usually involves trouble and there is no trouble apparent on this paced ECG.

The Nuts and Bolts of Paced ECG Interpretation, 1st edition. By Tom Kenny.
Published 2009 by Blackwell Publishing, ISBN: 978-1-4501-8404-5.

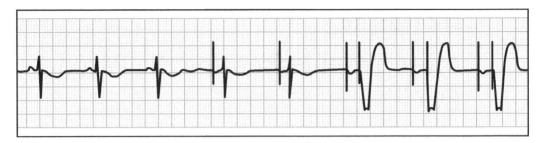

Figure 30.2

However, it is clinically prudent to check capture and sensing in both chambers ... even though there is evidence on the strip that things are appropriate. Capture tests involve forcing the pacemaker to pace. In a single-chamber pacemaker, the best way to force pacing is to increase the base rate. Do this gradually, in 10-ppm increments and making sure the patient knows that you are adjusting the device. In dual-chamber pacemakers, you can force atrial pacing by increasing the base rate in steps but there is a much better way to force ventricular pacing. Instead of changing the base rate, shorten the AV delay interval. You don't need to do this in steps; you can simply shorten the AV delay interval to 120 or 130 ms. This is likely to cause ventricular pacing.

When it comes to sensing tests, you have to get intrinsic activity to emerge. For single-chamber pacemakers or the atrial channel on dual-chamber pacemakers, just lower the pacing rate. Again, do this in 10-ppm steps, monitoring the patient as the rate decelerates. Even if no intrinsic activity appears on the strip, do not drop the rate below 30 or 40 ppm.

Ventricular sensing is best performed by extending the AV delay interval. Temporarily program the AV delay interval to 300 ms or higher. This often causes intrinsic ventricular activity to emerge.

More nuts and bolts of troubleshooting the paced ECG

- ECGs machines are not perfect and do not always work perfectly; as a result, you will sometimes see uneven or wavy or odd-looking baselines or artifacts. While it is imperative to check out the tracing carefully, not everything that looks unusual on a strip is really important – or even a real cardiac event.
- Focus on the steps of the system: rate, capture, sensing, and underlying rhythm.
- While comparing morphologies of sensed and paced waveforms may seem like an imperfect art, it is actually surprisingly reliable. In fact, late-generation devices are trying to imitate the human ability of matching patterns in waveform morphologies as an aid to detection.
- Even a small section of paced ECG can provide tremendous insight into a patient's paced activity and underlying rhythm, but be wary of generalizing too much based on short snippets of information.

- Let the tracing do as much work for you as you can but if you have only a very short tracing or limited data, it is prudent to test capture and sensing, even if you have some evidence that everything is appropriate.
- To test sensing, intrinsic activity has to emerge. The best way to do this for single-chamber devices or the atrial channel of dual-chamber devices is lower the base rate in 10-ppm steps (but not below 30 or 40 ppm). The best way to do this for the ventricular channel of a dual-chamber device is to extend the AV delay interval temporarily to 300 ms or more.
- To test capture, pacing must occur. For single-chamber devices or the atrial channel of a dual-chamber device, increase the base rate in 10-ppm increments while monitoring the patient. To force pacing on the ventricular channel of a dual-chamber device, temporarily shorten the AV delay interval to about 120 ms.

SECTION 31

Automatic Capture Algorithms

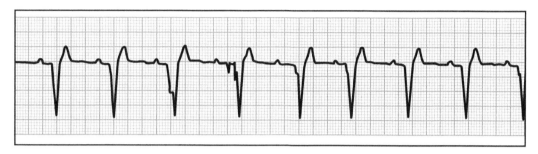

Figure 31.1

This paced ECG shows intrinsic atrial activity followed by a paced ventricular event in response in such a way as to preserve 1:1 AV synchrony. The ventricular pacing spikes on this particular strip are very small and almost imperceptible. While you can see a bit of a notch on the third, fourth and fifth ventricular events, the spike is all but invisible in some of the other complexes. So how do you know it's there?

The main reason to call all of the ventricular events paced is that the morphologies match and some of the events are clearly paced. The morphology shows distinctly that these ventricular events are all of the same type and originating from the same focus (or source). Thus, it looks like they are all paced.

However, looking at the pacing rate tells us another story. Normally, we would measure atrial automatic intervals but on this strip we do not have any examples of that. Measuring the first ventricular automatic interval (VP-VP) shows that the automatic interval is around 840 ms or 70 ppm. This interval marches through the strip with two exceptions.

The first exception is in the fourth complex. The pacing spike occurs at the right timing, but the fifth paced ventricular event is not timed to the fourth ventricular event or the preceding spike. The spike

is followed by another spike and a paced ventricular event.

The other trouble spot is the fifth complex. An intrinsic atrial event occurs, but the sensed AV delay is much too long. What's going on?

Based on morphologies and the visible pacing spikes, it appears that most of these complexes are AS-VP events. The odd appearance of the fourth and fifth complexes stands out. We need to figure out what is going on but based on how orderly the rest of the strip is, it looks like some kind of pacing algorithm or special pacemaker feature is in play.

The ventricular output spike appears in the fourth complex, fails to capture the ventricle, and then, almost immediately after it, a second ventricular spike occurs which successfully captures the ventricle. This is a very unusual paced ECG. Is this normal or is there a problem?

Test your knowledge

1 Is atrial capture and sensing appropriate?
2 Is ventricular capture and sensing appropriate?
3 Why do two pacing spikes appear rapidly, one right after the other, with only one capturing the ventricle?
4 Are both of these pacing spikes intentional?

The Nuts and Bolts of Paced ECG Interpretation, 1st edition. By Tom Kenny.
Published 2009 by Blackwell Publishing, ISBN: 978-1-4501-8404-5.

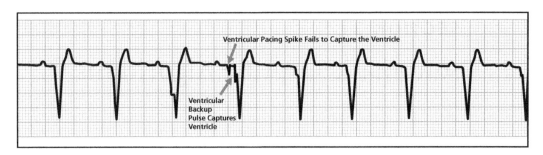

Figure 31.2

5 Why is the sensed AV delay in the next complex so long?

6 How can you troubleshoot this particular situation?

No matter how confusing a paced ECG may appear to you, it is always good practice to go through the basics systematically. First, we should check on atrial capture and sensing. There are no examples of atrial pacing in this strip, so it is not possible to evaluate atrial capture.

However, the presence of 1:1 AV synchrony and the fact that the atrial intrinsic beats appear to inhibit the atrial outputs indicate appropriate atrial sensing. This confirms that this is a dual-chamber device (because it times ventricular activity to the atrium and is therefore "seeing" what's going on in the atrium).

Ventricular capture appears appropriate in all of the complexes except the fourth one. Let's home in on the fourth complex. Based on the pacing rate, the first ventricular spike in the fourth complex (the one that fails to capture) was delivered appropriately, that is, it was timed to the preceding intrinsic atrial event. A second spike is delivered. This second ventricular output pulse is actually timed to the preceding, failed pulse. It is likely a higher-energy pulse because it is able to capture the ventricle while the first spike could not.

If this confuses you, you are not alone. Many clinicians seeing this kind of thing for the first time do not know what to make of the unusual appearance of a double ventricular pacing spike, one failed, one capturing. This strip comes from a patient with a device that offers the AutoCapture Pacing System™. This is an automatic capture algorithm that verifies capture on a beat-by-beat basis. Should a ventricular output fail to capture the heart, the pacemaker immediately delivers a backup safety pulse of sufficient amplitude to reliably capture the heart.

There are many automatic capture algorithms on the market and you will see such algorithms in paced ECGs. The big "tip off" that this is a capture algorithm is the pair of ventricular spikes, one failing and one succeeding. A capture algorithm uses a low amount of energy to capture the heart but, should capture not be achieved, the pacemaker automatically delivers another spike at a higher energy output.

That is exactly what is happening here. This strip shows the AutoCapture™ algorithm in action, and performing exactly as it ought to. Since the algorithm keeps pacemaker output parameter settings relatively low (which saves on battery life and may extend device longevity), the algorithm offers capture verification (for every beat) with the safety of a backup safety pulse.

Capture thresholds (the minimum amount of energy required to depolarize the heart) are not static and can change without warning. Sometimes even a subtle shift in capture threshold can be sudden and cause loss of capture in a patient who had capture previously. That's why capture was lost abruptly. The backup safety pulse was a larger-energy pulse and subsequent pacing reset the pacing output parameters to higher, more appropriate values.

That brings us to the other puzzling thing in this strip. Why is the sensed AV delay so long in fifth complex? The first clue is that the only time the AV delay is prolonged like this occurs right after AutoCapture™ pacing systems had to activate a backup pulse. That suggests this is part of the algorithm.

Whenever AutoCapture™ systems have to provide a backup safety pulse, the algorithm automatically extends the next AV delay in an effort to prevent possible fusion of the next beat. This so called "fusion avoidance algorithm" is automatic and temporary; by the sixth complex, the programmed AV delay interval is back in force.

When confronting any unusual strips of this nature, you may not always be able to figure out this sort of behavior on your own. Absent colleagues to help you figure out strips of this sort, you should feel free to access the technical support services of pacemaker companies or the pacemaker company representative. All major pacemaker companies operate round-the-clock telephone support services. Describing or faxing this sort of strip in to them would have resulted in a quick clarification of what is going on.

And, yes, this strip is normal. The device is performing appropriately.

The nuts and bolts of automatic capture algorithms

- When dealing with very unusual or puzzling ECGs, approach them with the same systematic style you use for more routine strips: analyze pacing and sensing in both chambers, check on the rate, and then explore unusual events.
- Bipolar pacemakers have characteristically small spikes that can be difficult to see on tracings.
- The AutoCapture Pacing System™ algorithm automatically checks for proper ventricular capture on a beat-by-beat basis and delivers an automatic backup safety pulse if capture is lost.
- The benefit of the AutoCapture Pacing System™ (which has been around for over a decade) is that it allows the pacemaker to use less energy to capture the heart while still providing patient safety. The net result is less battery drain, which can extend the service life of the device.
- The typical appearance of the AutoCapture™ Pacing Systems algorithm on an ECG is a ventricular pacing spike that does not capture followed immediately by a paced ventricular event.
- After the AutoCapture™ Pacing Systems, the next AV delay interval is extended as part of a "fusion avoidance algorithm."
- Pacemaker companies all operate 24/7 telephone technical support services that can help you interpret an unusual or confusing ECG or provide other information relevant to a specific type of device. Another good source of information is the representative of that particular pacing company. When in doubt, dig up the manual.
- It's a good idea to have the telephone technical support numbers for all companies handy if you deal with pacemakers, even occasionally. If you do not know them, they can also be obtained by calling the main number of the pacemaker manufacturer or from the manufacturer's website.

SECTION 32

Capture Testing

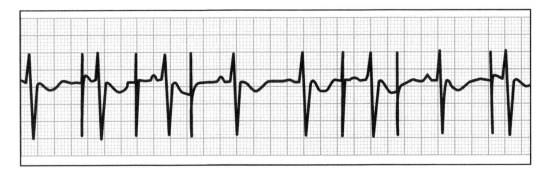

Figure 32.1

This is a paced ECG taken from a pediatric patient with a single-chamber pacemaker. Pacemakers are sometimes implanted in children, even neonates. One unique aspect to pediatric pacing that a clinician should know prior to an ECG evaluation is that pediatric heart rates are higher than adult heart rates. Thus, pacemakers in very young patients are often programmed to base rates of 90 ppm or above, much higher than you would see in an adult patient.

When looking at any strip, we need to remember the systematic approach. This is a single-chamber device, so we need only concern ourselves with the appropriateness of ventricular sensing and ventricular capture. The big pacing spikes indicate that the pacemaker is clearly generating output pulses. However, they never capture the ventricle. There is no spike followed immediately by a ventricular depolarization. This indicates a pretty serious problem: loss of capture.

However, there are some intrinsic ventricular events going on. If you put calipers to the intrinsic ventricular events only, it is apparent that the patient has a relatively stable (albeit imprecise) intrinsic ventricular rate that maps out to about 820 ms (73 bpm). This would be a good rate for an adult, but it is much too slow for a child.

If you measure the distance between ventricular pacing spikes (spike to spike), you get a pacing interval of 640 ms (about 94 ppm). The device is trying to pace at an appropriately high pediatric rate, but without capture, the patient is having to rely on his slower ventricular escape rhythm.

What about ventricular sensing? To check on ventricular sensing, you need to find the ventricular paced interval (from spike to consecutive spike) and then see if the escape intervals (from sensed event to next spike) are equal to or less than that. In other words, will a ventricular event get sensed and inhibit the output? The interval from an intrinsic ventricular event to next consecutive paced ventricular event should also be the same as the pacing interval. While that's true in a couple of places on the strip, look at the two complexes in the center.

These two complexes are completely intrinsic events (AS-VS). They are at the patient's underlying ventricular escape rate. But if the device was sensing appropriately, the first ventricular event would have been sensed and started the pacing interval timer. The next ventricular pacing spike should have appeared 640 ms later. It does not. It means some other event inhibited the pacemaker, which means the device sensed something that wasn't there (oversensing). There are also places that suggest under-

The Nuts and Bolts of Paced ECG Interpretation, 1st edition. By Tom Kenny.
Published 2009 by Blackwell Publishing, ISBN: 978-1-4501-8404-5.

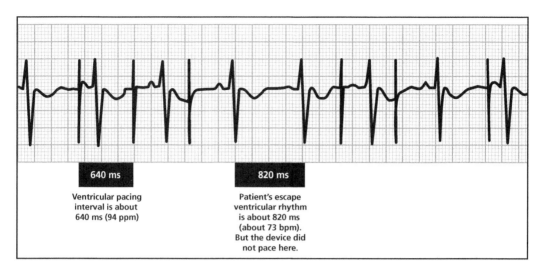

640 ms	820 ms
Ventricular pacing interval is about 640 ms (94 ppm)	Patient's escape ventricular rhythm is about 820 ms (about 73 bpm). But the device did not pace here.

Figure 32.2

sensing. So there is an intermittent problem with sensing, too.

Test your knowledge

1 How would you describe this patient's underlying rhythm?

2 How would you troubleshoot the loss of capture?

3 How would you troubleshoot the inappropriate sensing?

Not all paced ECGs reveal a lot about a patient's underlying rhythm, but this one does. This particular patient has a ventricular escape rhythm of about 73 beats per minute. This is the rate the heart would beat if it was not paced. This is much too slow for a pediatric patient.

However, loss of capture can be a devastating problem if the patient's underlying escape rhythm is very slow, erratic, or practically nonexistent. For so-called pacemaker-dependent patients, even a short episode of non-capture can provoke serious symptoms. While not all of the experts agree on how to define pacemaker dependency, the fact is that most pacemaker patients are going to suffer if they experience loss of capture, particularly for any length of time!

While the programmed rate is appropriate for this patient, there is no capture.

Troubleshooting capture is best done by conducting a threshold test (sometimes called a pacing test or pacing threshold test). This may be automatic or semi-automatic using the programmer. Basically, such tests use a step-down protocol, starting with a high output setting and gradually reducing it in small increments until capture is lost and then stepping it up to restore capture. The device reports the threshold value and recommends a safety margin. Conventional safety margins are 2:1 or 3:1. For example, if a patient has a ventricular pacing threshold of 1.5 V, then a good pulse amplitude value to program would be 3.0 V (2 × 1.5) or 4.5 V (3 × 1.5).

However, it's easy to see how you can sometimes get into some pretty high output settings to be sure to capture. If that is the only alternative, that's what you have to do. Nothing is more important in a pacemaker than capture.

Patients with high or erratic pacing thresholds can benefit from an automatic capture algorithm (see Section 31). The algorithm would verify capture every single beat and if a loss of capture occurred, an immediate higher-energy backup safety pulse would be delivered. There are two advantages to a system like this: first, it uses less battery energy than consistently pacing at a fairly high output setting and, second, the patient never "misses a beat" because of the safety net of the backup pulse.

If this patient had a device with an automatic capture algorithm, it would be useful to activate it. Not all devices are so equipped, but, when the tools are there, clinicians should take advantage of them.

What if this capture problem had nothing to do with the output settings? Rarely, loss of capture can be caused by other things. Those other "suspects" in a loss of capture problem are:

1 Lead problems (order a chest X-ray if this is suspected). A lead could become dislodged or pull out of the pulse generator. This is almost unheard of in a chronic system, but may happen rarely with acute devices. The lead might also be damaged in some way; that can happen in both acute and chronic systems.

2 There may be some sort of component issue. If you can rule out other causes of loss of capture, call the technical services hotline of the pacemaker manufacturer.

There appears to be inappropriate sensing on this strip as well. Using the programmer, conduct a sensing threshold test and then use the value to program the sensitivity. Since it looks like this device is oversensing (sensing events that are not there), you might be tempted to say the pacemaker is likely too sensitive. However, there is also undersensing. It is rare to encounter both as a sensitivity setting problem.

While many sensing problems can be managed by adjusting the sensitivity setting, but what about that rare case where sensitivity does not seem to be the issue? Sensing problems can sometimes be tracked back to a problem with the lead or a device component. Order a chest X-ray to determine if a lead has become dislodged or has visible damage. Call the technical services hotline of the manufacturer to discuss suspected component issues.

As this tracing shows both capture and sensing trouble, a lead problem could be the cause.

The nuts and bolts of capture testing

- Yes, pediatric patients can have pacemakers! These are the same devices adults use, but expect to see much higher programmed base rates.
- When looking at any ECG, approach it systematically and look at capture, sensing, and rates. It can be tempting to want to pursue the "oddity" on the strip rather than approaching the entire strip systematically.
- To troubleshoot any problem, look for the most likely culprit first. Most capture problems trace back to an insufficient pacemaker output pulse. That's why you should always run a pacing threshold test and look carefully at how the output parameters of the device (pulse amplitude and pulse width) are programmed.
- The most likely culprit for sensing problems is the sensitivity setting. Conduct a sensing threshold test and adjust the mV setting appropriately.
- Much rarer causes of sensing and capture problems are lead problems or (even rarer) component problems. These are so unlikely that you should exhaust the more obvious causes first before considering them.
- Lead problems are quite rare, but if a lead problem was to occur (which can impact proper sensing and pacing), it is more likely to occur in the acute phase of a device implant. A sudden problem in a chronic (and previously well performing) lead system is very, very unusual.
- When capture and sensing problems occur simultaneously, check the pacing lead.

SECTION 33

In Depth: Basic Troubleshooting Guide

Evaluating paced ECGs today goes hand-in-hand with device troubleshooting, a subject that can strike fear in the heart of an otherwise competent clinician. It is true that some troubleshooting involves very challenging and unusual case studies, and it is likely that those are the war stories you have heard from your colleagues. However, most troubleshooting involves "playing the odds," that is, looking at the most likely problems and the most likely solutions.

By far the two biggest troubleshooting problems a clinician will encounter when dealing with pacing are capture and sensing problems. Besides being the most typical problems, they can also be the most serious because devices that do not appropriately sense and pace cannot provide reliable pacing support.

Capture

The most severe capture situation you will ever see is a consistent loss of capture on a rhythm strip. If the patient has some underlying rhythm, this may not provoke serious symptoms, but total loss of capture (LOC) can be a very serious, even deadly, problem in a pacemaker-dependent patient. It is far more likely that patients experience intermittent LOC, that is, capture does not occur consistently. It can be hit-or-miss as to whether or not you will see this on a rhythm strip. For that reason, every pacemaker check-up should include a capture threshold test and a re-evaluation of pacemaker output settings. A pacemaker patient may be suffering from intermittent loss of capture that you do not see on a rhythm strip. Adjusting pacemaker output parameters is nothing out of the ordinary. It is not unusual for pacemaker output parameters to be adjusted many times over the patient's life.

Pacing thresholds (also known as capture thresholds) are not static values. They are known to fluctuate, even over the course of a day in a single patient. A lot of things can affect the pacing threshold:

drugs, disease progression, age, even whether or not the patient has just eaten and his posture! Since thresholds are notoriously variable, the threshold value obtained in a pacing test cannot be assumed to be the average. Instead, clinicians err on the side of caution and guess that this is the lowest threshold. A safety margin of 2:1 or 3:1 is typically built in to give an extra electrical "cushion" and assure capture.

I am a big fan of automatic capture algorithms for the simple reasons that they use less energy and still check up on every paced beat. There are a number of ventricular capture algorithms out there and there is a new atrial capture confirmation algorithm. These algorithms offer patient safety, can extend device longevity (by not unnecessarily taxing the battery with larger-than-necessary output pulses), and can help streamline follow-up because a lot of the "capture problem" are left to the device to regulate.

However, sometimes capture problems will occur that cannot be resolved by simply programming higher output parameter settings. The next likely suspect in capture loss is a lead problem. In new implants (acute systems) compared to older systems, it is far more likely that a lead will dislodge from where it has been fixated in the heart or that the lead will loosen or pull out of the pulse generator. Both situations, as you may suspect, can cause some loss of capture!

Chronic or long-term pacemaker systems are less likely to experience that kind of lead problem. Typically, once a lead is fixated and has several weeks to mature, fibrosis at the point where the lead interfaces with cardiac tissues will serve to secure the lead permanently. Leads firmly plugged into the generator do not suddenly pull away. Thus, it would be extremely unlikely to see that kind of thing in a chronic system. But one thing I know as a clinician: never say never!

However, acute and chronic pacing systems can experience problems if a lead is damaged. Lead dam-

The Nuts and Bolts of Paced ECG Interpretation, 1st edition. By Tom Kenny.
Published 2009 by Blackwell Publishing, ISBN: 978-1-4501-8404-5.

age includes nicks to the lead (insulation breach) or broken wires (conductor fracture). Older leads may be more likely to experience things like stress erosion cracking or fatigue. These problems are rare, but they can occur.

If you suspect a lead problem, it is good clinical practice to order a chest X-ray before proceeding. The X-ray may reveal if the lead is damaged, but it takes a trained eye to see such detail in the film. Then again, the problem may not show up on an X-ray. In such instances, it is typical to troubleshoot by ruling out the other causes and then deducing that the lead is damaged.

When leads are suspected as being the cause of a problem, check the impedance values of the pacing leads. These are available from the programmer and may also be contained in the patient's chart. Lead impedance values are typically stated as broad ranges for the particular lead with any value in the range technically "normal." For instance, many pacing leads will state that 300 to 1200 Ohms resistance is within specification. For that lead, an impedance value of 500 and an impedance value of 1100 would both be "normal."

Damaged leads are often out of specification

If you do not know the impedance value range for the lead(s) of a particular patient, check with the lead manufacturer (manual, representative, technical support line) to find out what values are acceptable.

However, don't assume that just because lead impedance values fall within range that all is well. A large or sudden change in impedance values also can suggest a lead problem. While there is no hard science to this, a good rule of thumb is that an abrupt change (up or down) of 200 Ohms or more is cause to investigate. "Abrupt" here means that the change happened since the last follow-up. Changes of less magnitude (say 50 Ohms) between follow-ups are not that unusual and do not suggest trouble. In fact, you will see variation in impedance values from check-up to check-up. If they are small, this is probably perfectly appropriate.

Sensing

When it comes to sensing problems, the best course

of action is to begin your troubleshooting with a sensing threshold test and a re-evaluation of the sensitivity setting. By far the vast majority of sensing problems can be solved with those basic steps. One caution with sensitivity adjustment: do not make big changes. If 2 mV is too sensitive, don't assume that 8 mV is the answer! It's true that 8 mV will solve your oversensing problems, but it will almost assuredly introduce undersensing problems.

When sensing problems persist, the next "likely culprit" is something going on with the lead. The same sorts of lead problems that can impact capture can also mess up sensing. In fact, if the lead is really at the root of the problem, it is likely that capture and sensing problems will appear together on one strip. (However, just because lead and capture problems occur on one strip does not mean it has to be a lead problem – it could be a sensitivity setting problem and too-low output parameters that happen together.)

Sensing problems may also be caused by inappropriate device programming. For instance, look at the refractory periods that are programmed. It is possible that the heart is contracting and the device is even seeing the events but the refractory periods prohibit device response. Look at PVARP and ventricular refractory period settings; it may be that you can program your way out of some sensing problems.

Do take advantage of contacting the representatives of the pacemaker manufacturer in tough cases of troubleshooting devices. Most manufacturers invest a lot of money maintaining a highly trained field force that is put in place specifically to help respond to situations like this.

Other problems

Other troubleshooting problems you can encounter include rate variations and pauses. When you see unusual rate activity (that is, pacing at a rate other than the programmed base rate), find out how the device is programmed. These features can cause pacing at rates other than the programmed base rate:

- Rate hysteresis (will often result in lower-than-base-rate pacing)
- Rate response (will often result in higher-than-base-rate pacing)
- Rest rate (lower than base rate)

• Atrial tracking (DDD and DDDR devices only, will cause the ventricle to be paced to maintain 1:1 AV synchrony with a rapidly beating atria up to a programmable maximum tracking rate)

Pauses sometimes show up mysteriously on paced ECG. The causes of pauses include:

• Loss of capture (the device thought it was pacing, but nothing happened)

• Oversensing (the device thought the heart was beating, but nothing happened)

When in doubt about troubleshooting, remember to keep it systematic. Look at capture, sensing, and the rate. Check out any unusual-looking activity. Consider the most likely causes and try to rule them out before you look at more unusual sources of the behavior. Most troubleshooting involves the basics.

The nuts and bolts of troubleshooting in depth

• Troubleshooting devices means looking at what is possibly inappropriate and trying to track down a cause and find the solution. When doing this, proceed systematically and play the odds. Look at the most likely causes first!

• The most common troubleshooting problems in the pacemaker clinic involve loss of capture and sensing problems (oversensing and undersensing). These sensing problems can occur consistently, but it is more likely that they will be intermittent.

• Don't assume that because a problem did not show up on a paced ECG that it could not be lurking in the background. During every pacemaker check-up in the clinic, evaluate pacing and sensing thresholds and check how these key parameters are programmed: pulse amplitude, pulse width, sensitivity, and rate.

• The most common cause of capture problems is that the pacemaker output pulse parameters (pulse amplitude and pulse width) are insufficient. They may need to be increased. It is more efficient to increase the pulse amplitude than the pulse width.

• The most common cause of sensing problems is an inappropriate sensitivity setting. Check the sensing threshold and reprogram the sensitivity, if necessary.

• When programming sensitivity, remember that a lower mV value makes the device more sensitive. Conversely, a higher mV value makes the pacemaker less sensitive.

• Other causes of pacing and sensing problems can be lead issues. Order a chest X-ray and look at recent lead impedance data if a lead problem is suspected. Damaged leads may require replacement (surgery).

• Rate variations can be puzzling. If you see paced activity at unexpected rates, check if the features such as rate response, hysteresis, rest rate, or atrial tracking (DDD or DDDR mode) are on.

• Pauses can appear on rhythm strips owing to oversensing or loss of capture.

• When in doubt about troubleshooting, do not hesitate to confer with a colleague or contact a representative of the device company.

SECTION 34

Navigating the Intracardiac Electrogram

Figure 34.1 is an atrial electrogram from a pacemaker patient with a relatively recent implant (<1 year) of a dual-chamber pacemaker. If you work with pacemaker patients for any length of time, you are going to encounter this sort of tracing, known as an intracardiac electrogram (also called an IEGM, EGM, electrogram, or even e-gram). In theory and form, it resembles the surface ECG. Like a surface ECG, an electrogram is a graphic depiction of the heart's electrical activity. While a surface ECG gets its electrical information from the heart through the skin, an EGM gets its electrical information from within the heart. Data for the EGM are picked up from the electrodes on the pacemaker leads.

Many clinicians unfamiliar with EGMs may find them a bit confusing. They look somewhat familiar, but start to study them, and you'll see they can be "different." Most electrograms tend to generate tracings that look more condensed, smaller, tighter, and more "smushed together" looking. Bear that in mind as you examine any EGM; it is rare to see large, crisp events that might occur on a surface ECG.

Since you can only get an electrogram from a pacemaker programmer (either in real-time, that is, "live," or downloaded as a stored EGM from the device's memory), they never appear the way you see this one. All EGMs you will work with in the clinic will be fully annotated and have even more device information at the top.

Thus, what we are going to start with here is a bit artificial. You won't get something like this in the clinic to work with. However, it is vitally important in working with paced tracings to view the tracing independently and *in isolation from the annotations*.

Annotations are markers on the tracing that show you what the pacemaker "saw" or how the pacemaker responded. Annotations are accurate in that they accurately tell you what the pacemaker "thinks" is going on. However, the pacemaker may not always be right! That's why you need to be able to assess the tracing independently. In most cases, happily, the tracing will match the annotations. But sometimes it will not, and when there is a discrepancy, clinicians need to realize that the tracing is indicative of what the heart is doing while the annotations are, at most, indicative of what the pacemaker is "thinking" or "doing."

Since this is an electrogram, you would typically see it annotated (we have deleted those for this first exercise). However, one special marking remains. The longest vertical line in the center of the strip is the "trigger." Electrograms are snapshots taken by the pacemaker when triggered by a specific event. In this case, something happened at that line that caused the electrogram to get recorded and stored in memory. The tracing to the left of the trigger line is called "pre-trigger." These are the events that led up to the triggering event; the post-trigger events are what happened afterward. In most cases, the pre-trigger waveforms are the more useful and interesting to the clinician.

There is one other bit of information you need to know to analyze an electrogram: the chamber. This particular electrogram happens to be an atrial electrogram (you know this from the annotations, which we'll go over in the next section). This means it is the view from the atrial electrode of a dual-chamber system. A dual-chamber pacemaker will also provide ventricular electrograms. Many pacemakers offer simultaneous atrial and ventricular electrograms (two tracings, one from each chamber, taken at the same time) and some will blend atrial and ventricular data in a way that produces one tracing but with information from both chambers. Electrograms have to be set up and programmed in advance; you cannot, for instance, program the pacemaker to record only the atrial electrogram but later obtain the ventricular electrogram for the same episode.

In this example, however, we have a conventional atrial electrogram from a dual-chamber pacemaker.

The Nuts and Bolts of Paced ECG Interpretation, 1st edition. By Tom Kenny.
Published 2009 by Blackwell Publishing, ISBN: 978-1-4501-8404-5.

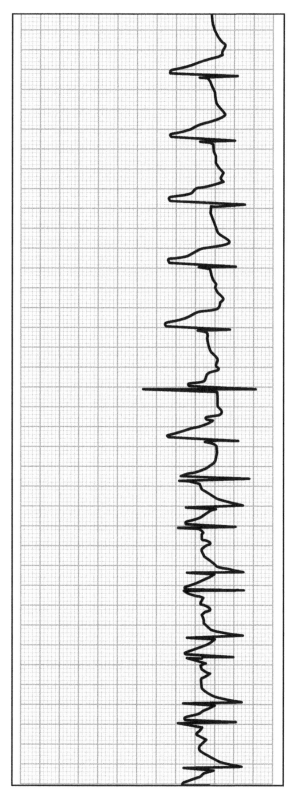

Figure 34.1

Using the trigger to get oriented in the electrogram, the next step is to approach this rhythm strip systematically. First we want to look for appropriate capture and sensing. At first glance, you may not be able to see anything that looks like a pacing spike! Electrograms usually show only small bumps or notches for spikes, even with unipolar systems.

Looking at the run of similar-looking post-trigger events, these complexes are actually paced atrial events that conduct down to the ventricle. Remember, this is an atrial electrogram, so we are going to see atrial events appear much larger than they would on a standard surface ECG. In fact, atrial events may appear as large as ventricular events! (This is not a hard and fast rule; just anticipate larger atrial events on an atrial electrogram than on a ventricular electrogram or a surface ECG.) The vertical lines are atrial output pulses and the large upward deflections are paced atrial events resulting in conducted ventricular beats.

These atrial events do not round out smoothly back to baseline. You'll notice a sort of notch or protrusion about one third down the downward slope. This is actually indicative of a sensed ventricular event. Thus, on the triggered half of the EGM, there is a run of paced atrial events that conduct down to the ventricle (AP-VS).

Bearing in mind that this is what a paced atrial event/sensed ventricular event looks like, you can see another one of them right before the trigger line.

On the post-trigger side, you may notice some bumps between complexes. If this were a surface ECG, those bumps might indicate rapid intrinsic atrial activity or interference. However, on an atrial electrogram, they indicate some sort of noise that is being picked up. Atrial events would show up as big events on this strip. These bumps might be distant ventricular noises, myopotentials, or (most likely) artifacts or stray signals generated by the electrogram.

Going to the pre-trigger side of the strip, starting at the trigger line, back up one complex. This is a wider event with a sharp notch at the top. If you back up another two events, you'll see a similar-looking complex. Back up two more, and there it is again. In-between these notched events are narrower, tighter, un-notched complexes. In fact, there is a pattern here of notched, unnotched complexes.

You can also see four downward "bumps" on the ECG that look almost like traditional P-waves. These downward rounded deflections are actually *ventricular pacing spikes*! The ensuing complex (tall but a bit wider than the others) is a paced ventricular event. The next very narrow complex after the paced ventricular event is a *paced atrial event*.

Thus, we're seeing a run of ventricular spike, ventricular depolarization, atrial spike, atrial depolarization. This is classic AP-VP behavior.

Coming back to basics, is there appropriate atrial sensing? We cannot determine that from this strip because there is only atrial pacing. Is there appropriate atrial capture? Yes, it looks like atrial pacing spikes consistently depolarize the atrium.

Is there appropriate ventricular sensing? Yes, intrinsic ventricular events appear to inhibit the ventricular output pulse. What about ventricular capture? Ventricular pacing spikes seem to be immediately followed by ventricular depolarizations. Note that on the pre-trigger side there is a bit of a lag between spike and depolarization, but this interval (fractions of a second) has more to do with how the electrogram is set up than time elapsing from spike to depolarization.

Here's how it works. When a spike is delivered, the device annotates it immediately and the electrogram responds with a pacing artifact called a spike. The sensed event on the tracing and on the annotations occurs after depolarization starts to occur. Since there is more distance for the signal to travel from ventricle to atrial electrode than ventricle to ventricular electrode, there will be a tiny time lag from ventricular output pulse to ventricular contraction *on an atrial electrogram*.

What about the pacing rate? On the post-trigger side, there are very consistent, easy-to-measure pacing intervals. The same pacing interval also "marches through" on the pre-trigger side. The rate is about 640 ms (94 ppm) which is somewhat rapid.

Test your knowledge

1 What are some reasons you might suggest for the patient's heart to be paced so rapidly? Is there any appropriate reason for this?

2 What was going on in the pre-trigger portion that triggered an electrogram?

3 Was this triggering appropriate?

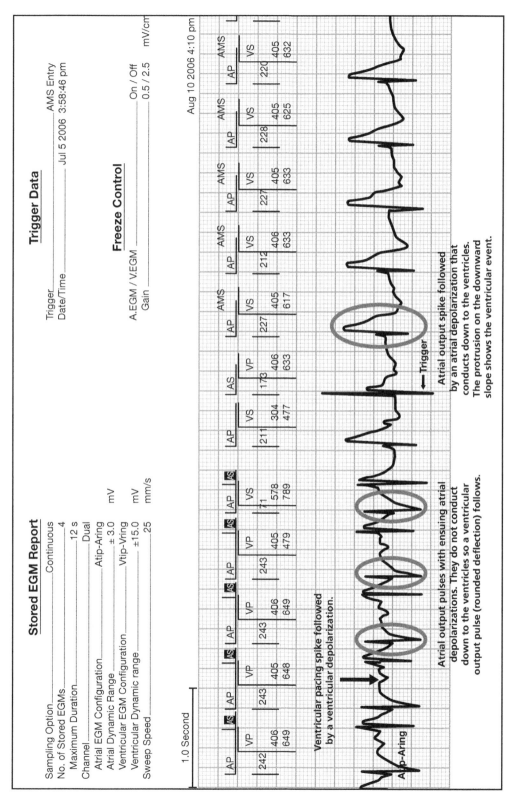

Stored EGM Report

Sampling Option	Continuous
No. of Stored EGMs	4
Maximum Duration	12 s
Channel	Dual
Atrial EGM Configuration	Atip-Aring
Atrial Dynamic Range	±3.0 mV
Ventricular EGM Configuration	Vtip-Vring
Ventricular Dynamic range	±15.0 mV
Sweep Speed	25 mm/s

Trigger Data

Trigger	AMS Entry
Date/Time	Jul 5 2006 3:58:46 pm

Freeze Control

A.EGM / V.EGM	On / Off
Gain	0.5 / 2.5 mV/cm

Aug 10 2006 4:10 pm

1.0 Second

Ventricular pacing spike followed
by a ventricular depolarization.

Atip-Aring

Atrial output pulses with ensuing atrial
depolarizations. They do not conduct
down to the ventricles so a ventricular
output pulse (rounded deflection) follows.

Atrial output spike followed
by an atrial depolarization that
conducts down to the ventricles.
The protrusion on the downward
slope shows the ventricular event.

← Trigger

Figure 34.2

This is a bit more like the typical electrogram you would see in the clinic (minus the circles and notes we added to the tracing). You'll notice some useful information spelled out at the top of the electrogram. Below the tracing and to the left, it says Atip-Aring which means the electrogram was taken from the perspective of the *atrial tip* electrode to the *atrial ring* electrode. It is always a good idea to verify the type of electrogram you're evaluating from the tracing itself; an atrial electrogram looks different than a ventricular one!

By the way, the type of electrogram available for download depends on how the device was programmed. If you did not program a particular trigger or set up a certain type of electrogram, it will not be available in memory later on. For that reason, it is good practice to think about what types of electrograms might be useful for a patient and to program them carefully. It is tempting to want to program everything just so all electrograms will be handy if you need them – but electrograms consume memory in the pacemaker. If you program too many triggers, you may wind up with more electrogram data than the pacemaker can store. In such cases, the pacemaker will either overwrite old data (this is called "continuous," where the oldest data are overwritten by the newest data) or simply stop recording once it's full (this is called "freeze"). A new option in advanced pacemakers from St. Jude Medical allows the clinician to prioritize electrograms so that high-priority electrograms are saved while low-priority ones get overwritten if the memory reaches capacity.

Off to the right, the device reports what the trigger line was. For now, we will ignore this and see if we cannot figure out from the tracing what is going on. This information is good for verification purposes, but we do not need it for our systematic analysis.

First, let's look at the pacing rate, which we already determined to be about 90 ppm. This patient does not have an intrinsic rate of 90 ppm (which might occur in the event of a sinus tachycardia, an atrial tachycardia, or exertion which sped up the intrinsic atrial rate); he has a paced rate of 90 ppm.

Although we have no notation to this effect on the top of the strip, the first thing to suspect is that the device is rate responsive. The patient may have been active enough at that time to drive up the sensor rate to 90 ppm. That is not a particularly high sensor-driven rate and would be appropriate in many patients doing ordinary things like household chores, going up steps, taking a walk, and so on. Checking on the device parameters, it is found that the pacemaker is indeed a rate-responsive device. Thus, this rate appears to be appropriate.

Now let's look at what the pacemaker *thought the heart rate was doing*. Paced atrial events on the pre-trigger side are properly annotated and recognized as paced events. The ventricular output pulses (spikes) are annotated as VP, again appropriate. But after the ventricular output pulse, the ensuing ventricular contraction is annotated AS in a black box (meaning it occurred in the refractory period).

This means the pacemaker "thought" that paced ventricular activity was actually an intrinsic (non-paced) atrial event!

This kind of behavior does show up in some dual-chamber systems. In fact, it even has a name. It's called far-field R-wave sensing (or far-R). Far-R occurs when something on the ventricular channel (even something paced) shows up on "atrial radar" and is inappropriately counted as an intrinsic atrial event.

While the tracing showed the patient had 1:1 AV synchrony (one atrial event for each and every ventricular event), the pacemaker "thought" there were two atrial events for each ventricular event. In other words, the pacemaker was seeing atrial activity at about twice the paced rate or around 180 bpm! Any time events are miscounted in this pattern, it can be termed double-counting. Double-counting can cause the pacemaker to make inappropriate decisions.

The pacemaker thought that there was high-rate intrinsic atrial activity which ended up causing the device to mode switch, triggering the electrogram. But it is an inappropriate mode switch! Look closely and you'll see that the patient's paced rate does not drop when he enters AMS (and it would if there was genuinely high-rate intrinsic activity going on).

The problem traces back to the device seeing ventricular events as atrial events. Troubleshooting this kind of problem should start with a test of atrial sensitivity. It may be that the atrial channel is overly sensitive. Sometimes making the atrial channel less sensitive can reduce far-field R-wave sensing, but not always. (And it may not be appropriate to reduce sensitivity! It is possible for the atrial lead to be programmed to an appropriate sensitivity setting and still pick up far-field signals.)

Another troubleshooting approach might be to make the ventricular output pulse less powerful. Run a ventricular capture test and verify that the output parameters are not overly high. If you can safely reduce them, that might reduce far-R sensing. It is possible that the ventricular output is appropriately programmed.

What next? In some cases, the reason that far-field R-wave sensing occurs in the first place has to do with the physical proximity of the atrial electrodes and the ventricular electrodes. Although it is a serious step, lead revision may be required to rectify a particularly stubborn far-R problem.

There is a new atrial bipolar lead on the market with 1.1 mm spacing between the atrial tip electrode and the atrial ring electrode. This unique spacing has been shown to help dramatically reduce the incidence of far-R sensing because it narrows the "antenna" that the atrial signal has to pick up signals. If a lead revision is required, the leads might be repositioned or the atrial lead could be replaced with this new type of atrial lead.

One last thing. If you look on the pre-trigger side of this electrogram, you may notice the annotations show AS and then AP in very close proximity. Does the nearness of a paced atrial event so soon after a sensed atrial event indicate a problem with atrial sensing as well?

The answer is: not necessarily. After any ventricular event, the pacemaker automatically starts a special post-ventricular atrial refractory period (PVARP) timing cycle. A typical PVARP setting is 250 ms, but it is programmable. During PVARP, the atrial channel is refractory to atrial activity. Using calipers set to 250 ms, it is clear that these sensed atrial events fall in the PVARP. This means that the pacemaker was prohibited from responding to these atrial events.

But don't think that an AS event in the PVARP does not count. It does count! The pacemaker still "saw" the AS event and counted it toward legitimate atrial activity. It just could not respond to it, that is, it could not use it to inhibit the next atrial output pulse.

The PVARP timing cycle is actually divided into two sections. The PVARP actually starts out with the post-ventricular atrial blanking period (PVAB). During PVAB, no atrial events can even be seen by the pacemaker. Any atrial event that occurs during PVAB will not get annotated or counted or responded to. Once PVAB expires, however, the pacemaker starts to see and count atrial activity, even if it does not respond to it.

This EGM shows AMS entry. However, upon careful analysis (*and viewing the tracing as distinct from the annotations*) it is clear that it is inappropriate mode switching and that far-field oversensing is going on.

By the way, this mode switch was from DDDR to DDIR, which explains the presence of atrial paced beats. Many older systems mode-switched to VVIR, but it is more common today to see atrial tracking (but not atrial pacing) turned off, thus, the switched mode is likely to be DDI or DDIR.

The nuts and bolts of navigating the intracardiac electrogram

- Electrograms (EGMs) are "inside" looks at cardiac activity. They resemble surface ECGs but they are taken using the electrodes on the pacing leads. Expect to see more condensed, tighter, smaller looking complexes.
- EGMs can be atrial, ventricular, both together, or both blended, depending on how the device is programmed. Devices can be easily reprogrammed for different types of electrogram storage.
- EGMs can be obtained "live" (in real time) or stored in device memory and downloaded. When electrograms are stored, a trigger is needed to launch the storage. Triggers may be automatic (default values in the device) or programmable or both. Typical EGM triggers are premature ventricular contractions (PVCs), high-rate intrinsic atrial activity, ventricular tachycardia, and mode switch entry and exit.
- On an atrial electrogram, atrial activity will appear as large or larger than ventricular activity!

- EGMs typically show very small pacing spikes; in fact, they may look more like bumps or protrusions than the spikes commonly seen on surface ECGs.
- When evaluating an annotated EGM or any annotated rhythm strip, never rely on the annotations alone. Always view the tracing in isolation. If the tracing does not line up with the annotations, count on the tracing to show you what the heart is actually doing.
- Atrial events that occur in the PVARP can be counted even if the device is prohibited from responding to them. Only atrial events that occur during the PVAB portion of the PVARP are not seen.
- This particular example shows an inappropriate mode switch but it is one that the patient was unlikely to have noticed. That's why a thorough understanding of paced ECGs and EGMs can help clinicians solve problems before they become symptoms!

SECTION 35

Tracings from a Programmer (Combining E-grams with the ECG)

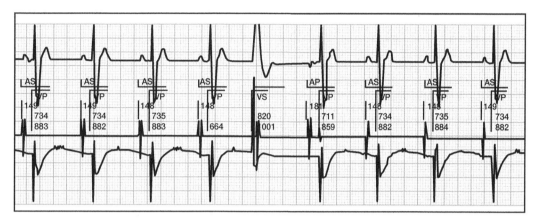

Figure 35.1

This is an electrogram from a dual-chamber pacemaker. The top tracing shows the atrial electrogram and the bottom tracing shows the ventricular electrogram. Dual electrograms like this can be programmed for most dual-chamber pacemakers but they use up a lot of memory space for storage. However, they provide the most comprehensive data of what was actually going on in the heart. This electrogram was stored in the pacemaker memory, so some sort of remarkable event triggered it.

In this electrogram, the annotations appear between the tracings. While annotations are useful, it is important in electrogram analysis to allow the tracings to tell the story of what is going on in the heart, while the pacemaker annotations report how the device perceived the events.

As is typical with electrograms, atrial events appear larger on the atrial electrogram (top) and ventricular events appear large on the ventricular electrogram (bottom). In fact, it is somewhat hard to see atrial activity at all on the ventricular strip. That is fine, since we have the atrial electrogram above to fill in the gaps.

Atrial sensing appears appropriate on the strip. On the atrial electrogram, distinct atrial sensed events can be seen. Look down on the ventricular strip and you'll notice these same sensed atrial events appear as vertical lines on the ventricular strip. Atrial sensing seems appropriate because the atrial events inhibit atrial output pulses.

There is only one atrial paced event on the strip, best viewed as the downward-deflecting P-wave on the upper strip. The pacing spike is not clear here (it often is not easy to see spikes on electrograms) but the different morphology coupled with the AP annotation show that the device delivered an atrial spike which caused an immediate atrial depolarization. This is evidence of appropriate atrial capture.

On the ventricular channel, there are mostly paced ventricular events. Large ventricular pacing spikes are evident on the lower tracing and confirmed by the VP annotations. The immediate ventricular depolarization is good evidence of capture.

There is only one sensed ventricular event, and it occurs in the middle of the strip. Ventricular sensing appears appropriate in that this ventricular event inhibited a ventricular output.

Measuring the interval from one consecutive ventricular pacing spike to the next, the interval appears consistent at 880 ms (about 68 ppm) with one

---

The Nuts and Bolts of Paced ECG Interpretation, 1st edition. By Tom Kenny.
Published 2009 by Blackwell Publishing, ISBN: 978-1-4501-8404-5.

exception. The sensed ventricular event should have caused a paced ventricular event to come in at 880 ms. Instead, the interval from sensed ventricular event to the next paced ventricular event is about 1000 ms. This is too long for the programmed base rate.

Furthermore, right after this overly long interval, the pacemaker paces the atrium although the patient otherwise appears to have a steady intrinsic atrial rate.

This "odd beat" in the middle of the strip is the trigger for the electrogram.

Test your knowledge

1 Is there anything unusual about the ventricular event in the middle of the strip (the one with the VS annotation)?

2 What would cause the pacemaker to generate one overly long interval?

3 Was the pacemaker performing appropriately?

4 Would you troubleshoot this situation, and, if so, how?

The event circled on the EGM is a premature ventricular contraction (PVC) rather than just an ordinary sensed ventricular event. Some programmers would even have annotated it PVC (or also PVE for premature ventricular event) rather than just VS. A pacemaker defines a PVC as any two ventricular events without an intervening atrial event. Since the

earlier portion of this strip showed good 1:1 AV synchrony, suddenly having a ventricular beat appear without a preceding atrial beat caused the device to treat it as a PVC.

PVCs are not all that unusual; they appear on paced and non-paced rhythm strips and occur all of the time, even in otherwise healthy patients. An abundance of PVCs can be a cause for concern, but an occasional PVC is not necessarily indicative of anything in particular. However, in a pacemaker, a sudden PVC can sometimes trigger a pacemaker-mediated tachycardia. For that reason, many pacemakers have special algorithms to help manage PVCs.

In this device, the pacemaker responds to a PVC by extending the PVARP timing cycle. Upon PVC, the PVARP is automatically set to 480 ms for that one cycle. The PVARP actually consists of two phases: the first portion is the post-ventricular atrial blanking period or PVAB (150 ms in this case) and the second portion is sometimes called the relative refractory period or RRP. In this case, the RRP is 330 ms. The PVAB and RRP are shown in Figure 35.3 (PVAB is the lighter bar, RRP the darker).

A normal PVARP is about 250 ms, with a PVAB and an RRP. This prolonged PVARP occurs only right after a PVC if this particular PVC option algorithm is programmed on.

During the PVAB, the pacemaker will not see or respond to an atrial event. During the RRP, however, the pacemaker will not respond to atrial activity al-

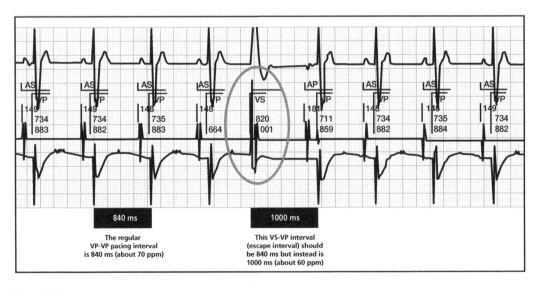

Figure 35.2

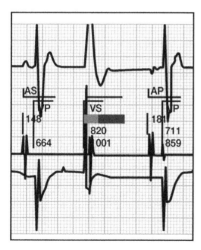

Figure 35.3

though it can see it and will count it. The reason for the extended PVARP is that a PVC is likely to initiate a pacemaker-mediated tachycardia only if an atrial event manages to begin the cycle. These are sometimes called "retrograde P-waves" and can result in a pacemaker-mediated tachycardia. An extended PVARP means the device will ignore any atrial events in a fairly long period of time.

The algorithm is also set up to automatically pace the atrium if an intrinsic atrial event is sensed during the RRP portion of the pacemaker. The RRP means the pacemaker will not respond to it, but if the intrinsic atrial event is perceived it will launch the automatic atrial paced event. In this particular case, no atrial activity was perceived during the RRP portion of the PVARP.

When the prolonged PVARP expires, the device goes into its atrial alert mode. When no intrinsic atrial event occurs in the atrial alert mode, the device paces the atrium at a rate which, if the paced AV delay were applied, would maintain the VP-VP rate.

Although this algorithm will sometimes automatically pace the atrium after a PVC and prolonged PVARP (only if a sensed atrial event occurs in the RRP portion of the PVARP), in this particular case it did not. The paced atrial event occurred because the PVARP timed out and the atrial alert period timed out.

If you see from the chart or programmer that a PVC option is programmed on, this is certainly appropriate device behavior. Even without such verification, this is likely the cause of such a precise deviation from otherwise classic paced activity. No troubleshooting is required.

The one caveat to that last remark is that PVCs are not worrisome unless they occur frequently. If the patient is known to be susceptible to PMTs, PVCs can be more serious, in that they are a common trigger for PMTs in susceptible patients. Most pacemakers offer downloadable diagnostic reports that can give you a count (absolute or percentages) of total PVC activity since the last follow-up.

The nuts and bolts of combining e-grams with the ECG

- Pacemakers define a PVC as two consecutive ventricular events (the second one sensed) without an intervening atrial event.
- Some EGMs will annotate PVCs as such, but not all of them do that. Sometimes the device will count a PVC but annotate just VS.
- PVCs are usually not in and of themselves harmful (unless they are very abundant) but they can trigger pacemaker-mediated tachycardias (PMTs) in some pacemaker patients.
- Most pacemakers offer PVC options to help manage PVCs automatically. When you see a PVC on a paced strip and then unusual device behavior for one cycle, you should suspect that a PVC option is in play.

- There are several different PVC options on the market; they differ slightly by manufacturer and even by device by one manufacturer. When in doubt, consult the manual, manufacturer website, or manufacturer's representative.
- In this example, the PVCs automatically extended the PVARP to help "blot out" any atrial activity following too closely in the wake of the PVC. When the PVARP timed out, the atrial alert period followed.
- However, had an atrial event been picked up during the RRP (relative refractory period) or latter portion of the PVARP, the pacemaker would have automatically paced the atrium.

SECTION 36

Stored Electrograms

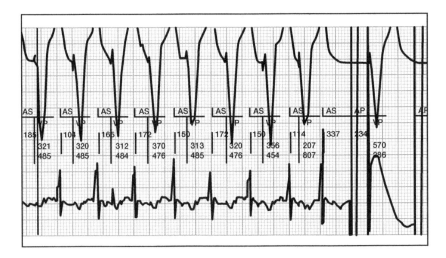

Figure 36.1

In the clinic, electrograms are typically downloaded only when you already know what has triggered them. In this particular case, this dual-channel electrogram from a DDDR pacemaker was downloaded as a PMT option algorithm. PMT stands for pacemaker-mediated tachycardia. In this case, a PMT is already going on as the strip begins.

A PMT is a special type of tachycardia which is abetted by the pacemaker. It sets up an endless loop which causes a "backward" relationship of ventricular event to atrial event; in fact, the atrial events are sometimes called retrograde. For the pacemaker, a PMT is diagnosed when it sees a stable VP-AS relationship at an interval of around 666 ms (90 ppm). The pacing should be higher than base rate (nominally, the PMT rate cutoff is 90 ppm but can be programmed differently) and the VP-AS pattern should be very stable. The device actually looks to see that the variation in these intervals is less than 16 ms! (That's less than half of one little box on the grid!)

The PMT algorithm works by counting a programmable number of such fast, stable VP-AS intervals and then goes into effect. In this example, the

PMT diagnosis was reached after the eighth complex on this strip. At that point, the pacemaker responded by withholding a ventricular output after the intrinsic (retrograde) atrial event and paced the atrium 330 ms after the intrinsic atrial event. This resulted in a paced ventricular event after the paced AV delay expired. The PMT was broken and it is quite likely the patient never noticed anything unusual.

Test your knowledge

1 The EGM shows an atrial and a ventricular channel. Which is which?
2 Do the annotations match up with what is going on in the tracing?
3 Based on a PMT algorithm as described above, did the device perform appropriately?
4 Would you leave this PMT option programmed on in this patient? Why or why not?

This is one of those "expensive" EGMs with a separate atrial and ventricular tracing. These sorts of EGMs use up a lot of memory (which is getting

The Nuts and Bolts of Paced ECG Interpretation, 1st edition. By Tom Kenny.
Published 2009 by Blackwell Publishing, ISBN: 978-1-4501-8404-5.

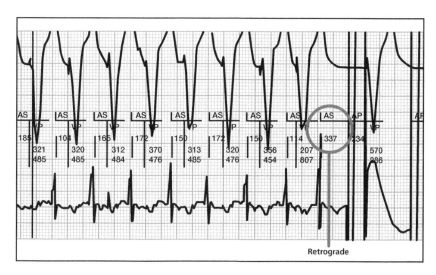

Retrograde

Figure 36.2

larger with each new generation of devices but still is finite) but offer the clinician the most information. The ventricular channel is on top and the atrial channel is on the bottom.

The atrial channel will show large atrial events, sometimes (as in this example) larger than the ventricular activity. The bottom strip shows large atrial sensed events followed by more rounded, smaller ventricular events. The upper strip shows very large ventricular events that obscure the atrial events. Had a clinician only had the ventricular electrogram to work with, it would have been very hard to see what was going on.

The annotations align well with the tracings. Atrial sensed events appear, ventricular pacing spikes and resulting depolarizations are evident. Everything looks to be in the right place. This is typical for an electrogram; most of the time, the pacemaker "sees" what is going on and interprets it properly. Nevertheless, a clinician should always check out the EGM carefully.

This particular example required eight intervals with a stable, fast VP-AS interval to diagnosis PMT. Using fewer events is not recommended, since variability requires a run of several complexes to ascertain, plus an occasional unusual event does not necessarily mean the patient is experiencing a PMT. On the other hand, a prolonged PMT can subject the patient to symptoms. A run of eight complexes at this rate (about 480 ms or 125 ppm) would last

less than 4 seconds (480 × 8 = 3840 ms or 3.84 seconds). That brief a period of rapid pacing is unlikely to provoke severe symptoms.

Once PMT is diagnosed, the next retrograde AS event (circled) will cause the pacemaker to withhold a ventricular output pulse. This essentially breaks the PMT because the pacemaker ceases to contribute to it! A timing cycle of 330 ms is launched, starting with the retrograde AS event (circled). After 330 ms, an atrial output pulse is automatically delivered. The 330 ms timing cycle is long enough to allow the atrium (which just depolarized) to emerge from its refractory period and become vulnerable again. This means the atrial pacing output that is delivered will find responsive tissue and cause an atrial depolarization which, in fact, is exactly what has occurred.

The atrial output pulse launches the paced AV delay. When that expires (which it does), a ventricular output pulse is delivered, causing a ventricular contraction. The patient has come out of the PMT.

In this example, the pacemaker performed appropriately and as expected. Although the EGM cuts off here, it is likely that this terminated the PMT successfully.

Not all patients are susceptible to PMTs, but many are. PMTs can occur suddenly, without warning, even in pacemaker patients that had never had them previously. In this particular case, the clinician has proof positive that this particular patient is indeed susceptible to PMTs. For that reason, the algorithm should be left programmed ON. In fact, unless there are compelling reasons to do otherwise, it is good clinical practice to program PMT options ON for most patients. If the patient never develops a PMT, the algorithm will simply never go into effect. On the other hand, if the patient gets a PMT, having an automatic termination algorithm launch into effect can spare the patient (and clinician) some pain!

The nuts and bolts of stored electrograms

- A pacemaker-mediated tachycardia (PMT) is an endless loop tachycardia that is sustained, in part, by the pacemaker. It involves a backward relationship of the ventricular paced event (VP) to the sensed atrial event (AS). The VP-AS interval in a PMT is fast and very stable (variation is less than 16 ms from cycle to cycle).
- Although a PMT is sustained in part by the pacemaker, it feels like a real VT to the patient and can provoke symptoms.
- Many dual-chamber pacemakers offer automatic PMT options to help diagnose PMTs and terminate them. There are variations in these algorithms, of course, but in our example the pacemaker evaluated a run of VP-AS intervals for rate (> 90 ppm) and stability (variation < 16 ms) and count (eight such events in a row). When PMT was diagnosed, the pacemaker responded by withholding a paced ventricular event after a sensed atrial event and then, 330 ms following the sensed atrial event, delivering an atrial output pulse.
- There may be a lot of programmability in the PMT algorithm including rate, interval stability variation, and how many consecutive intervals must occur for the diagnosis. PMT algorithms should be programmed ON unless there is good reason not to use them.
- Not all patients are susceptible to PMTs, but it is impossible to know who is and who is not until a patient gets a PMT. A patient who has ever had a PMT can get another one.
- Stored electrograms are usually downloadable from the device by trigger; in other words, the clinician knows the triggering event before even seeing the EGM. Despite having advance information, view the EGM with unbiased eyes to determine if the events are really what the pacemaker says they are!

In Depth: Electrograms

If you have much exposure to pacemakers and other implantable cardiac rhythm management devices, you will eventually run into EGMs or electrograms. Many clinicians take an instant dislike to EGMs, particularly those healthcare professionals who have spent a lot of time working with classic surface ECGs.

An intracardiac electrogram or EGM is the same thing as a surface ECG in theory, it is just that the heart's electrical information is transmitted from electrodes inside the heart rather than electrodes stuck on the skin. Because of memory constraints and how the device works, EGMs tend to be more condensed, grainier, and can seem squashed together. Pacing spikes almost disappear on an EGM. You can sometimes see them as little tabs or notches but often they are all but invisible.

An EGM is recorded from a pacing lead. A dual-chamber pacemaker can transmit an atrial electrogram, a ventricular electrogram, or both. Some devices offer ways to blend atrial and ventricular information together into one tracing that actually tends to more closely resemble a surface ECG. When viewing an atrial or ventricular electrogram, realize that the tracing's point of view can cause events to look disproportionately large. For example, on an atrial electrogram, atrial events may be as large or larger than ventricular events.

The type of EGM recorded is the result of how the device is programmed. Clinicians can set up the device to record a certain type of EGM. Unfortunately, you cannot switch formats when you are ready to download data. If you previously set up the pacemaker to provide you with ventricular EGMs, you will not get atrial information. (By the way, you need a lead to get an electrogram. A VVI pacemaker cannot provide atrial electrograms because it does not have an atrial lead.)

EGMs are stored in pacemaker device memory, which is finite. Every year, it seems, new genera-

tions of pacemaker products hit the market with expanded memory capacity. EGM storage is much greater now than it was even 5 years ago. However, no matter how you slice it, memory capacity is still limited.

Thus, pacemaker clinicians have to balance the need for complete information (dual-channel EGMs for every possible trigger) versus memory capacity. EGMs are recorded based on triggering type events (such as PMT, PVC, mode switching, high-rate activity, and so on). Programming a trigger will cause all such events to store an EGM. Thus, the more triggers you program, the more electrograms are likely to be stored. For some patients, this can use up memory capacity quickly.

What happens when the memory fills up? Most devices are set up so that the oldest information is overwritten with the newest information (this is called "continuous" storage). Thus, when stored EGMs are retrieved from memory, the clinician gets the latest EGMs only. Although it is not as frequently programmed, some pacemakers let the clinician "freeze" electrograms. This means when memory fills up, the device stops recording electrograms.

A new device now offers preferential EGM storage. This feature allows clinicians to flag which types of EGMs (based on triggers) are of greater value and which are of lesser value. Then when the memory fills up, the device overwrites lower-priority electrograms first.

For a patient with known atrial tachyarrhythmias, mode switching and high-rate intrinsic atrial activity is likely of more interest than PVC or PMT activity. By programming the proper mode switch triggers and using preferential storage, the clinician can minimize the risk that an especially valuable EGM is discarded in favor of a less-useful one.

Another factor influencing EGM storage is pre-trigger data. Most EGMs allow the clinician to record a specific amount of pre-trigger data (buffer data). These are the events immediately preceding the point at which the trigger is reached. In most cases, pre-trigger data are actually more useful than post-trigger data. The post-trigger data show you how the device responds (which is important). The pre-trigger data tell you what was going on in the patient's heart that provoked a device response (very useful for diagnostic purposes). Most EGMs allow you to set up how many seconds of pre-trigger data are desired, but pre-trigger data cost memory. Again, it is a balancing act to weigh the benefits of many seconds' worth of pre-trigger data against the limitations of memory capacity.

The nuts and bolts of dual-chamber electrograms in depth

- The terms electrogram, intracardiac electrogram, IEGM, EGM or even e-gram all mean the same thing. It's an electrical recording or tracing of cardiac activity taken from within the heart courtesy of the pacemaker's electrodes.
- A dual-chamber pacemaker can provide atrial electrograms, ventricular electrograms, both together (dual), or sometimes even blended electrograms (one tracing with data blended from the atrial and ventricular channels). However, you are limited to what you can download by the type of electrograms previously programmed. Thus, if you programmed ventricular electrograms to be stored, you cannot download atrial electrograms at the next follow-up.
- Electrograms store cardiac data in device memory, which has limited capacity. This can be managed by continuous storage (oldest electrograms are overwritten by newest ones when memory capacity is reached) or by freezing the electrograms (when the memory is full, nothing more is recorded). New devices from St. Jude Medical allow for preferential electrogram storage, that is, tracings can be designated as higher or lower priority so that high-priority electrograms are preserved but lower priority ones may be overwritten.
- Electrograms can be challenging for clinicians used to surface ECGs. Electrograms can be more compact and grainier than standard surface ECGs. Pacing spikes are small or even imperceptible. The electrogram also takes on the viewpoint of where it is recorded. For example, on an atrial electrogram, atrial events may appear as large or larger than ventricular events.
- Triggers are events that launch electrogram storage. Typical triggers include AMS entry, AMS exit, PVC, ventricular tachyarrhythmias, high-rate atrial activity, PMTs, and so on. The more triggers you program, the more likely electrograms will be stored (and fill up memory). Careful programming of triggers can go a long way to easing memory problems with electrogram storage.
- Pre-trigger or "buffer" data are the events immediately preceding the trigger. For most cases, pre-trigger data are more interesting and useful for diagnostic purposes than post-trigger data. The amount of pre-trigger data recorded is programmable.

SECTION 38

Conclusion

Whether you are the rookie in a pacemaker clinic or work in a general practice, it is hard to avoid coming into contact with paced ECGs. With device implantation on the rise all over the world, paced ECGs will soon become fairly common fare for all healthcare professionals. Yet most of us are mildly (or extremely) disconcerted when we first run into these strange-looking paced ECGs.

Even if you eventually get used to them, that feeling of being on familiar ground will soon slip away! That's because with advanced device features and some unusual device behavior patterns, even experienced pacemaker clinicians can sometimes get tripped up.

In fact, if you ever attend a specialty society meeting or pacing symposium, you may notice that a very favorite topic on the roster always appears to be something like "Challenging ECGs" or "Difficult Tracings." Even experts can sometimes disagree about what is going on in a paced ECG.

My approach has always been to keep your approach systematic, stick with the basics, and to look for the most likely causes before going out on a limb with some exotic scenario. I realize unusual cases happen all of the time in medicine, but what makes them unusual is the fact that they are infrequent. Day in and day out, most paced ECGs deal with the same basic issues.

It is crucial to paced ECG interpretation that you can properly observe capture and sensing and determine if it is appropriate or inappropriate. Pacemakers really can do only two things: capture and sense. Always check those two functions out very carefully.

Look at the rate next and remember to convert intervals to ppm and back again. Pacemaker programming is done in pulses per minute, but the pacemaker (and the ECG) "think" in intervals. As a

pacemaker clinician, you need to be able to translate one to the other quickly and fluently.

Rate variations occur more often than you might think. The most likely reasons for rate variations are special features, like rate hysteresis, rate response, mode switching, overdrive pacing, and rest rate.

Pauses can sometimes confound a clinician, but on a paced ECG, a pause is likely to be the result of loss of capture or oversensing (sensing something that is not there). Pauses should always make you suspect a sensing problem, specifically oversensing.

DDD and DDDR devices are very sophisticated but also quite common. In the US, it is the most frequently implanted pacing system and global popularity of DDD(R) devices is on the rise. These devices can sometimes cause unusual-looking (but appropriate) upper-rate behavior if the patient's intrinsic atrial rate gets high and the pacemaker tries to track the atrium by pacing the ventricle at the same rate to maintain 1:1 AV synchrony.

If you see such odd-looking paced ECGs, check out the intrinsic atrial rate and see if the device is just encountering problems as it tries to keep up with a rapid native atrial rate.

This book purposely does not discuss a great deal about device programming or troubleshooting, although those topics are briefly introduced since they go hand-in-hand with paced ECG evaluation. For those working more closely with pacemakers or other implanted devices, I recommend my other books: *The Nuts & Bolts of Cardiac Pacing, The Nuts & Bolts of ICD Therapy,* and *The Nuts & Bolts of Cardiac Resynchronization Therapy.* Those books describe a great deal about the features and functionality of those devices but not so much about analyzing paced ECGs.

Remember: **you see only what you look for, you recognize only what you know.**

The Nuts and Bolts of Paced ECG Interpretation, 1st edition. By Tom Kenny.
Published 2009 by Blackwell Publishing, ISBN: 978-1-4501-8404-5.

PART II
Workbook

Introduction to Workbook

In this next section, I've compiled 100 tracings from a variety of sources to challenge you and continue the learning experience. First, you'll see the large tracing without a lot of extraneous information. The idea is to let the tracing speak for itself. By going through the systematic approach and applying many of the things you've learned in this book so far, you should be able to analyze the tracing.

I admit that some of these tracings are pretty challenging. Many were selected specifically to introduce certain concepts. As you make your way through the workbook, I want to encourage you to keep at it, even if you are occasionally stumped by something you have not seen before.

We've grouped the tracings by difficulty into Easy, Moderate, and Tough tracings, but our categorizations are subjective. No doubt, some people will disagree with how I've arranged them. In the last section, Scramble, we present a whole range of ECGs, from the easiest to the most challenging in no particular order. In some ways, I think the Scramble section best mirrors what actual clinical practice can be like!

To help reinforce the systematic approach, we organized the workbook analysis into six steps. You may find this a bit repetitious, but my purpose is to make this become second nature when you approach an ECG. You want to assess:

- Mode
- Rate
- Capture
- Sensing
- Underlying rhythm
- What to do next

This is my particular favored order. The actual order is not as important as the fact that you use a systematic approach.

"What to do next" covers the next step following ECG analysis. We're assessing these tracings with a purpose in mind, namely to provide the patient with optimal pacemaker therapy. When it comes to "next steps," you must be able to verify proper function of capture and sensing. Many programmers offer automatic or semi-automatic tests for these functions, but I think it is still important to know how to test manually or at least understand how the programmer conducts one of these tests.

The table below provides a good overview of how to "set the stage" to test for proper atrial and ven-

Desired Test	Steps
Atrial capture	To verify atrial capture, you must see atrial pacing. If there is no atrial pacing, increase the base rate in 10 ppm increments until atrial pacing occurs.
Ventricular capture	To verify ventricular capture, you must see ventricular pacing. *Dual-Chamber Pacemakers:* shorten the AV delay to about 120 or 130 ms. *Single-Chamber Pacemakers:* increase the base rate in 10 ppm increments until ventricular pacing occurs.
Atrial sensing	To verify atrial sensing, you must have intrinsic atrial activity. Decrease the base rate in 10 ppm increments until intrinsic atrial activity appears. This may or may not happen. Some patients have such compromised sinus nodes that it may not be possible to observe intrinsic atrial activity. Do not go below 30 or 40 ppm.
Ventricular sensing	To verify ventricular sensing, you must have intrinsic ventricular activity. *Dual-Chamber Pacemakers:* extend the AV delay to 350 ms. *Single-Chamber Pacemakers:* decrease the base rate in 10 ppm increments until intrinsic ventricular activity occurs. Do not go below 30 or 40 ppm.

tricular capture and sensing. Despite the clinician's best efforts, sometimes it is not possible to see atrial pacing or intrinsic ventricular activity or force some other condition to occur temporarily for testing purposes. In such instances, that should be noted in the chart and the clinician should do his or her best to work around the situation. Pacemaker patients may have severely compromised hearts with limited cardiac function. Not all tests will be possible in all patients.

During testing in the clinic, remember you are treating the patient, not treating the pacemaker! If you decide to drop the pacing rate in a VVI pacemaker to see if you can coax intrinsic ventricular activity to occur, lower the base rate in gentle 10-ppm increments and check with the patient to see how well he or she tolerates it. Most pacemaker clinicians would never go below 30 or 40 ppm base rate settings for such testing, but don't jump from 60 ppm to 30 ppm; that's too sharp a transition, even for a temporary test.

Obviously, single-chamber pacemakers require testing in only one chamber. If you are dealing with a dual-chamber pacemaker, please resist the temptation to temporarily program it to VVI or AAI to run the atrial and ventricular tests. A dual-chamber pacemaker is more than just an atrial and a ventricular single-chamber pacemaker slapped together. In dual-chamber systems, it is crucial that the atrial and ventricular channels interact and work together. If you temporarily program a DDD device to VVI and run ventricular capture and sensing tests, you're really not seeing how the ventricular channel of a dual-chamber pacemaker functions. You'll only be testing how the device works in VVI mode.

The tracings we are presenting in this section were all redrawn by an artist. We did that in part to assure that nothing detracted from the tracing itself and that you could see everything clearly. In the clinical setting, you may have to work with tracings that look rougher or grainier. Furthermore, for the purposes of this book, we only provide you with very brief snippets of an ECG. You will be making your evaluation based on about 6 seconds of ECG. This is far less than you'll usually be working with in the clinic, so please accept this as an artificial device we had to use to create a book like this.

Last of all, I want to stress that ECG interpretation is well named in that clinicians take the evidence on the strip and "interpret" it. There are many strips in the workbook section that could be interpreted more than one way. In such instances, I tried to state the likely interpretations and to give reasons to support my interpretation. By and large, my interpretations are based on likelihood. Knowing the most likely causes of certain pacemaker behavior is something that clinicians gain only with experience. So please accept my encouragement that the more intensely you are involved with paced ECGs and pacemaker patients, the better your interpretative skills will become. This is largely a matter of learning some of the telltale clues for the most common pacemaker issues. In this workbook, I tried to introduce you to "all of the usual suspects."

Easy

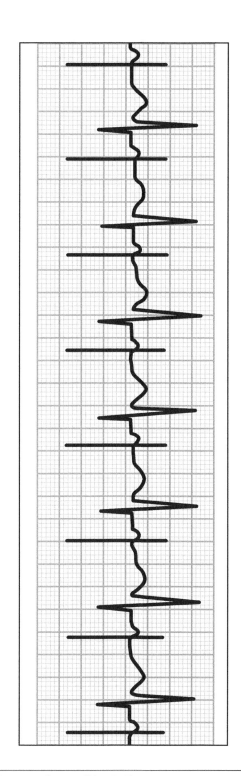

The Nuts and Bolts of Paced ECG Interpretation, 1st edition. By Tom Kenny.
Published 2009 by Blackwell Publishing, ISBN: 978-1-4501-8404-5.

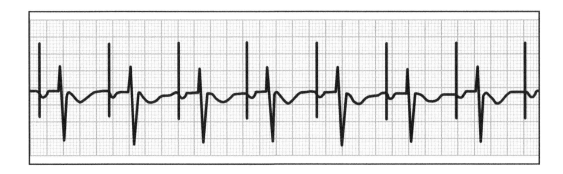

Mode

There are pacemaker spikes associated with atrial activity. There is apparent association between atrial pacing and ventricular activity. In fact, at a glance, it looks like the atrial pacing is driving the rate. This pacemaker is functioning in AAI mode and could be either a single-chamber pacemaker or a dual-chamber pacemaker that just does not need to pace the ventricle at this time.

Rate

To measure the rate, use calipers to assess the atrial pacing interval (AP-AP).

> **The nuts and bolts of paced ECG interpretation: measuring the pacing rate**
>
> • Pacing rate in a DDD or AAI device refers to the rate of pacing in the atrium. Find the pacing rate by measuring the atrial pacing interval (AP-AP).
> • Pacing rate in a VVI device refers to the rate of pacing in the ventricle. Find the pacing rate by measuring the ventricular pacing interval (VP-VP).

We don't know if this is an atrial pacemaker or a dual-chamber pacemaker, but we do know that the pacing interval in this case is the distance between two consecutive atrial paced events. Dual-chamber devices are more common, so this is more likely (in terms of probability) to be a dual-chamber system.

However, at this point in our analysis we have no "hard evidence" either way.

With calipers, the atrial pacing interval measures to 840 ms. That converts to a pacing rate of about 71 ppm. Since calipers are always a bit inexact, this would reasonably correspond to a base rate of 70 ppm. The pacing rate is consistent throughout the strip.

> **The nuts and bolts of paced ECG interpretation: appropriate rate ranges**
>
> In the clinic, you'll frequently be confronted with rhythm strips and have no information on the programmed base rate. So how do you assess appropriate rate if you don't even know what it is supposed to be?
>
> As a rule of thumb, the most common base rates are:
> • 60 ppm (1000 ms) for dual-chamber devices
> • 70 ppm (857 ms) for single-chamber devices
>
> If rates out of this range occur, that should make you suspicious. Keep digging!
>
> While it is possible to program pacemakers to other base rates, they are uncommon. The exception to this rule is pediatric pacing, where it is not unusual to see permanently programmed base rate pacing at 100 ppm (600 ms) or higher.

Capture

Atrial capture appears appropriate in that every atrial pacing spike is followed by an immediate atrial depolarization. These depolarizations all have a similar morphology, indicating they are the same "type" of event. While that *suggests* appropriate capture, we should take a step further. It appears that each paced atrial event conducts and leads to a sensed ventricular event. If these atrial events are truly captured and conducting over the AV node and causing a ventricular depolarization, then we are going to see *consistent PR intervals*. In this case, the PR interval is actually measured from the atrial paced event to the onset of the intrinsic ventricular event (AP-VS interval).

Using calipers, this PR interval (AP-VS) measures 240 ms consistently. It's the consistency rather than the exact length that's important. This is evidence that the ventricles are timing themselves to the atrial activity. That gives us stronger evidence to say that we have appropriate atrial capture.

Ventricular capture cannot be assessed in this strip, since there is no ventricular pacing.

Sensing

Atrial sensing cannot be evaluated from this strip, because there is only atrial pacing going on.

Ventricular sensing is a bit more tricky. We know the pacemaker is functioning in AAI mode and we know it is possible that this is a single-chamber AAI device. However, what if it was actually a dual-chamber device acting in AAI mode? In that case, the pacemaker should sense the ventricles.

In a dual-chamber pacemaker, the atrial pacemaker spike would start the paced AV delay interval. If no intrinsic ventricular event occurred during the paced AV delay interval, the pacemaker would deliver a ventricular pacing spike. A typical paced AV delay interval setting is around 200 ms. We already know the PR interval (which would correspond to the sensed AV delay) is 240 ms.

It could be that this is a dual-chamber pacemaker with a long programmed AV delay. If the patient has intact AV conduction but a long PR interval, it would be wise to program a long AV delay. Here's why:

- A long AV delay would give the patient's ventricles maximum opportunity to contract on their own; this encourages intrinsic activity and avoids unnecessary right-ventricular pacing

- A long AV delay is only prudent if the patient has reliable intact native conduction; that seems to be the case here

If this device is indeed a dual-chamber pacemaker with a long AV delay, ventricular sensing is appropriate because the intrinsic ventricular events inhibit ventricular pacing spikes. However, it cannot be stated with certainty whether this is a dual-chamber or single-chamber pacemaker.

Underlying rhythm

Since the paced atrial events seem to be driving the rhythm and there is an intrinsic ventricular event at a consistent interval after each paced atrial event, this patient has intact AV conduction. The PR interval suggests that the patient might have a form of delayed AV conduction, which is accommodated nicely in this rhythm strip by allowing a slightly longer-than-normal interval between atrial event and corresponding ventricular event. If this patient is paced in DDD mode with a paced AV delay interval of 200 ms, there would be consistent AP-VP pacing. Since the patient is likely getting the rate support he needs plus avoiding unnecessary right-ventricular pacing with the longer AV delay, this looks good. If this is indeed a DDD device, it is an example of good programming to meet the individual needs of the patient.

What to do next

Use the programmer to get more details on the pacemaker; the programmer should report if this is a dual-chamber or single-chamber pacemaker.

If it is a dual-chamber pacemaker, ventricular capture should be assessed. To do that, ventricular pacing must occur. The best way to encourage ventricular pacing is to shorten the AV delay (while you're at the programmer, verify the AV delay setting, namely that it is at or above 240 ms). Shorten the AV delay to 120 or 130 ms. Ventricular sensing seems appropriate, but a ventricular sensing threshold test is prudent.

Regardless of whether this is a dual-chamber or single-chamber pacemaker, an atrial sensing test should be performed. For an atrial sensitivity evaluation, intrinsic atrial activity must occur. The best way to try to get intrinsic atrial activity to appear is to lower the base rate. Do this in gradual 10-ppm steps to avoid abrupt rate transitions. Talk to the patient about what you're doing as you temporarily lower the pacing rate, since patients may feel any number of symptoms during such programming changes (even brief ones). Lower the pacing rate until one of three things happens:

1 Intrinsic atrial activity (even intermittent) occurs

2 The patient does not tolerate the rate

3 You reach 30 or 40 ppm

It is my opinion that for the purposes of an atrial sensing test, the pacemaker should not be programmed – even temporarily – to a rate lower than 30 or 40 ppm for any patient. Some patients are pacemaker dependent and may not tolerate a rate of even 40 ppm. Lower the base rate gradually and with special attention on the patient!

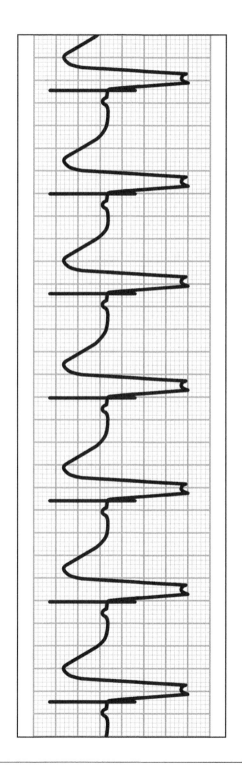

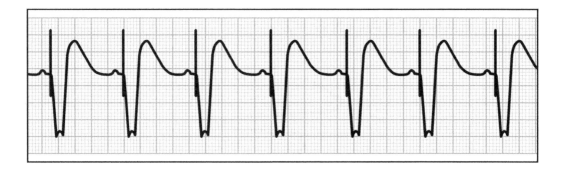

Mode

Ventricular pacing is evident from the prominent pacemaker spikes. There are intrinsic atrial events on the strip as well. But do the atrial events have a relationship with the ventricular events? If they do, this is a dual-chamber pacemaker. To assess a possible relationship between atrial and ventricular activity on this strip, measure the sensed AV delay interval (AS-VP) on the strip. If it is consistent, then the pacemaker is sensing the atrial activity and timing the ventricular spikes to the intrinsic atrial events. Using calipers, you can see that the sensed AV delay measures roughly 120 ms … consistently across the strip. This is a dual-chamber pacemaker.

Rate

The ideal way to measure the base rate in a dual-chamber pacemaker is to measure the atrial pacing interval (AP-AP). In this particular strip, we don't have any atrial pacing intervals! We will have to make do with the ventricular pacing interval (VP-VP), which on this particular strip will serve us just as well. Using calipers, the ventricular pacing interval is about 920 ms (that's four large boxes on the grid and three small ones or 800 + 120 = 920). A pacing interval of 920 ms translates into a pacing rate of about 65 ppm. That falls within the range of appropriate rates for a dual-chamber pacemaker.

Capture

Atrial capture cannot be assessed from this strip because there is no atrial pacing.

Ventricular capture appears to be appropriate. Every time a ventricular output pulse occurs (spike),

there is an immediate ventricular depolarization with the characteristic widened, bizarre morphology of a paced ventricular event. Notice that every ventricular event shares the same morphology; they are all the same type of event.

Sensing

Atrial sensing is appropriate on this strip. The key reason for this determination is the fact that all of the ventricular pacing spikes are timed to the atrial event. The pacemaker sensed the intrinsic atrial event, inhibited the atrial output pulse, and launched the sensed AV delay. The sensed AV delay appears to be about 120 ms. This is short but within the range of programmable AV delay values.

Ventricular sensing cannot be assessed from this strip because no intrinsic ventricular events occur.

Underlying rhythm

This patient appears to have reasonably good sinus node function but AV conduction is compromised.

What to do next

To approach this systematically, we need to conduct tests to verify appropriate atrial capture (increase the base rate in 10-ppm steps to force atrial pacing) and ventricular sensing. The best way to try to encourage intrinsic ventricular activity to appear to test ventricular sensing is to extend the sensed AV delay. Right now, the AV delay appears to be set to about 120 ms; I would extend it to 300 or higher for testing purposes.

If a longer AV delay interval allows intrinsic ventricular activity to appear, it may be that this patient has intact AV conduction but at a rate slower than the programmed sensed AV delay of 120 ms. For such patients, it is a good idea to observe native conduction times and adjust the AV delay appropriately. For instance, if this patient conducts reliably at around 220 ms, I would program the sensed and paced AV delay to 250 ms. This gives the ventricles ample opportunity to contract on their own and may actually help avoid some unnecessary right-ventricular pacing.

On the other hand, this patient may not exhibit intrinsic ventricular activity even at an AV delay of 350 ms. If that is the case, the next way to try to encourage some intrinsic ventricular activity to appear is to program the device temporarily to VVI mode and then lower the programmed base rate. Do

not do this abruptly. Tell the patient what you are doing and decrease the rate in steps of 10 ppm down to 30 or 40 ppm. As the rate slows, intrinsic ventricular activity may appear. One word of caution: only lower the base rate if you have already extended the AV delay and failed to see intrinsic ventricular activity!

What happens if you try both methods and you cannot get intrinsic ventricular activity to appear? In such cases, note it on the chart, check the programmed output settings (pulse amplitude and pulse width) and confirm that they seem adequate. There will be times in the clinic when you cannot conduct all of the desired tests because the patient "won't allow it."

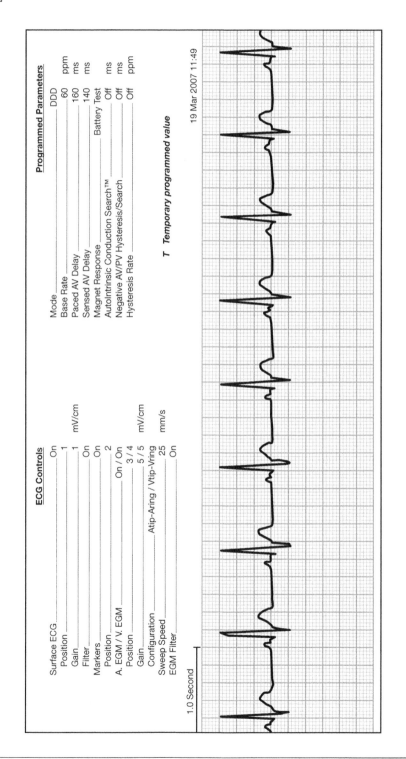

ECG Controls

Surface ECG	On	
Position	1	
Gain	1	mV/cm
Filter	On	
Markers	On	
Position	2	
A. EGM / V. EGM	On / On	
Position	3 / 4	
Gain	5 / 5	mV/cm
Configuration	Atip-Aring / Vtip-Vring	
Sweep Speed	25	mm/s
EGM Filter	On	

1.0 Second

Programmed Parameters

Mode	DDD	
Base Rate	60	ppm
Paced AV Delay	160	ms
Sensed AV Delay	140	ms
Magnet Response	Battery Test	
AutoIntrinsic Conduction Search™	Off	ms
Negative AV/PV Hysteresis/Search	Off	ms
Hysteresis Rate	Off	ppm

T *Temporary programmed value*

19 Mar 2007 11:49

The Nuts and Bolts of Paced ECG Interpretation, 1st edition. By Tom Kenny.
Published 2009 by Blackwell Publishing, ISBN: 978-1-4501-8404-5.

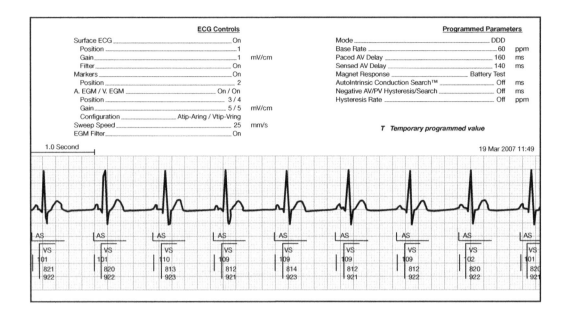

Mode

If you had only the tracing to evaluate, it would be impossible to say for sure whether or not this patient even had a pacemaker, much less what type of pacemaker it was! The strip shows only native cardiac activity. However, from the printout information at the top, it is clear this patient has a DDD pacemaker set to 60 ppm.

The annotations are very helpful in that they report what the pacemaker has done and how the pacemaker interprets various events. In this case, the AS and VS annotations indicate the pacemaker has sensed atrial and ventricular activity.

Rate

Annotated tracings are both a blessing and curse to clinicians. They are a great help because they give us a fast, easy way to get information. They can be liabilities when clinicians tend to "read the annotations" and forget about the tracing. As far as I'm concerned, the annotations only report what the pacemaker interprets. The tracing itself tells us what the heart is doing. For that reason, focus on the tracing and see if it matches what's going on in the annotations … not vice versa.

There is no pacing interval at all to measure, but there is an atrial interval (AS-AS) which measures to

be around 920 ms with calipers. This is confirmed by the more accurate intervals at the bottom of the strip which show values ranging from 921 to 930 ms. That translates to a rate of around 65 ppm.

From the printout, we know that the base rate has been programmed to 60 ppm. Even if we did not have the printout, that is the "most likely" rate for a dual-chamber pacemaker. Since the intrinsic activity is occurring at around 65 ppm, it inhibits the pacemaker.

Capture

Capture cannot be assessed for either chamber because there is nothing but intrinsic activity on the strip.

Sensing

Atrial sensing is likely to be appropriate because the intrinsic atrial events inhibit the atrial output pulse and show up on the annotations as AS. Every intrinsic atrial event seen on the tracing can be accounted for on the annotations.

Ventricular sensing is also appropriate for the same reasons.

Underlying rhythm

This patient has a very good-looking rhythm! Many

pacemaker patients have intermittent arrhythmias, that is, they may have one or more serious cardiac arrhythmias but nothing that affects them permanently. It is likely that this patient is between arrhythmic episodes. The patient has intact AV conduction and good sinus function – at least at this moment. This strip provides no solid clues as to this patient's rhythm disorder.

What to do next

To run through our basic checklist, it is important to evaluate proper atrial and ventricular capture. Both require pacing in order to make an evaluation. To observe atrial pacing, increase the base rate first to 90 ppm and, if that doesn't work, continue to increase it in 10-ppm steps until the pacemaker starts to pace the atrium.

In order to force ventricular pacing, the preferred method is to shorten the programmed AV delay. It is currently set to a paced AV delay of 160 ms and a sensed AV delay of 140 ms. Reduce these to around 110 ms.

If that does not cause ventricular pacing to occur, temporarily program the pacemaker to VVI mode and then increase the base rate, starting at 90 ppm and, if that doesn't force pacing, ramp up the base rate in 10-ppm steps. One important caution for ventricular pacing: shorten the AV delay first and only increase the base rate if shortening the AV delay fails.

Does this patient even need a pacemaker? It is unclear from this strip, but not every patient with an arrhythmia has an arrhythmia every moment of the day. Information from the patient's chart or previous check-ups may give you clues as to the nature of the rhythm disorder. The best interpretation of this strip is that whatever this patient's arrhythmia(s) happen to be, they are intermittent.

The nuts and bolts of paced ECG interpretation: normal rhythm

The short snippets of rhythm strips in this book are a convention we used to demonstrate basic principles of paced ECG interpretation. In actual clinical practice, you can and should look at much longer tracings to determine cardiac rhythm. Since many patients have intermittent arrhythmias, you will frequently see normal-looking ECGs from device patients. Try to look at as much ECG as is reasonable to give you a good overview of the patient's rhythm and how the patient and device are interacting. While a few cardiac events can often give you major clues about what's going on with a pacemaker patient, avoid basing your complete evaluation on just a few waveforms!

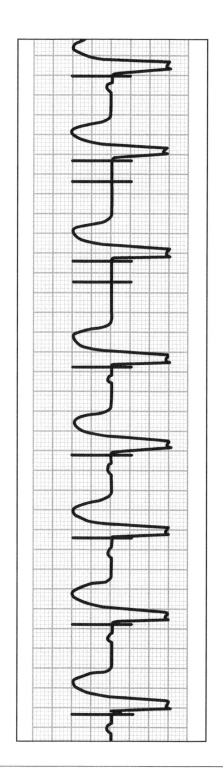

The Nuts and Bolts of Paced ECG Interpretation, 1st edition. By Tom Kenny.
Published 2009 by Blackwell Publishing, ISBN: 978-1-4501-8404-5.

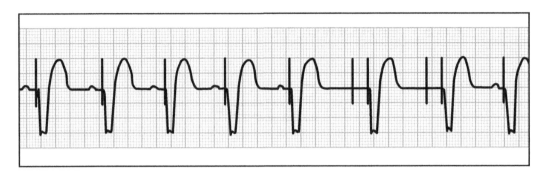

Mode

The presence of both atrial and ventricular pacing spikes means that this is a dual-chamber pacemaker. However, in the first few complexes of this strip (AS-VP events) you can see that this is a dual-chamber device in that the ventricular spike is clearly being timed to the intrinsic atrial event. The proof of that is in the consistent sensed AV delay interval.

Rate

In a dual-chamber device, pacing rate is measured by the atrial pacing interval (AP-AP). There is one atrial pacing interval (AP-AP) on this strip and it measures 1000 ms (60 ppm), which is an appropriate rate for a dual-chamber device.

Capture

While there are two atrial pacing spikes on the strip, neither captures the atrium.

On the other hand, ventricular capture looks appropriate. Every ventricular pacing spike is followed by an immediate ventricular depolarization with the characteristic widened bizarre morphology of a paced event.

Sensing

When evaluating atrial sensing in a dual-chamber device, it is a good idea to review the sensed AV delay. This is the timing cycle imposed by the pacemaker for AS-VP events. This strip has several AS-VP complexes and they should all be using the same sensed AV delay interval. In other words, we should see a consistent interval between the atrial sensed event and the ventricular pacing spike (the "electronic PR interval") if the atrial event is being properly sensed. While calipers are not the most precise measuring tool for such small intervals, even with calipers it appears that the sensed AV delay is consistent, measuring about 200 ms. That, along with the fact that the sensed atrial events inhibit atrial output pulses makes a strong case for appropriate atrial sensing.

The nuts and bolts of paced ECG interpretation: AV delay

Dual-chamber pacemakers impose a forced time delay between an atrial event and the next ventricular event, known as the AV delay. There are two types of AV delay: **the sensed AV delay** (which follows a sensed atrial event and creates an AS-VP complex) and **the paced AV delay** (which follows a paced atrial event and creates an AP-VP complex).

The sensed and paced AV delays may be the same length or they may differ; it is often recommended that the sensed AV delay be programmed to a slightly shorter value than the paced AV delay, usually about 25 ms less. The reason for a shorter sensed AV delay is that the pacemaker takes about 25 ms from the true onset of an intrinsic atrial event before it can properly sense it and launch the AV delay timing cycle. An atrial paced event launches the paced AV delay immediately

When AS-VP complexes appear on a strip, one way to verify if the device is sensing the atrium correctly is to see if the pacemaker is taking its timing cues from the atrial event and imposing the sensed AV delay. With proper atrial sensing, you should see a consistent AV delay interval. Typical AV delay settings are around 200 ms but can range from 150 to 350 ms.

Ventricular sensing cannot be assessed from this strip since there are no intrinsic ventricular events.

Underlying rhythm

This patient appears to have some atrial activity, but it does not conduct via the AV node down to the ventricles. This indicates the patient has slow AV conduction.

What to do next

Atrial capture must be restored, which means an atrial threshold test should be conducted. This will result in determination of the required atrial output parameters (pulse amplitude and pulse width) necessary for reliable, consistent capture. (The atrial pacing threshold is determined and then a "safety margin" of 2:1 or 3:1 is typically applied; many programmers will show recommended programmed settings on the screen.)

If the currently programmed atrial output settings are too low, reprogramming new, higher output settings will likely restore proper atrial capture. This should be verified before moving on.

But what if the currently programmed output settings are already appropriate? Too-low output settings are one of the most likely causes of loss of capture, but they are certainly not the only ones! You may need to troubleshoot the source of loss of atrial capture (see box).

While lead problems are comparatively rare, they are always important to consider (and hopefully rule out). In this case, the fact that atrial sensing seems reliable makes a lead problem less likely. When leads are compromised, it usually affects both sensing and capture. In fact, when you see both capture and sensing problems on the atrial or ventricular channel, it should make you suspect a lead problem.

In this case, loss of capture is most likely caused by inappropriately low output settings. This may not be inappropriate programming. Pacing thresholds are not static values; they can change over time, with disease progression, as a result of drug interactions or changes in pharmacotherapy, or even just over the course of the day!

As a rule of thumb, pacing output parameters should be set to at least a 2:1 safety margin. That means if the pacing threshold is 1.3 V at 0.4 ms, the device should be programmed to at least 2.6 V at 0.4 ms. Safety margins should be generous, so in this case, I would probably set the pacemaker to 3 V at 0.4 ms. The patient's capture threshold should be

---

The nuts and bolts of paced ECG interpretation: troubleshooting capture problems

Capture problems are very serious and demand our immediate and full attention. Finding the solution to a capture problem means identifying what is at the root of the problem. When it comes to capture, these are the "usual suspects":

Lead problems
- Lead dislodgment is more likely in acute implants
- However, lead fractures or damage to insulation can occur at any time

Output problems
- The output parameter settings (pulse amplitude and pulse width) may not be adjusted to high enough values either from improper programming or the fact that the pacing threshold may have changed
- There may be a problem with the output from the device (hardware problem)

---

given some room for the normal fluctuations that are bound to occur.

If the pacemaker has an automatic capture function (such as A-Cap Confirm), that can be enabled. This is one of the safest and most reliable ways to manage capture.

Ventricular sensing should also be evaluated. In order to do this, intrinsic ventricular activity has to emerge. In a dual-chamber device, the better way to force ventricular intrinsic events to appear on the ECG is to temporarily prolong the AV delay. As a rule of thumb, I would extend the sensed and paced AV delay to 300 ms or higher and see if any intrinsic ventricular events occurred. If that worked, a sensing test could be conducted.

If (and only if) that fails, the next choice is to program the device temporarily to VVI mode and then lower the base rate in 10-ppm steps while telling the patient what you are doing. Go down to about 30 or 40 ppm (no lower) and see if ventricular activity starts to occur on its own.

It is not always possible to evaluate sensing for all patients; however, every reasonable attempt should be made to do so before throwing in the towel!

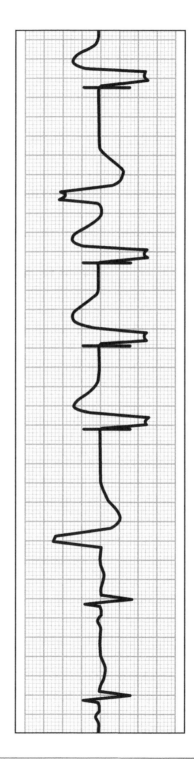

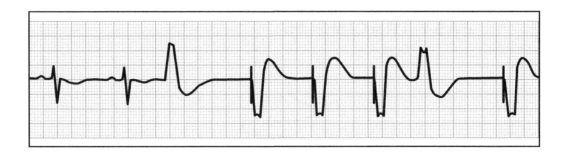

Mode

This is a VVI strip.

Rate

The ventricular pacing interval (VP-VP) measures 880 ms with calipers (about 70 ppm), which is an appropriate rate. However there are two large unusual-looking intrinsic ventricular events on the strip (premature ventricular contractions or PVCs). The escape interval following these events is longer than the pacing interval. Measuring with calipers from the onset of the PVC to the next ventricular pacing spike, the interval is 1200 ms (50 ppm). The most common reason for an escape interval to be longer than pacing interval is hysteresis. Since both intervals time out to rates that would be quite appropriate for base rate and hysteresis rate, hysteresis is very likely activated.

Capture

Ventricular capture looks appropriate.

Sensing

Ventricular sensing is appropriate in that intrinsic ventricular activity (whether "normal" or in the form of a PVC) inhibits the ventricular pacing spike and resets device timing.

Underlying rhythm

This patient has sinus node dysfunction and may have AV block. He is also prone to PVCs.

What to do next

This pacemaker appears to be functioning appropriately and is well programmed to meet this particular patient's needs. Ventricular capture and sensing are the two most important things to evaluate and both can be seen to be working appropriately from this strip.

The nuts and bolts of paced ECG interpretation: let the strip do the work!

There are many things to keep in mind during a systematic evaluation of paced ECGs. The more work the strip can do for you, the better. Use the strip to get all of the information you can. In some cases, like this example, you can evaluate both sensing and capture from the tracing.

EASY TRACING #6

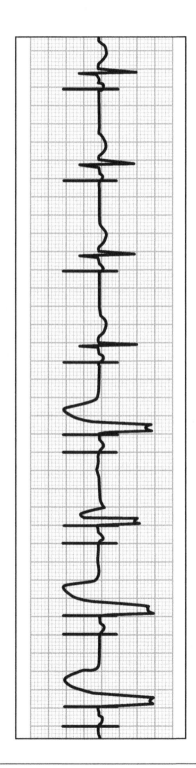

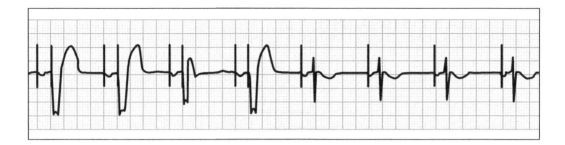

Mode

The presence of both atrial and ventricular pacing spikes means that this has to be dual-chamber pacing.

Rate

Dual-chamber devices measure their rate based on the atrial pacing interval (AP-AP). Using calipers from one atrial pacing spike to the next reveals 1000 ms pacing intervals (60 ppm), which run consistently through the strip. The rate is appropriate for a dual-chamber system.

Capture

Atrial pacing spikes are consistently followed by an atrial depolarization. All of these atrial events have the same morphology. While these suggest appropriate atrial capture, atrial capture can be confirmed in AP-VS pacing by a consistent interval (representing the conduction time of the AP event to the ventricles). The last four complexes on this strip show a consistent AP-VS interval of about 160 ms. Atrial capture is appropriate.

Ventricular activity is a little bit more unusual. Notice that there are three different ventricular morphologies on this small section of strip! The first two ventricular events are wide, notched complexes right after a ventricular output spike. The last four events on the strip are smaller, narrow ventricular complexes without a spike; these are intrinsic ventricular events. So what are the third and fourth ventricular events?

When you evaluate ventricular waveform morphology, consider the T-wave as well as the QRS complex. Looking at the T-waves, it is clear that the fourth complex on this strip more closely resembles the two paced ventricular events than the third

event. That makes me think that the third event is fusion (a cross between true capture and intrinsic) but the fourth event is a paced ventricular beat.

Fusion occurs when an output spike occurs just as the heart was depolarizing on its own. Both the pacemaker spike and the intrinsic depolarization contribute to the event. Fused beats are not uncommon to see in clinical practice, but do require some special awareness.

Fusion is not just one kind of event; fused beats occur over a spectrum. Thus, it is not unusual to see fused beats that look slightly different from each other. For that reason, it is possible that both the third and fourth beats are indeed fusion, just that one is more intrinsic (the third) and the other more paced (the fourth).

The nuts and bolts of paced ECG interpretation: fusion

Fusion is a timing issue; it happens when a pacemaker output occurs just exactly at the same moment that the heart was starting to depolarize on its own. Both the pacemaker output pulse and the native depolarization contribute to the beat. That's why fused beats look like a cross between a true paced and a true sensed event.

Although fused beats may look a bit unusual, if they occur occasionally, they are not a source of concern. The patient does not feel fusion when it occurs and it does not harm the natural cardiac contraction. At worst, it is wasteful of pacemaker battery energy since the output pulse was not needed.

One thing many clinicians do not always realize: *fused beats confirm capture*. The output pulse "changed" the intrinsic morphology, indicating capture.

Ventricular capture in this strip seems to be appropriate. The paced ventricular events and the fused beat(s) confirm capture.

Sensing

Atrial sensing cannot be evaluated from this strip because all of the atrial events are paced.

Ventricular sensing appears appropriate in that the intrinsic ventricular events at the end of the strip inhibit the ventricular output. To confirm ventricular sensing, use the AV delay. Measure the paced AV delay at the beginning of the strip with calipers; it is 200 ms. If the pacemaker sensed the last three ventricular events, it means they had to have occurred within that 200-ms window. Using calipers, it is clear that all three ventricular events at the end of the strip occurred just before the paced AV delay timed out. Thus, ventricular sensing is appropriate.

Underlying rhythm

This patients has sinus node dysfunction and slow AV conduction.

What to do next

First, atrial sensing should be tested. This requires intrinsic atrial events to emerge. By temporarily reducing the base rate in 10-ppm steps, intrinsic atrial events should appear on the ECG and atrial sensitivity testing can be conducted. Some patients have very erratic or even no atrial activity (silent atria) so it may not always be possible to evaluate atrial sensing.

The patient also has at least one fused complex on this strip. Occasional fusion beats are not uncommon and no reason for concern. In fact, it would be tough to find a pacemaker patient who did not occasionally experience a fused beat. But fusion is something we should always investigate a bit.

Fusion is a timing issue – it is not a capture or sensing issue. Since we know this patient has intermittent AV conduction, the fusion occurs because an intrinsic ventricular event is happening just at the moment the pacemaker's timing cycles are telling it to beat. In other words, the pacemaker is competing with the patient's AV conduction.

The best fix for this situation is to extend the AV delay. With calipers, it looks like the AV delay is approximately 200 ms. Extending that to 240 ms or even longer will give the ventricles more opportunity to depolarize on their own before delivering the pacemaker spike.

EASY TRACING #7

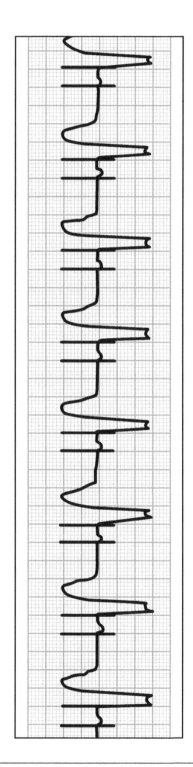

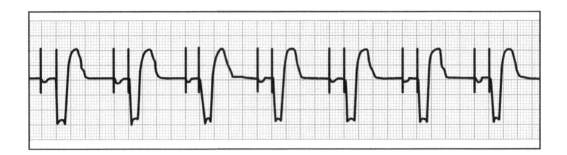

Mode

Atrial and ventricular spikes mean this is a dual-chamber pacemaker.

Rate

Measure the rate in a dual-chamber pacemaker based on the atrial pacing interval (AP-AP); in this case it is 1000 ms (60 ppm), which is appropriate. This is a very consistent strip; every complex is the same.

Capture

Every atrial spike is followed by an atrial depolarization with the same morphology; this suggests appropriate capture. Likewise, every ventricular spike is followed by a ventricular depolarization with the same morphology, also suggesting appropriate capture. This particular QRS morphology is typical of a paced beat in that it is widened, notched, and bizarre looking.

Sensing

Neither atrial nor ventricular sensing can be evaluated from this strip because all of the events shown are paced.

Underlying rhythm

This patient has sinus node dysfunction (he required consistent atrial pacing) and slow AV conduction.

The nuts and bolts of paced ECG interpretation: pacemaker dependency

The term pacemaker dependency is complex and a bit controversial, but the concept is simple. There are patients who simply depend on the presence of a pacemaker. The controversy over pacemaker dependence is based on how dependency is determined. Patients who may be pacemaker dependent are those who are very frequently, if not 100 percent, paced. As such, a patient presenting with this ECG might well turn out to be pacemaker dependent.

My own rule of thumb for pacemaker dependency is that any patient whose escape rhythm is under 40 bpm should be treated as pacemaker dependent.

Such patients should be monitored closely and their devices replaced in plenty of time to assure there is no interruption in pacing support. Pacemaker tests that temporarily suspend pacing or slow it down may be inappropriate for such patients.

In some clinics, the files of pacemaker-dependent patients are stickered or prominently labeled to that effect to avoid pacemaker tests that might temporarily interrupt their needed pacing support.

What to do next

Sensing in both chambers should be evaluated. I always start with atrial sensing, not because there is any scientific reason to review atrial sensing prior to ventricular sensing, but because it keeps things systematic. The systematic approach actually makes things faster and helps avoid errors of omission.

To test atrial sensing, intrinsic atrial activity has to emerge. The best way to encourage this is to slow the base rate in 10-ppm steps, which will reduce the rate at which the pacemaker paces the atrium. Reduce the base rate in small steps until intrinsic atrial activity occurs. Explain to the patient what is going on; some patients become symptomatic at even slightly reduced pacing rates. Even if no intrinsic atrial activity appears, do not go lower than 30 or 40 ppm.

Reducing the base rate may be inappropriate if the patient is pacemaker dependent. Furthermore, there will be some cases in which atrial sensing simply cannot be evaluated.

Assuming you can evaluate atrial sensing, you would then go back and check the atrial sensitivity settings and be sure that they are appropriate in view of the atrial sensing threshold. Any changes in the sensitivity should be carried out in small, incremental steps. Big swings in sensitivity settings can sometimes solve one problem but cause new ones.

Next, evaluate ventricular sensitivity. Again, the theory is to encourage intrinsic ventricular activity. The preferred method to accomplish this is to extend the paced AV delay. The atrial rate will pace at the normal rate, but you can temporarily allow the paced AV delay to be 300 ms or more. (There is really no need to extend the AV delay in increments; change it to 300 or 350 ms and observe whether or not intrinsic ventricular events appear.) If that does not cause intrinsic ventricular activity to appear on the ECG, you may temporarily program the pacemaker to VVI mode and reduce the base rate in 10-ppm steps down to about 30 or 40 ppm (providing the patient can tolerate it).

In my opinion, the AV delay extension should always be done first and is by far the better method. Always try to evaluate dual-chamber pacemakers in dual-chamber modes. (There is another advantage to extending the AV delay. If you see that the patient has intrinsic ventricular activity with a prolonged AV delay setting, measure the AV conduction interval. You may be able to reprogram the permanent AV delay interval setting to something that will encourage more intrinsic conduction – good for the patient and good for the pacemaker battery.)

Presuming the ventricular sensing threshold can be ascertained, this threshold should be used to adjust the ventricular sensitivity setting, if necessary.

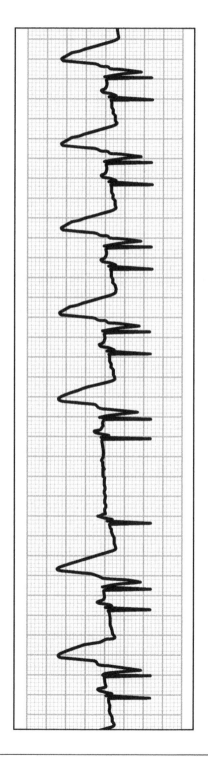

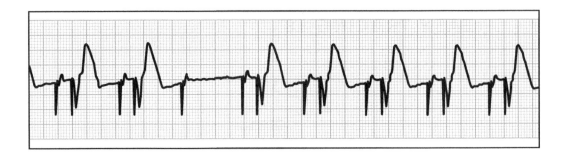

Mode

The atrial and ventricular pacing spikes show that this is a dual-chamber strip.

Rate

Dual-chamber rates are measured by the atrial pacing interval (AP-AP). In this case, the atrial pacing rate is about 68 ppm (880 ms). This is an appropriate rate.

Capture

Atrial spikes are followed by atrial depolarizations with similar morphology, so atrial capture seems appropriate. Ventricular spikes are followed by ventricular depolarizations with the same morphology, so ventricular capture seems appropriate, too.

But notice the pause on the strip. The third paced atrial event is followed by a long pause, after which AP-VP pacing resumes. There is not a loss of capture because although we can see where the paced ventricular event should appear, there is no ventricular pacing spike. For now, let's note this pause and proceed with the systematic review.

Sensing

Every atrial event on this strip is paced, so it is not possible to evaluate atrial sensing.

We cannot evaluate ventricular sensing based on the series of paced ventricular events, but there is one spot on the strip where the pacemaker inhibited the ventricular output – it's the "missing ventricular event" from the pause. The pacemaker withheld a ventricular output pulse, and we need to figure out why that happened.

There are actually any number of possible reasons that this could happen. The first, and most common, is a phenomenon called oversensing.

The nuts and bolts of paced ECG interpretation: oversensing and undersensing

Oversensing occurs when the pacemaker senses something that is not there. Undersensing occurs when the pacemaker fails to sense something that is there.

The concept is pretty easy to understand. However, it shows up on a paced ECG this way:

Oversensing leads to under-pacing
Undersensing leads to over-pacing

But there are other causes for pauses. They include intermittent lead fracture (that is, a problem with the lead that only manifests some of the time); crosstalk inhibition (when the pacemaker's ventricular channel "hears" something it thinks is a ventricular event but which, in truth, is an atrial event); or it could be noise.

Noise is a general term given to all kinds of pacemaker interference. Notice how wavy the baseline is during the pause. That may be an artifact from the ECG machine, or it could be that the pacemaker is picking up stray signals.

The nuts and bolts of paced ECG interpretation: noise

Noise or interference refers to stray signals picked up by the pacemaker. The body is actually a pretty noisy place in terms of electrical signals, so all pacemakers are equipped with standard filters to help block out regular body and muscle noise. However, some patients will experience myopotential noise (muscle noise) that the pacemaker can pick up and inappropriately "sense" as cardiac activity.

Interference can also come from outside the body. Certain electronic devices and environmental atmospheres can produce noise that interferes with pacemakers. Common culprits include high-power lines, arc welding equipment, very large magnets, and certain in-store theft detection systems.

Noise will show up on an ECG in several ways. Most commonly, it causes oversensing which appears on the ECG as paused or "missing beats." If you had an annotated strip, you would see annotations for sensed activity that does not appear on the actual tracing. Noise can show up as bumps or odd, very low amplitude waves on the tracing.

When the pacemaker is in the presence of noise for an extended period of time, the device may automatically revert to a safety pacing mode. Manufacturers have different names for this reset function, but basically the pacemaker reverts to basic asynchronous ventricular pacing in the presence of noise. The purpose of this is to make sure the patient is being paced even in the presence of what appears to be noise (which can cause the device to not pace at all). The originally programmed parameters can be restored in a simple programming step.

From the information we have, it appears that the pacemaker is oversensing as a result of noise or interference. The evidence of oversensing is the pause; I suspect interference is involved because of the appearance of the tracing.

Underlying rhythm

This patient has sinus node dysfunction and slow AV conduction.

What to do next

Atrial sensing should be evaluated, which means dropping the base rate in 10-ppm increments to force intrinsic atrial activity to emerge, if possible. Drop the base rate gradually and make sure the patient tolerates it, but do not go below 30 or 40 ppm, even if no intrinsic activity appears and the patient seems to be doing fine.

Ventricular sensitivity should also be tested, but the best way to do that is to prolong the AV delay to 300 ms or more and see if native ventricular events appear.

The real "issue" on this strip is figuring out the cause of the "missing ventricular event." If possible, obtain an annotated strip to see if the pacemaker "thought" it saw one or more VS events in the pause area. That would prove that the pacemaker was oversensing. The bumpy baseline would lead me to believe that there was some kind of noise or interference going on. If this strip was obtained in-clinic, the source of the interference would likely be muscle noise.

A good basic test for muscle noise involves observing the ECG as you have the patient do some upper-body isometric exercises. Moving the arms around is likely to produce some myopotentials. If this shows up as more missed ventricular beats (oversensing leading to under-pacing), then that would confirm this is oversensing due to noise.

On the other hand, if you cannot simulate myopotential noise, this is cause to suspect some kind of lead problem. The likely next step is to order a chest X-ray to verify lead integrity.

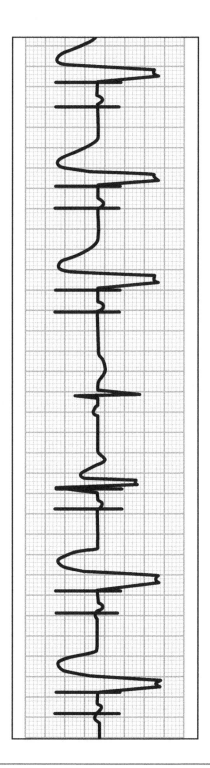

The Nuts and Bolts of Paced ECG Interpretation, 1st edition. By Tom Kenny.
Published 2009 by Blackwell Publishing, ISBN: 978-1-4501-8404-5.

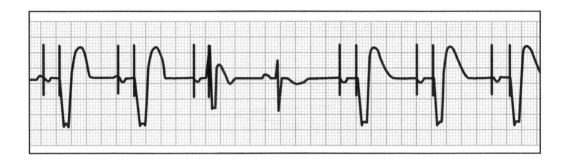

Mode

This has to be a dual-chamber pacemaker because there are atrial and ventricular spikes on the ECG.

Rate

The atrial rate "drives" pacing in a dual-chamber system. The atrial pacing interval (AP-AP) here measures 1000 ms (60 ppm). The rate is appropriate.

Capture

Atrial pacing spikes are followed by downward-deflecting P-waves that differ in morphology from the lone intrinsic atrial event that appears on the middle of the strip. Atrial capture seems appropriate.

Ventricular capture is a little more complex. There are three very distinct QRS morphologies on this strip! In the middle of the strip there is an intrinsic ventricular event. Note its typical narrow, sharp morphology.

The first two and last three complexes on the strip show a ventricular output pulse followed by a wider, notched, bizarre looking QRS complex. These are paced ventricular events and they all share the same QRS and T-wave morphology. These events show appropriate capture.

The unusual-looking third beat is ventricular fusion (where both spike and intrinsic activity contribute to a single depolarization), even though some clinicians might be inclined to call it pseudofusion (where the spike lands on an intrinsic event but makes no contribution to the depolarization). In general, pseudofusion morphology resembles an intrinsic event with a spike. Fusion looks like a cross between a paced and sensed event.

If intrinsic QRS morphology changes to any degree, then the beat is fusion. Fusion exists across a spectrum, so some beats can looked "more fused" than others … but since this QRS morphology in this third complex is not identical to the intrinsic morphology of the fourth complex, this is an example of fusion rather than pseudofusion.

When confronted with fusion and pseudofusion events, the T-wave can also provide valuable clues. Pseudofusion beats should have T-wave morphology identical to intrinsic T-waves. Fused beats have T-waves that look like a hybrid between the T-waves of an intrinsic and paced complex. That convinces me the third beat is fused.

This strip shows appropriate ventricular capture with one fused ventricular event. Remember that fusion confirms capture.

Sensing

Atrial sensing is appropriate in that the intrinsic atrial event inhibits the atrial output and resets device timing. Of course, this is based on one single event, but that is all we have to work with.

Ventricular sensing is also based on one single intrinsic event; it appears to be appropriate because the ventricular event inhibits ventricular pacing and resets device timing.

Underlying rhythm

This patient has sinus node dysfunction and slow AV conduction.

What to do next

Besides mode and rate, there are four things to check when evaluating a dual-chamber pacemaker (sensing and capture in both chambers). This strip has evidence of appropriate behavior for all four categories. However, it would be prudent to test atrial and ventricular sensitivity in that our initial evaluation is based on one single event. Sensing problems can be intermittent and may not show up in every single sensed complex.

The presence of fusion should also be investigated. In strict clinical terms, fusion is not a problem. It does not hurt the patient and is, at most, wasteful of device battery energy. Many pacemaker patients occasionally experienced fused beats. However, fusion occurs because the patient's intrinsic rate is competing with the programmed base rate. In other words, fusion is a matter of timing. If the patient experienced frequent fusion, it might be worthwhile to program hysteresis on or even lower the base rate slightly. However, if fusion is an occasional event, no special steps need be taken.

EASY TRACING #10

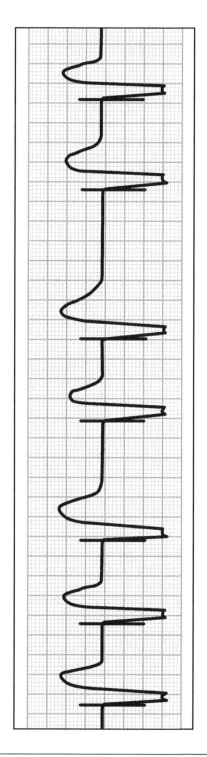

The Nuts and Bolts of Paced ECG Interpretation, 1st edition. By Tom Kenny.
Published 2009 by Blackwell Publishing, ISBN: 978-1-4501-8404-5.

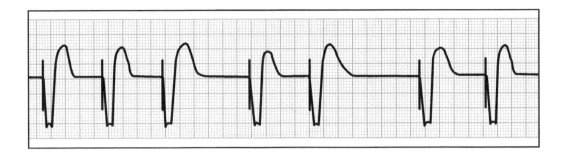

Mode

This is a VVI pacemaker; that's clear from the fact that there are neither intrinsic nor paced atrial events.

Rate

The ventricular pacing interval (VP-VP) provides the rate in a VVI strip and on the left end of the strip, it measures to be 840 ms (about 70 ppm), which is an appropriate rate. But the rate is inconsistent. There are pauses (of different lengths) between the third and fourth complexes and between the fifth and sixth complexes.

Capture

Since this is a VVI device, we can only evaluate capture in the ventricle. Every single ventricular event on this strip is paced and judging from the spike and the QRS morphology, it appears as if ventricular capture is appropriate.

Sensing

With nothing but ventricular pacing, we cannot evaluate appropriate ventricular sensing using this strip. However, the pauses suggest something is inappropriate about ventricular sensing. To evaluate this strip, the pauses must be explained.

Set calipers to the ventricular pacing interval (840 ms). Putting one leg on the fourth ventricular spike, use the calipers to measure backward toward the third spike and place the other caliper leg on the spot where the pacemaker "thought" it sensed a ventricular event. It occurs on the QRS complex.

This is an example of oversensing or sensing a ventricular event that really was not a true ventricular event.

Using this same technique for the second pause, it appears that the pacemaker also oversensed a nonexistent event that occurred during the baseline!

> ### The nuts and bolts of paced ECG interpretation: the causes of pauses
>
> Pauses occur in both the intrinsic and paced cardiac rhythm, but they are often indicative of some kind of problem. When pauses occur in a paced rhythm strip, the clinician must account for them and it is likely that corrective action will be warranted.
>
> The main causes of pauses are oversensing (sensing something that really isn't there and resetting the device timing); variations caused by hysteresis; or a problem with the hardware (device or leads) such that the output is not delivered.

Lead or hardware problems (such as no-output from the pulse generator) can cause pauses, but such events are quite rare. When they do happen, there is usually more evidence of problems than occasional pauses. Since this strip shows good ventricular pacemaker function except for these pauses, I would rule out a lead or hardware problem.

Hysteresis can cause pauses, but hysteresis goes into effect after intrinsic events, not after paced events. Thus, this is ventricular oversensing.

Underlying rhythm

This patient has silent atria. It is possible he is

pacemaker dependent. My working definition of pacemaker dependency is a patient without an escape rhythm of 40 bpm or higher. Therefore, I would treat this patient as pacemaker dependent.

What to do next

Ventricular sensing should be evaluated to eliminate oversensing. Since the strip already shows one interval of 1520 ms (40 ppm), it is probably impossible to provoke intrinsic ventricular activity in this patient. The pacing rate could be lowered in 10-ppm increments, but since it should never be dropped below 30 or 40 ppm, I suspect that it may not be possible to evaluate ventricular sensing in this patient.

If it is possible, obtain the ventricular intracardiac electrogram. This will reveal what the pacemaker is seeing and where.

In cases like this, we may want to approach the ventricular sensitivity issue from a different angle. Even if we cannot force intrinsic ventricular activity to appear, we may still be able to improve ventricular sensing. Make the ventricular sensitivity of the device slightly less sensitive (increase the mV setting)

and observe the patient's ECG. Keep making small changes to see if it clears up the sensing problem.

When making adjustments to sensitivity, take very small steps. Large changes in sensitivity values can solve one problem but cause another.

The nuts and bolts of paced ECG interpretation: sensitivity

Sensitivity defines the size an intrinsic cardiac signal has to be before the pacemaker can detect it. If a pacemaker is set to 2 mV sensitivity, that means that an intrinsic cardiac waveform has to be 2 mV or greater for the pacemaker to "see" and sense it.

The higher the mV setting, the more insensitive the pacemaker. For example, a pacemaker set to a sensitivity value of 5 mV would only sense signals that were 5 mV or greater.

This creates the sometimes confusing programming situation where to *increase sensitivity*, you have to *lower the mV setting*. To *decrease sensitivity*, you have to *increase the mV setting*.

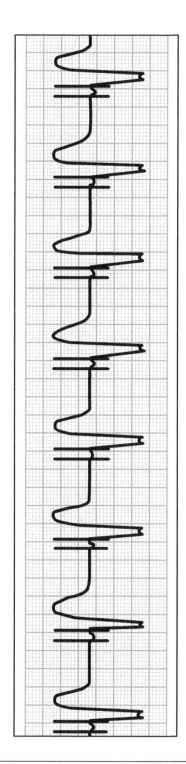

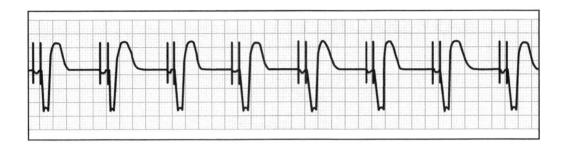

Mode

This is a dual-chamber pacemaker.

Rate

In a dual-chamber system, the atrial channel "sets the pace." The atrial pacing interval (AP-AP) provides the rate. Here that interval is 1000 ms (60 ppm). This rate is appropriate for a dual-chamber pacemaker.

In evaluating rate, it is always a good idea to check out the AV delay setting. This is particularly important when there is a lot of AP-VP activity, since sometimes a change to the AV delay interval can encourage more intrinsic ventricular activity (AP-VS activity), which is generally agreed to be better for the patient. A typical AV delay value might be anywhere from 150 to 250 ms. Using calipers, it appears that this AV delay interval is about 110 or 120 ms. That is very short and bears further scrutiny.

Capture

Every atrial spike is followed by an atrial depolarization with a similar downward-deflecting morphology. Atrial capture seems appropriate.

Ventricular capture also looks appropriate; note that every ventricular spike is followed by a ventricular depolarization and all the ventricular events share the same widened, notched morphology.

Sensing

With nothing but constant atrial and ventricular pacing, we cannot evaluate appropriate sensing in either chamber.

Underlying rhythm

This patient has sinus node dysfunction. It is unclear from this strip whether the patient has slow AV conduction since the AV delay interval is so short that even a patient with normal AV conduction would be paced at these parameter settings.

What to do next

Atrial and ventricular sensing should be evaluated. To test atrial sensitivity, decrease the base rate in 10-ppm steps to cause intrinsic atrial activity to emerge. Monitor the patient as you decrease the rate gradually and do not go below 30 or 40 ppm.

For ventricular sensitivity, temporarily extend the paced AV delay to 300 ms or more and see if native ventricular events appear.

While the AV delay is temporarily set to a long value, observe whether or not the patient has intrinsic conduction. If the patient has intrinsic ventricular activity at, say, about 200 ms following the atrial paced event, the paced AV delay could be programmed to 240 or 250 ms to encourage more intrinsic ventricular activity and discourage unnecessary right-ventricular pacing.

Why is the AV delay interval so short? While a very short AV delay might be permanently programmed (very unusual but possible), this is more likely the result of a special algorithm like safety pacing to ensure ventricular pacing in the presence of noise or interference. Verify whether or not the pacemaker is pacing in a safety mode. If so, program the device back to normal pacing and the originally programmed AV delay interval. You may still need to adjust the AV delay to better suit the patient's intrinsic conduction timing, if possible.

EASY TRACING #12

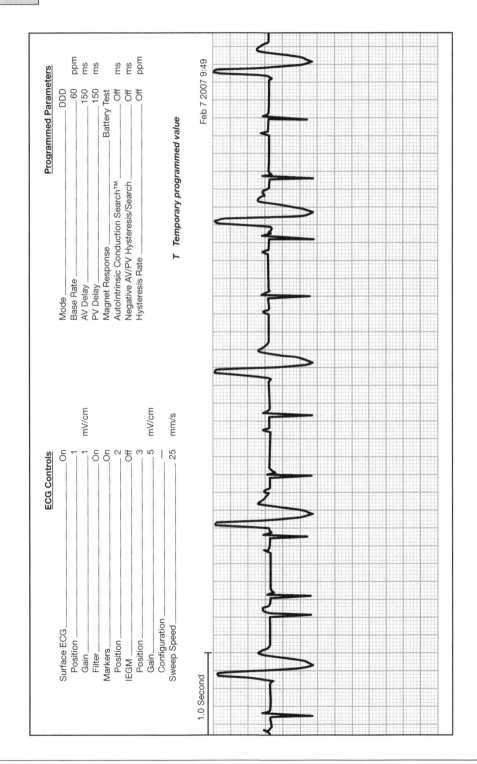

ECG Controls

Surface ECG	On	
Position	1	
Gain	1	mV/cm
Filter	On	
Markers	On	
Position	2	
IEGM	Off	
Position	3	
Gain	5	mV/cm
Configuration	—	
Sweep Speed	25	mm/s

Programmed Parameters

Mode	DDD	
Base Rate	60	ppm
AV Delay	150	ms
PV Delay	150	ms
Magnet Response	Battery Test	
AutoIntrinsic Conduction Search™	Off	ms
Negative AV/PV Hysteresis/Search	Off	ms
Hysteresis Rate	Off	ppm

T   Temporary programmed value

Feb 7 2007 9:49

1.0 Second

The Nuts and Bolts of Paced ECG Interpretation, 1st edition. By Tom Kenny.
Published 2009 by Blackwell Publishing, ISBN: 978-1-4501-8404-5.

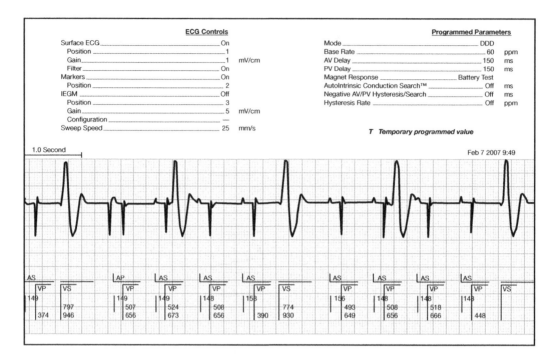

Mode

The printout reveals that this is a dual-chamber strip, but that is evident looking at the atrial and ventricular pacing spikes. If the exact nature of the events confused you, the annotations and strip reveal that there is one atrial pacing spike, some intrinsic atrial events (AS), some ventricular pacing spikes (VP), and five intrinsic ventricular events, of which only three are annotated (VS).

Rate

In a dual-chamber device, the rate is controlled by the atrial channel. However, this strip does not offer any atrial pacing intervals (AP-AP) to measure the rate. We could measure ventricular pacing intervals (VP-VP), but the presence of intrinsic atrial events keeps resetting the timing. (Remember, a dual-chamber device takes its rate cues from what's going on in the atrium.)

Capture

There is only one atrial paced event with appropriate atrial capture. However, I would hesitate to pronounce atrial capture appropriate based on just one event.

The ventricle is more problematic. The wider, larger QRS complexes are intrinsic ventricular events. The sharp narrow downward deflections on the strip that align with the VP annotations are not ventricular events at all; they're just pacing spikes. There is no ventricular capture on this strip. (This is a great example of why you can't trust annotations to tell you the whole story; look at the tracing and then check it against the annotations. Whenever they don't agree, the tracing wins!)

How can we be sure these rather large spikes aren't just unusual-looking paced ventricular events? Look at the third ventricular pacing spike and notice that right after the spike, the ventricles depolarized on their own. Had the first spike captured the ventricle, the ventricles would have been physiologically refractory and could not have depolarized. There is no appropriate ventricular capture on this strip at all.

Sensing

Atrial sensing appears to be appropriate in that intrinsic atrial events inhibit the atrial output and reset device timing. When an intrinsic atrial event occurs, a ventricular output pulse is delivered (in the case of AS-VP events) at the point at which the sensed AV delay times out (150 ms). Atrial sensing is functioning properly.

Ventricular sensing is more complicated. Go to the first sensed ventricular event on the strip. There is an annotation VS, indicating it was sensed. This resets timing because the next VP occurs about 950 ms after that sensed event (which is compatible with a 60 ppm rate). Thus, this VS event was properly sensed and reset timing.

The second intrinsic ventricular event is more problematic. It occurs right after the VP annotation and there is no VS annotation to indicate that the pacemaker "saw" it. An intrinsic atrial event occurs right after it, which is properly sensed and launches the sensed AV delay. So the second intrinsic ventricular event is not properly sensed.

Whenever something is not sensed, you must ask, "Should it have been sensed?" There are times when a pacemaker is behaving appropriately and not sensing events, for example, during a refractory period. The pacemaker imposes a refractory period right after a pacing spike. The second intrinsic ventricular event occurred within 200 ms of the ventricular pacing spike. That means this ventricular event "fell into the refractory" and was not sensed. This is called functional non-sensing and it actually is not a sensing problem at all.

These examples repeat themselves across the strip; there are five intrinsic ventricular events in this strip and the first is properly sensed; the second is not sensed (functional non-sensing); the third is properly sensed; the fourth is not sensed (functional non-sensing); and the fifth one is properly sensed. Functional non-sensing is not a sensing problem, in that the pacemaker is sensing appropriately. For that reason, ventricular sensing is actually appropriate.

Underlying rhythm

This patient has intrinsic atrial activity at an erratic but relatively fast rate. AV conduction is slow or delayed.

The nuts and bolts of paced ECG interpretation: functional non-sensing

Whenever the pacemaker does not sense something properly, it is important to determine "should it have sensed this event?" The reason to ask this question is that events that occur during refractory period timing cycles are, by definition, appropriately *not sensed*. When an intrinsic events "falls into the refractory period" and is not sensed, the proper term for this is "functional non-sensing," meaning the non-sensing is actually the appropriate function of the device.

Functional non-sensing is not a sensing problem at all. (Depending on the situation, it may be a timing problem.)

What to do next

Although there is one example on this strip of appropriate atrial capture, atrial capture should be evaluated. It is quite possible that everything is fine and atrial output settings are appropriate. Increase the base rate in 10-ppm increments (starting at about 90 ppm) to force pacing. This will likely work well in this patient, in that there is already an example of atrial pacing on the strip.

Ventricular capture is more urgent; it must be restored. Ventricular capture should be tested by conducting a ventricular pacing threshold test and reprogramming output parameters (ventricular pulse amplitude and pulse width). It is likely that increasing the energy of the output pulse can restore proper ventricular capture. When capture is restored, the issue of functional non-sensing will become a non-issue.

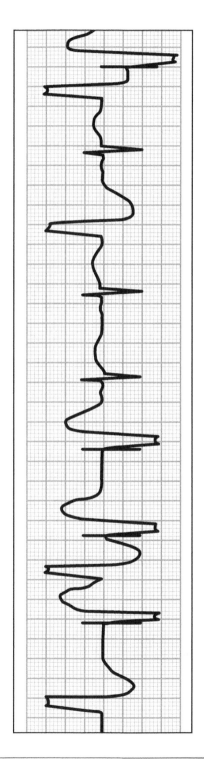

The Nuts and Bolts of Paced ECG Interpretation, 1st edition. By Tom Kenny.
Published 2009 by Blackwell Publishing, ISBN: 978-1-4501-8404-5.

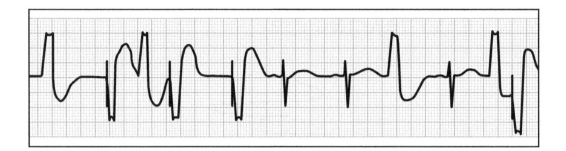

Mode

This is a VVI strip.

Rate

In a VVI strip, rate is measured from the ventricular pacing interval (VP-VP) which is about 880 ms as measured with calipers (around 68 ppm). This is an appropriate rate.

The nuts and bolts of paced ECG interpretation: types of intrinsic ventricular events

This strip has two different types of intrinsic ventricular events: there is a narrow, pointed morphology of a true intrinsic ventricular depolarization and there are four examples on this strip of upward-deflecting tall widened intrinsic ventricular events that are actually premature ventricular contractions of PVCs.

The reason that the PVC has a different morphology from the other intrinsic ventricular event is that the narrow ventricular events are conducted from an intrinsic atrial impulse and depolarization, while the PVCs originate from a ventricular focus.

While many pacemaker patients experience occasional PVCs, PVCs are of concern to the clinician in that they can trigger a pacemaker-mediated tachycardia or PMT in susceptible patients and may trigger potentially lethal ventricular tachyarrhythmias.

Capture

Ventricular capture appears appropriate in that every ventricular spike is followed by a ventricular depolarization with the characteristic widened, bizarre look of a paced QRS. Notice that the ventricular depolarizations following spikes have a completely different morphology from the intrinsic ventricular events on the strip.

Sensing

As far as the pacemaker is concerned, a PVC is an intrinsic ventricular event. The first event on this strip is a PVC and it is properly sensed in that it resets device timing (the first ventricular spike on this strip is timed to the preceding PVC). However the second PVC is not sensed; notice that the interval between the two ventricular pacing spikes before and after the second PVC is about 880 ms or the pacing interval. That means the second PVC was not sensed.

The clinician might ask whether this intrinsic ventricular event should have been sensed or if it "fell into" the refractory period initiated by the ventricular pacing spike. Although we don't know the refractory period parameter settings, calipers show that there is about a 440 ms interval from the ventricular spike to the onset of the PVC. It is highly unlikely the ventricular refractory period is that long! This PVC did not occur during the device's refractory period and should have been sensed. This is undersensing.

The other intrinsic ventricular events on this strip are properly sensed with the exception of the last PVC. A ventricular sensed event occurs, then a PVC, and then a pacing spike. The spike is timed to the first ventricular sensed event. That means the pacemaker did not properly sense the PVC, which occurred well outside of the refractory period.

Diagnosis: intermittent ventricular undersensing.

Underlying rhythm

This patient has sinus node dysfunction, slow AV conduction, and appears prone to PVCs. While occasional PVCs are normal in both paced and non-paced patients, the presence of frequent PVCs is of concern for pacemaker patients in that PVCs can trigger pacemaker-mediated tachycardias (PMTs) and lead to potentially lethal ventricular tachyarrhythmias.

What to do next

Ventricular sensing should be evaluated and reprogrammed, if necessary. From the rhythm strip, it appears that PVCs are very large events, so it may seem odd to you that the pacemaker seems to be able to reliably sense the relatively small "true" intrinsic ventricular events that conduct down over the AV node from the atrium, yet it undersenses the large PVCs. This may be a matter of perspective.

Bipolar pacemakers sense cardiac events by detecting the difference between electrical potential picked up at the two electrodes on the pacing lead. If the ventricular wavefront travels through the heart in such a way that there is a large differential, the signal is sensed. However, a PVC and a conducted ventricular depolarization originate from different points in the heart and travel along different pathways. If the PVC hits the bipolar electrodes "head on," there may be very little potential difference on the two electrodes even though the electrical energy of the waveform can be quite substantial.

Actually, it is not at all unusual to see bipolar pacemakers undersense PVCs. While sensitivity should definitely be checked and possibly reprogrammed, there is another strategy that can sometimes help when PVCs are not properly sensed. If the patient

has a bipolar system, the ventricular pacing lead polarity could be changed. For instance, if the patient has a bipolar ventricular lead programmed to unipolar, it can be programmed to bipolar; likewise, if the lead is programmed to bipolar, it can be changed to unipolar. Changes in polarity configuration may improve sensitivity.

The nuts and bolts of paced ECG interpretation: polarity configurations and sensing

The polarity of a pacing lead is defined by the number of electrodes that are on the lead tip itself; a unipolar lead has only one tip electrode (and forms a circuit with the pulse generator can), while a bipolar lead has one tip electrode and a ring electrode, both of which are on the end of the lead.

The lead senses the cardiac waveform by measuring the difference in electrical potential from one pole of its circuit to the next. While this is normally pretty straightforward, sometimes the way the electrical energy travels through the heart and the relative position of the lead make it so that some signals are missed. This is sort of like an electrical "blind spot" because the wavefront hits the poles so head-on that there is not sufficient potential difference to measure. In such cases, a change in polarity (that is, a change in how the electrical poles on the circuit are arranged) may restore proper sensing. This can only be done with a bipolar lead (a unipolar lead only has one electrode on the lead tip and so cannot be reprogrammed to operate as a bipolar lead).

While changing polarity configurations can help make the device more sensitive to PVCs, it may also make the pacemaker too sensitive to other signals, such as myopotential noise or interference. If you do decide to change polarity settings to better sense PVCs, make the change and observe as much device function as you can to verify appropriate operation.

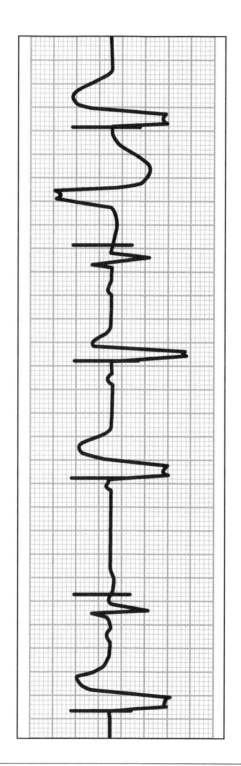

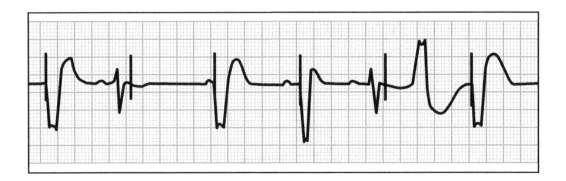

Mode

This is a VVI strip.

Rate

Rate is measured on a VVI strip by the ventricular pacing interval (VP-VP). The best spot to measure on this strip would be the third and fourth spikes. It measures a pacing interval of 1000 ms (60 ppm), an appropriate rate.

Capture

Moving from left to right, the first ventricular pacing spike appears to capture the ventricle; a widened, notched QRS complex follows the spike. The second spike is a different story; it does not capture. However, is it reasonable to expect it to have captured? Notice that it falls right after an intrinsic ventricular event. The myocardium is physiologically refractory at this point; no amount of electrical stimulation could cause a depolarization at that particular moment. This is an example of functional non-capture, which is actually an issue we will revisit when we look at sensing below. (Functional non-capture is usually the result of a *sensing problem*.)

The third spike appears to be appropriate capture, but the fourth spike is a bit of a puzzle. There is a spike with an immediate ventricular depolariza-

tion, but the QRS morphology is not the same as the previous two ventricular paced events.

This fourth spike is an example of fusion, which occurs when both an intrinsic depolarization and a pacing spike contribute to one event. The result is a QRS morphology that looks like a cross between a true paced ventricular event and a true intrinsic ventricular event. Fusion actually confirms capture, in that the pacing spike clearly played a part in the depolarization. However, fusion is a coincidence of timing; the spike and the patient's intrinsic depolarization happened almost simultaneously.

The fifth spike shows functional non-capture and the last spike captures properly. Overall, this strip reveals intermittent functional non-capture, which suggests a sensing problem.

Sensing

Starting at the left, there is a paced ventricular event followed by an intrinsic ventricular event and then a spike. The spike is an example of functional non-capture, but the real question for the clinician is: why is that spike there? If you set the calipers to 1000 ms and measure the first and second spikes, it is clear the intrinsic ventricular event was not properly sensed and, therefore, did not reset the device timing. This is an example of ventricular undersensing. This occurs again with the fifth spike.

The nuts and bolts of paced ECG interpretation: things that go together

While a systematic approach is by far the best way to interpret a paced rhythm strip, it can also be useful to think of certain things that "go together" as you work through the steps.
- **Pauses go together with oversensing**
- **Too much pacing goes together with undersensing**
- **Functional non-capture suggests undersensing**
- **PMTs are associated with loss of atrial capture and PVCs**
- **Fusion and pseudofusion are timing problems (base rate is competing with the intrinsic rate)**

Underlying rhythm

This patient has slow AV conduction and may be prone to PVCs.

What to do next

Functional non-capture is not a capture problem; here, like most cases, it's actually a sensing problem. Ventricular sensing should be checked and adjusted so that intrinsic ventricular events are properly sensed. With proper ventricular sensing, the problem of functional non-capture should disappear.

This patient has some intrinsic activity, so it would be useful to activate hysteresis. Since the base rate is 60 ppm, setting hysteresis to 50 bpm would encourage more intrinsic ventricular activity to occur. Notice that this patient's native ventricular activity is not slow. It is likely that hysteresis could help reduce the total amount of ventricular pacing in this patient.

The nuts and bolts of paced ECG interpretation: hysteresis

The pacing rate is the rate at which the pacemaker will pace the heart in the absence of intrinsic activity. Hysteresis sets a second limit, below the base rate, that allows the patient's intrinsic rate to prevail. Typically the pacing rate and the hysteresis rate are close, usually no more than 10 or 15 beats apart. If a patient had a pacing rate of 60 ppm and a hysteresis rate of 50 bpm, the pacemaker would be inhibited as long as the patient's intrinsic rate was 50 bpm or higher. As soon as the patient's intrinsic rate dipped below 50 bpm, the pacemaker would resume pacing at the programmed pacing rate of 60 ppm.

One advantage of hysteresis is that it allows sufficiently fast pacing for the patient but still defers to the intrinsic rate, if the intrinsic rate is reasonably close to the pacing rate. If the base rate was programmed to 50 bpm, that might be too slow for the patient over the course of the day.

Thus, hysteresis is a "best of both worlds" algorithm in that it allows the patient to be paced at an appropriate pacing rate but still encourages the intrinsic rate to take over. Generally speaking, pacemaker patients are better off with an intrinsic rhythm than a paced rhythm, so every effort should be made to encourage intrinsic activity. (This does not apply to cardiac resynchronization patients, who should be paced as much as possible.)

Another reason to activate hysteresis is that the algorithm only goes into effect if the patient has a sufficiently fast intrinsic rhythm.

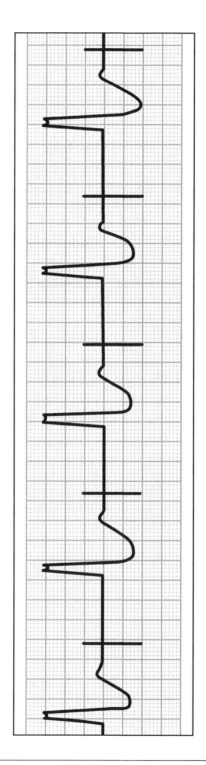

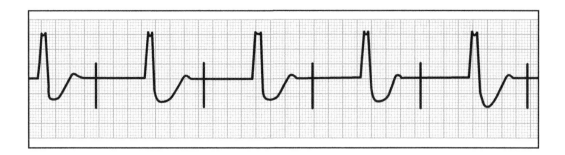

Mode

This is a VVI strip.

Rate

Rate is measured on a VVI strip by the ventricular pacing interval (VP-VP). However, this strip has no ventricular pacing intervals. The intervals here are ventricular escape intervals (VS-VP). Because this strip is so symmetrical, you may be tempted to measure the distance between spikes; that would come up to a 1520 ms interval or a pacing rate of 40 ppm. That is a very unlikely pacing rate! Instead, measure from the onset of one intrinsic ventricular event to the next pacing spike. That yields an 840 ms interval or a 70 ppm pacing rate. That's an appropriate rate.

Capture

Every single ventricular spike on this strip fails to capture. The next question to ask is whether we ought to expect such spikes to capture. Do they "fall into" the physiological refractory period? Looking at the strip, it is clear that they should have captured. Thus, we have consistent loss of ventricular capture.

Sensing

The intrinsic ventricular events on the strip are all properly sensed, in that they all reset the timing. Ventricular sensing is appropriate.

Underlying rhythm

This patient is currently relying on a ventricular escape rhythm of about 40 bpm. He has no intrinsic atrial activity at all.

What to do next

The consistent loss of ventricular capture is an urgent problem, so a ventricular capture test must be performed. The two most likely causes of the loss of ventricular capture are insufficient energy delivered to the heart (output parameters are too low) or a lead problem. The former is the more likely scenario and can be addressed by increasing the output settings (pulse amplitude and pulse width). Lead problems are less likely but are very serious and should always be considered. However, in this particular case, there is another reason to think that the real issue is output. If the problem was a lead, it would typically affect both capture and sensing. In this patient, sensing appears consistently appropriate.

The nuts and bolts of paced ECG interpretation: lead issues

When a pacing lead is compromised in some way, it typically will manifest in unusual device behavior. Crushed, fractured, or otherwise damaged leads will often result in a loss of capture and inappropriate sensing. Such problems may be intermittent, particularly if the lead damage is not extensive. While lead problems are relatively uncommon, they do occur; since the first clues of lead compromise usually appear on the ECG, it is important to consider the integrity of the pacing lead when you see sensing and capture problems.

Lead problems often affect both capture and sensing. It is not typical to have a lead problem impair capture but allow appropriate sensing or vice versa. Other signs of possible lead damage include sudden changes in capture or pacing behavior, sudden changes in lead impedance values, or very large changes in lead impedance.

If the sensing or capture problems can be addressed by adjustments to parameter settings, that suggests that lead problems can be ruled out.

If the problems persist despite such adjustments or if you see further evidence of damaged leads, a chest X-ray should be ordered.

Lead problems are more common in acute than chronic implants but can occur at any time over the life of a pacing system.

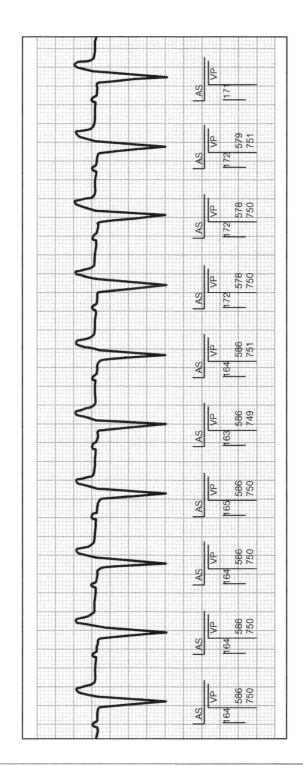

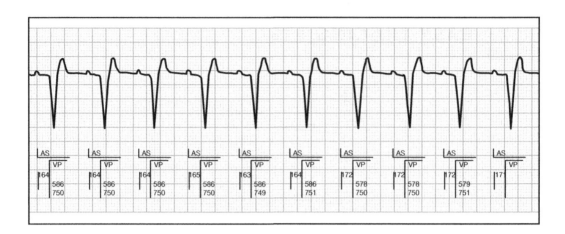

Mode

Even without the annotations and the lack of a prominent pacemaker spike, there is good evidence that this strip comes from a dual-chamber pacemaker. Notice that the intrinsic atrial events have a consistent sensed AV delay interval before the widened ventricular events. This strongly suggests that the atrial events are being sensed and used to time a ventricular output pulse.

Rate

A dual-chamber device takes its timing cues from the atrium, but all of the atrial activity on this strip is sensed. That means the device is tracking the atrium or timing ventricular pacing to accommodate the patient's intrinsic atrial rate. A dual-chamber pacemaker will track the atrium up to the programmed maximum tracking rate (MTR), which is typically set to about 120 ppm. Thus, the pacing rate cannot be ascertained from this strip. If you measure the interval between *sensed atrial events*, it's about 760 ms (78 bpm), which is well above the base rate to which the pacemaker would be programmed. However, this would be appropriate for atrial tracking.

Capture

Atrial capture cannot be assessed from this strip, since all atrial events are intrinsic.

Evaluating ventricular capture may seem difficult because there is no clear ventricular pacing spike. However, the annotations serve the same function

as a spike in that it tells you when a pacemaker output pulse was delivered. Thus, pacing can be confirmed by checking out whether the VP annotations align with the ventricular events on the strip.

A further confirmation that ventricular pacing occurred is found in the QRS morphology. The QRS here has the characteristic widened, bizarre look of a paced complex. Every VP annotation (spike) aligns with a QRS complex of the same morphology. Thus, even without spikes, it is clear that the pacemaker is pacing the ventricle and that capture is appropriate.

The nuts and bolts of paced ECG interpretation: spikes

When it comes to paced ECGs, the old rule of thumb was that unipolar devices had big pacing spikes and bipolar devices had smaller (maybe even scarcely visible) pacing spikes. While this is still true of paced ECGs obtained from a programmer, many ECG monitors and other equipment today offer spike enhancement. This enlarges the pacemaker output spike so that even bipolar systems offer clinicians very prominent pacing spikes.

Sensing

Atrial sensing is appropriate. The intrinsic atrial events in the strip inhibit atrial pacemaker outputs and launch a consistent sensed AV delay interval of about 170 ms. Since the pacemaker inhibited atrial outputs and timed ventricular pacing to these intrinsic atrial events, atrial sensing is functioning properly.

Ventricular sensing cannot be evaluated from this strip since all ventricular events are paced.

Underlying rhythm

This is a classic example of atrial tracking. This patient currently has a reliable intrinsic atrial rhythm that fails to conduct over the AV node to the ventricles. The use of a dual-chamber device provides this patient with 1:1 AV synchrony.

What to do next

Atrial capture must be assessed. To do this, atrial pacing must occur which can generally be forced by increasing the base rate (starting at about 90 ppm) in small 10-ppm steps.

Ventricular sensing also should be evaluated. To evaluate ventricular sensing, extend the AV delay (temporarily program the AV delay to 300 ms or more) and observe if ventricular activity occurs.

Right now, the intrinsic atrial rate is not very high and the patient probably tolerates this atrial tracking well. However, it is possible that the patient will experience occasional episodes of high-rate intrinsic atrial activity. It would be worthwhile to evaluate the setting of the maximum tracking rate (Max Track Rate or MTR). Typically, the MTR is set to 120 ppm. It can be set to whatever value the patient can reasonably tolerate. If 120-ppm ventricular pacing is uncomfortable for the patient, it should be programmed to a lower setting than 120 ppm.

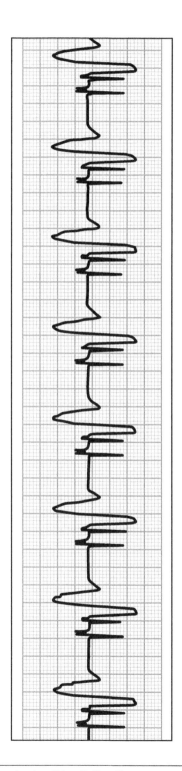

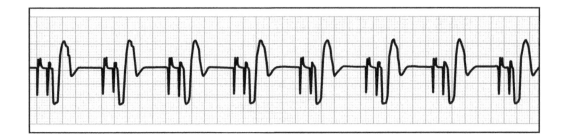

Mode

The presence of atrial and ventricular spikes means that this is a dual-chamber pacemaker.

Rate

To assess rate in a dual-chamber paced strip, measure the atrial pacing interval (AP-AP). The atrial pacing intervals measures 1000 ms or 60 ppm, an appropriate rate.

Capture

The atrial pacing spike is followed by an atrial depolarization and morphologies are consistent across the strip. Atrial capture is appropriate.

There is a prominent ventricular spike followed by a ventricular depolarization. All of these ventricular events share the same morphology. Ventricular capture seems appropriate.

Sensing

Neither atrial nor ventricular sensing can be evaluated using this tracing since all of the events are paced.

Underlying rhythm

The patient has sinus node dysfunction and slow AV conduction.

What to do next

This strip shows classic dual-chamber paced activity (AP-VP events), but we still need to check some pacemaker functions.

Atrial sensing should be evaluated. The best way to do that is to reduce the base rate in steps of 10-ppm until intrinsic atrial activity breaks through. Lower the base rate gradually and monitor the patient for any signs of discomfort. Even if native atrial activity fails to appear, do not drop the base rate below 30 or 40 ppm.

Ventricular sensing can be evaluated by extending the AV delay to 300 ms or higher and then observing the ECG to see if native ventricular activity occurs. While some clinicians try to encourage ventricular activity by temporarily programming VVI mode and then lowering the base rate, in my opinion, that should be avoided except as a last-ditch attempt to try to coax ventricular activity to emerge. An extended AV delay is not only easier, it will also provide good information on the patient's intrinsic conduction interval which may be used to better program an appropriate AV delay interval. Test the dual-chamber pacemaker in the dual-chamber mode!

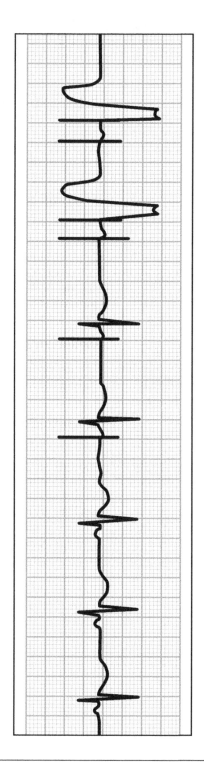

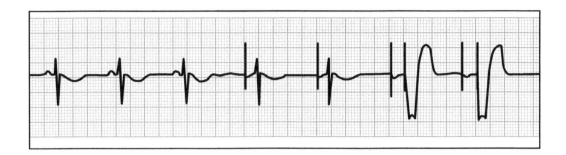

Mode

From the atrial and ventricular spikes, it is clear that this pacemaker is dual chamber.

Rate

The atrial pacing interval (AP-AP) measures 1000 ms (60 ppm), which is an appropriate rate for this kind of system.

Capture

There are four atrial pacing spikes, all of which result in an atrial depolarization with the same morphology. The first two conduct, leading to AP-VS events. The AP-VS interval is consistent in both, measuring approximately 160 ms with calipers. A stable AP-VS interval is further proof of appropriate capture.

The next two atrial paced events do not conduct (AP-VP events) but still appear to have captured the atrium properly. Thus, atrial capture is appropriate.

There are just two ventricular pacing spikes and both are associated with a widened, notched, "paced-looking" QRS complex that differs marked-ly from the intrinsic ventricular events on the strip. Ventricular capture is appropriate, too.

Sensing

Atrial sensing seems appropriate in that the intrinsic atrial events in the first three complexes inhibited the atrial output and reset device timing.

Ventricular sensing also looks appropriate, in that ventricular intrinsic activity inhibited pacing and reset timing.

Underlying rhythm

This patient has sinus node dysfunction and slow AV conduction.

What to do next

This strip indicates everything is functioning appropriately. This is one of those rare examples where the strip demonstrates appropriate capture and sensing in both chambers. However, if possible, it would be good clinical practice to evaluate capture and sensing thresholds for both chambers as part of a routine check-up.

EASY TRACING #19

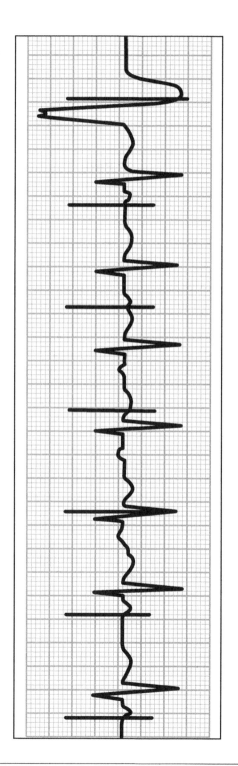

The Nuts and Bolts of Paced ECG Interpretation, 1st edition. By Tom Kenny.
Published 2009 by Blackwell Publishing, ISBN: 978-1-4501-8404-5.

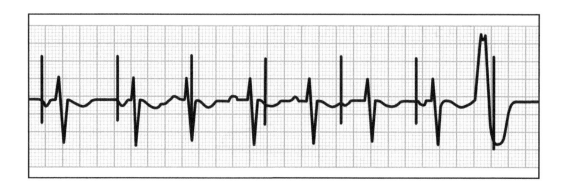

Mode

Sometimes it can be tough to even tell what mode the device is operating in! This is one of those strips.

If this was a dual-chamber pacemaker, we would see consistent dual-chamber activity, that is, if there was an atrial spike there would be a closely related sensed or paced ventricular event. If there was a ventricular spike, we would expect to have a preceding paced or sensed atrial event. These spikes occur alone, so this is a single-chamber system.

But is it an atrial or ventricular pacemaker? Ventricular single-chamber pacemakers are far more common, but AAI pacemakers still turn up at the clinic. To evaluate what kind of pacemaker this is, the best tactic is to look at each individual pacing spike and see what it did.

In the first two complexes, the spike occurs before an atrial depolarization which is followed by an intrinsic ventricular event. Later on in the strip, the spike occurs in closer proximity to ventricular activity. How can we tell if this really atrial pacing? Evidence of atrial capture includes an atrial waveform morphology that differs from the morphology of an intrinsic atrial event, an atrial depolarization immediately after the spike, and a consistent AP-VS interval in the case of AP-VS pacing. All three of these are present in the first two complexes. This spike has to be atrial.

In the next four complexes, the pacing spike occurs on top of, after, and between ventricular events and the sixth spike again captures the atrium. That means the last output pulse is not the dangerous R-on-T phenomenon, but rather harmless atrial pacing during the T-wave.

This pacemaker has to be a single-chamber atrial pacemaker.

Rate

The atrial pacing interval (AP-AP) gives us the rate; it's 880 ms or 68 ppm, measured with calipers.

Capture

The first two atrial spikes capture the atrium; note the morphology of these two events compared to the upward-deflecting of the intrinsic atrial events in the middle of the strip. These are two examples of proper atrial capture (distinctive waveform morphology, depolarization after the spike, and consistent AP-VS intervals).

The third atrial spike is a bit puzzling. If you look at the other waveforms, you can see that this third event is unique. My interpretation of this event – and this may be subject to disagreement among my colleagues – is that the ventricles depolarized intrinsically at the same moment that the pacemaker paced the atrium, resulting in an aberrant-looking QRS. This would be what I would call pseudo-pseudofusion (it looks like pseudofusion but it really isn't!)

Moving on, the fourth atrial spike fails to capture. The atrium was not physiologically refractory at this point. The spike should have captured the atrium, so we will have to call this inappropriate.

The fifth spike may look like it might be atrial capture, but do not let it fool you. If this was true atrial capture, it would have conducted down over the AV node to the ventricles, and the AP-VS interval would be consistent with the AP-VS intervals of previous atrial capture events. It is not, so this is atrial non-capture.

The sixth atrial spike did capture properly; notice the P-wave morphology and AP-VS interval match previous captured atrial events.

The seventh pacing spike looks like it is "R-on-T" or pacing into the T-wave. That's actually an optical illusion. An atrial spike happens to occur simultaneously with the T-wave portion of a premature ventricular contraction (PVC). The PVC is so large that it overwhelms the ECG. Even if this atrial spike captured the atrium, the resulting atrial depolarization would have been too small to show up on the ECG. We cannot really tell what happened in the atrium with the seventh spike.

There is intermittent loss of capture in the atrium.

The nuts and bolts of paced ECG interpretation: why it's called ECG interpretation

Reading a paced ECG may seem like science, and certainly there is a lot of science behind it, but it also involves the ability of the clinician to interpret or give meaning to what the strip shows. Paced ECGs show remarkable variability and, at times, the best we can do is say what we think is the most likely event that is represented on the ECG.

Many scientific meetings have lively sessions during which experts debate what specific tracings might mean. Even some of the key opinion leaders in the world in cardiac rhythm management can disagree heatedly on specific ECGs or electrograms. I do not expect all of my colleagues to always agree with my assessments in this book or in my classes. My approach is to look at strips systematically and to try to have solid reasons for my interpretations. But sometimes that's all they are: my interpretations!

Sensing

There are two prominent intrinsic atrial events in the middle of this strip and neither one is sensed properly. If you measure out the pacing spikes, you can see that atrial pacing "marches through" at the pacing rate and without resetting to accommodate sensed events. Thus, there is atrial undersensing. In fact, the functional mode is actually AOO.

Underlying rhythm

This patient has sinus node dysfunction and what appears to be intact AV conduction. The large event at the end is a premature ventricular contraction or PVC.

What to do next

Atrial capture and sensing have to be restored.

Since intrinsic atrial events appear even on this strip, it should not be difficult to conduct an atrial sensing threshold test and adjust atrial sensitivity.

Atrial capture should also be evaluated. Atrial pacing must occur, which should not be difficult to achieve.

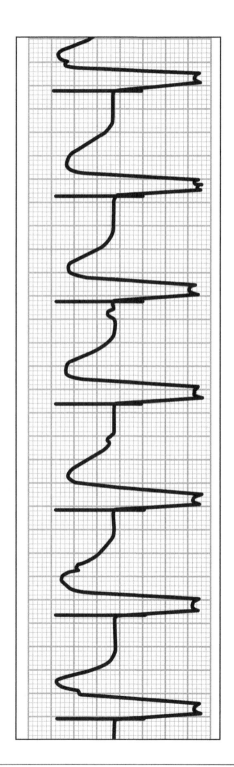

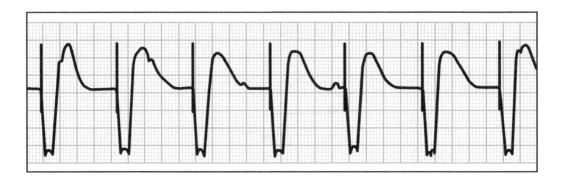

Mode

This is a VVI pacemaker. There is no relationship between the intrinsic atrial activity and the ventricular pacing spikes.

Rate

The ventricular pacing interval (VP-VP) is consistent at about 920 ms (65 ppm), an appropriate and expected rate for a single-chamber system.

Capture

Ventricular capture appears to be appropriate; notice that all of the ventricular complexes have similar morphology.

Sensing

Ventricular sensing cannot be evaluated since there are no intrinsic ventricular events.

Underlying rhythm

This patient has sinus node dysfunction and slow AV conduction.

What to do next

Test ventricular sensing by reducing the pacing rate in 10-ppm increments so that intrinsic ventricular events appear. Drop the rate gradually, observing the patient, and do not go below 30 or 40 ppm even if no intrinsic activity occurs.

The nuts and bolts of paced ECG interpretation: morphology

Waveform morphology on a tracing varies greatly depending on where the electrical energy causing the depolarization originates. A paced ventricular event is a beat that originates from the pacemaker electrode. That's why a paced ventricular complex looks different than an intrinsic ventricular event, which originates from energy conducted over the AV node from the atrium.

Morphology also varies by patient. For some patients, sensed and paced beats will look extremely different, but for others, the differences will be more subtle. While you cannot interpret paced versus sensed complexes solely from waveform morphology, the morphology is a great clue.

The nuts and bolts of paced ECG interpretation: help – I can't make intrinsic events show up!

It may be that you want to evaluate ventricular sensing in a patient who is consistently paced but even when you reduce the pacing rate (VVI or AAI device) or extend the AV delay (DDD device), intrinsic activity does not occur.

The fact is that some patients do not have a reliable intrinsic rate, even a very slow one. Other patients may have an escape rhythm you could test but they become highly symptomatic even experiencing short spells of such slow rates. There will be cases where you will not be able to evaluate sensing. In these cases, check the sensitivity settings and everything else you can check, and note in the chart that sensing function could not be assessed and why.

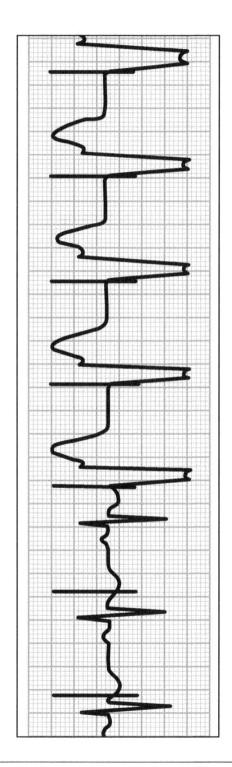

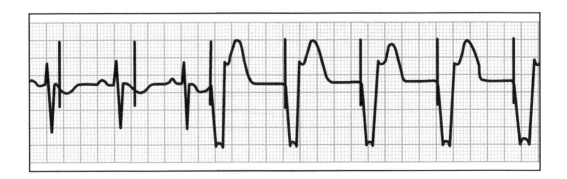

Mode

This is a strip from a patient with a VVI pacemaker.

Rate

The ventricular pacing interval (VP-VP) is about 880 ms or 68 ppm. (Since this was measured with calipers, it is approximate.) That is appropriate and expected for VVI pacing.

Capture

The first two spikes on the strip do not capture the ventricle. Whenever we observe unexpected device behavior, we have to ask how we expected the device to behave. Should these output pulses have captured the ventricle? Since both of them occur right after an intrinsic ventricular event (while the ventricular myocardium would still be physiologically refractory), the answer is no. This is an example of functional non-capture. Functional non-capture is not a true capture issue; it's almost always an indication of something not right with sensing. This is something we can revisit when we look at sensing.

After the two functional non-capture events, there is a series of paced ventricular activity. Since a depolarization of distinct morphology immediately follows the pacing spikes, these reflect appropriate capture. This patient has appropriate capture with functional non-capture.

Sensing

A ventricular spike occurs right after an intrinsic ventricular event in the first two complexes. This would only happen if those intrinsic ventricular events were not sensed. The third complex shows an intrinsic ventricular event which also does not reset device timing or inhibit the output pulse (note that the third ventricular spike is timed to the prior spike, not the intervening intrinsic ventricular event). Clearly, this is ventricular undersensing.

Underlying rhythm

This patient has some intrinsic atrial activity and slow AV conduction.

What to do next

The most crucial first step is to restore appropriate ventricular sensing. Conduct a ventricular sensing threshold test, adjust ventricular sensitivity settings, and observe how the ECG activity responds. This should solve both the undersensing and the functional non-capture, which are both symptoms of inappropriately programmed sensitivity.

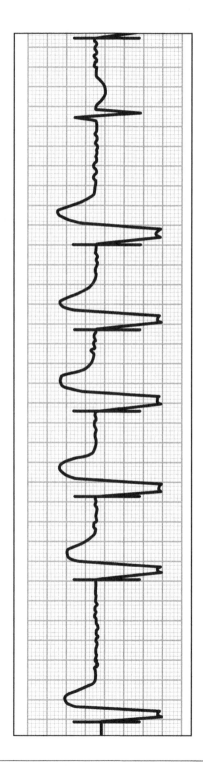

The Nuts and Bolts of Paced ECG Interpretation, 1st edition. By Tom Kenny.
Published 2009 by Blackwell Publishing, ISBN: 978-1-4501-8404-5.

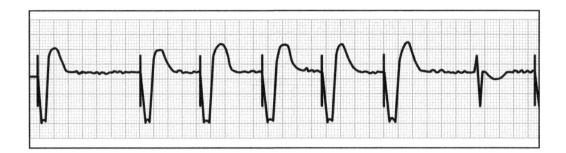

Mode

This is VVI pacing.

Rate

The ventricular pacing intervals (VP-VP) in the middle of the strip are about 880 ms or 68 ppm, which is appropriate. However, there are some pauses. Note the long interval between the first and second pacemaker spikes and the long pause after the last spike on this strip and the next sensed ventricular event. We will need to investigate the causes for these pauses.

Capture

Every ventricular spike is associated with an immediate ventricular depolarization of similar morphology. These events have a different morphology than that of the intrinsic ventricular event at the end of the strip. Capture is appropriate.

Sensing

The pauses tip us off to a potential issue with sensing. Set calipers to 880 ms (the ventricular pacing interval) and then put one leg of the calipers on the second spike and measure backward. The calipers will show where the pacemaker "thought" it sensed something and reset its timing. This same thing happened at the end of the strip. The pacemaker inhibited a ventricular output and reset its timing

because it "sensed" a ventricular event that actually was not there. This is classic ventricular oversensing.

What caused the oversensing? The ECG does not always reveal what the pacemaker oversenses. It might be tempting to look at the bumpy baseline and wonder if the pacemaker oversensed that. This baseline indicates the presence of a lot of high-rate intrinsic atrial activity. The patient has atrial tachycardia, perhaps even atrial fibrillation (AF). It is not at all unusual to observe AF in pacemaker patients. However, the AF did not contribute to the ventricular oversensing. Atrial activity like this would almost never be misinterpreted by the pacemaker's ventricular electrode as possible ventricular activity.

Underlying rhythm

This patient has some form of atrial tachyarrhythmia. He also has slow AV conduction.

What to do next

Ventricular sensing should be evaluated and ventricular sensitivity adjusted. That should solve the oversensing problem and get rid of the pauses.

The atrial activity, though problematic, is not something for this pacemaker to address. The first line of defense for this sort of atrial arrhythmia is drug therapy, which is beyond the scope of this book. The pacemaker is doing its job, which is providing reliable ventricular pacing support.

The nuts and bolts of paced ECG interpretation: atrial fibrillation in paced patients

Atrial fibrillation (AF) is a common rhythm disorder, which means you will see it in the clinical setting, probably more often than you would care to.

AF is a complex and progressive condition that often starts out in paroxysmal form (starting suddenly, resolving on its own) but deteriorates over time to a chronic arrhythmia. AF is appropriately first treated with pharmacological therapy. More persistent cases may require chemical or electrical cardioversion. There are also surgical as well as RF ablation approaches to AF, but such interventions are considered more invasive steps to a troublesome arrhythmia that resists other treatments.

Some pacemakers offer special algorithms to help suppress high-rate atrial activity before it starts.

Ironically, most AF symptoms are not caused by the rapid beating of the atria but rather by the ventricular rate. When AF conducts to the ventricles, it results in "rapid ventricular response," which shows up on an ECG as a characteristically erratic but rapid rhythm.

In this particular case, the patient's VVI pacemaker can – by nature of the device – only ignore the atrial rhythm and pace the ventricle.

EASY TRACING #23

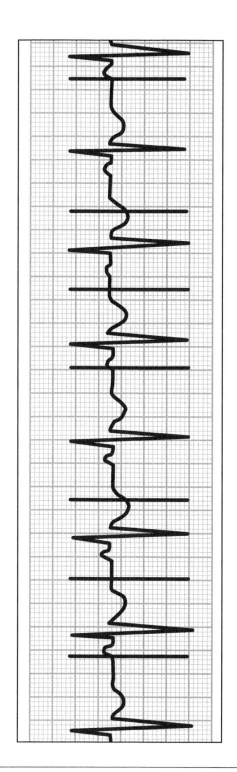

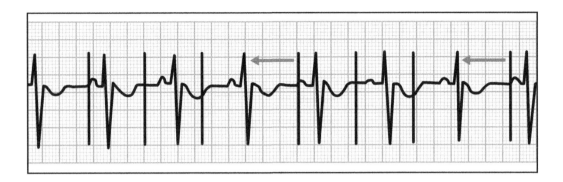

Mode

This is single-chamber pacing but it may take a moment to figure out in which chamber the spike belongs (AAI or VVI device).

Notice the two arrows, indicating pauses in the strip where the pacemaker timing was reset by an intrinsic complex. Using calipers, it is apparent that the rate is setting itself to the intrinsic QRS complex, not the intrinsic atrial event. Although there are a couple of spots on this strip where it appears that the spike "captures" the atrium, that is just a coincidence. This is a ventricular single-chamber pacemaker. Another clue that there is no atrial pacing going on is the fact that the intrinsic P-wave morphology does not vary between "seemingly paced" and intrinsic events.

Rate

The ventricular pacing interval (VP-VP) is very short, about 680 ms or 88 ppm. Pacing at such a high rate would be typical in pediatric patients or with a rate-responsive system (VVIR). If this is an adult who is not exercising, it could also be an example of an inappropriately high programmed pacing rate.

Capture

The pacing spike never once captures the ventricle on the whole strip. Ventricular capture is not appropriate.

Sensing

The two intrinsic ventricular events shown by the arrows are properly sensed in that they inhibit the ventricular output pulse and reset device timing. However, all of the other intrinsic ventricular events on this strip are not sensed. This is intermittent ventricular undersensing.

Underlying rhythm

This patient actually has a pretty good-looking intrinsic rhythm. He has consistent atrial activity which reliably conducts down and over the AV node to the ventricles, resulting in a consistent ventricular depolarization. The patient's intrinsic rate is about 800 ms (75 bpm).

What to do next

Ventricular sensing must be evaluated and restored. Ventricular capture must be tested and restored. This most likely will result in the reprogramming of ventricular sensitivity (making the device more sensitive or lowering the mV setting) and reprogramming of the ventricular output settings (pulse amplitude and pulse width) to deliver more energy in the output pulse.

The pacing rate is also inappropriately high. Unless there is a good reason for such a fast pacing rate, it should be reduced to a base rate of 60 or 70 ppm. Since the patient has an intrinsic rhythm of around 75 bpm, a base rate of 70 ppm would result in device inhibition – which is a good thing because it means the patient's intrinsic rhythm would be encouraged to take control.

The nuts and bolts of paced ECG interpretation: pacing threshold fluctuations

The pacing threshold is defined as the minimum amount of energy required to reliably pace the heart. It is typically obtained in a pacing threshold test (sometimes called a capture threshold test) and reported as a single setting in two parameters (a pulse width and a pulse amplitude).

This is a bit misleading, because the pacing threshold is not a static value.

Even in one patient, even in a brief period like the course of one day, the pacing threshold fluctuates. Furthermore, many factors, including drugs and disease progression are known to affect the pacing threshold.

For that reason, pacing thresholds should be checked routinely at every follow-up session. Adequate safety margins should be allowed to provide a "cushion" for threshold variations (2:1 or 3:1 safety margins are standard).

This is why loss of capture can sometimes occur intermittently and loss of capture may occur suddenly in a patient even when output settings had not been changed.

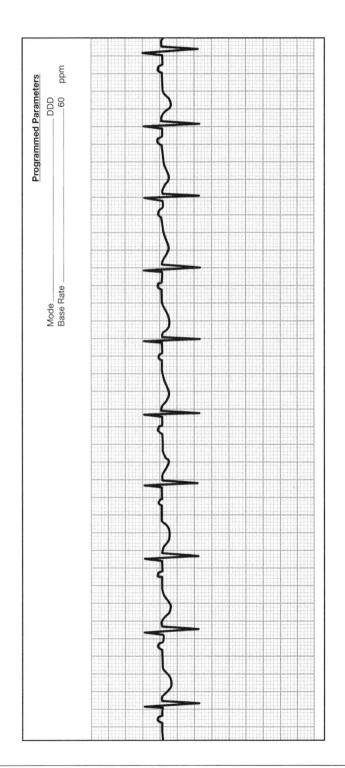

Programmed Parameters

Mode _____ DDD

Base Rate _____ 60 ppm

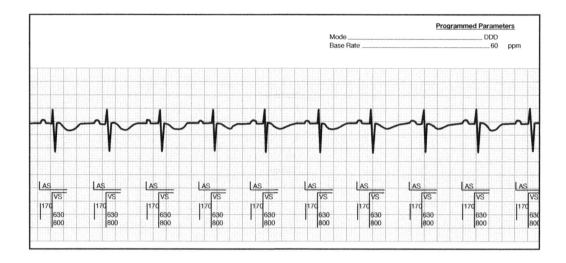

Mode

If you only had the tracing, you could not say with certainty if the patient even had a pacemaker. But the printout reveals it's a DDD device. The annotations reveal that the pacemaker is sensing events on both channels.

Rate

The printout reveals the pacing rate is set to 60 ppm, an appropriate rate. The intrinsic atrial rate is about 800 ms (75 bpm) which is doing what one would expect – inhibiting the output pulses.

Capture

Capture cannot be evaluated from this tracing.

Sensing

Atrial sensing is appropriate in that every atrial event inhibits the atrial output spike. Evaluate sensing by looking first at the tracing and then verifying that the annotations agree with what appears on the rhythm strip.

Ventricular sensing is likewise appropriate.

Underlying rhythm

This patient has a good and stable underlying rhythm as seen by the AS-VS complexes at around 70 ppm.

What to do next

Capture should be evaluated in both chambers. To do so, it will be necessary to force the device to pace. For atrial capture, increase the base rate in small steps of 10 ppm, starting at 90 ppm. Monitor the patient and keep increasing the rate gradually until the device starts to pace.

To evaluate ventricular capture shorten the AV delay setting. This need not be done incrementally; a temporary setting of 110 or 120 ms is fine. If that does not work, the device can be temporarily programmed to VVI and the base rate increased in 10-ppm steps starting at 90 ppm. The first method is far superior in that it allows you to evaluate the device as a true DDD system, not in a different mode. In my opinion, testing ventricular capture by temporarily programming a faster rate in VVI mode should only be done if shortening the AV delay fails to result in ventricular pacing.

The nuts and bolts of paced ECG interpretation: does this patient even need a pacemaker?

Sometimes in the clinic, you will encounter pacemaker patients with ECGs that show no pacing and no apparent need for pacing. Before you wonder why this patient ever got a pacemaker in the first place, remember that many arrhythmias are intermittent. If you download pacemaker diagnostics, you will often find that pacemaker patients are paced only a percentage of the time. For a great many patients, this percentage may be as low as 30% or 40% of the time … which means that the majority of the time, such patients require no pacing. In fact, patients who are paced 100% of the time are rare.

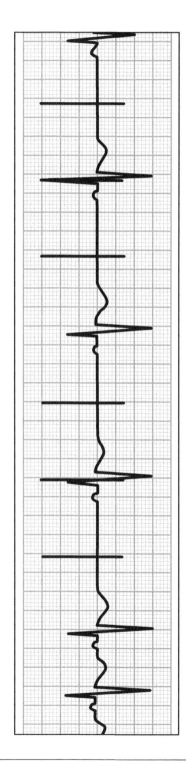

The Nuts and Bolts of Paced ECG Interpretation, 1st edition. By Tom Kenny.
Published 2009 by Blackwell Publishing, ISBN: 978-1-4501-8404-5.

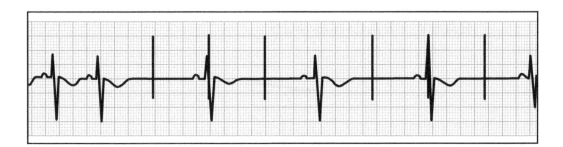

Mode

This is a single-chamber pacemaker and, since the spikes affect the ventricular complex, it must be a VVI pacemaker.

Rate

The ventricular pacing interval measures 800 ms (75 ppm). While this is a bit faster than most strips you'll encounter in the clinic, the rate is still appropriate.

Capture

There are four ventricular pacing spikes on this strip that fail to capture, and there is no physiological reason they should not have resulted in a ventricular depolarization. Thus, ventricular capture is inappropriate.

Notice that two ventricular spikes in this strip occur on top of a ventricular event that has the general morphology of an intrinsic ventricular depolarization. Is this capture or failure to capture? Actually, it is pseudofusion.

The spike occurs after the ventricle has already depolarized on its own. While this does not "hurt" the heart rhythm, it is wasted energy from the device since the ventricular spike makes no contribution to the depolarization. Pseudofusion is a timing issue (the intrinsic rate is bumping into the pacing rate). Since the pacemaker output does not contribute to the depolarization, it neither confirms nor refutes appropriate capture.

Pseudofusion, like fusion, is not a capture problem – it has to do with timing. The pacemaker spike and the patient's intrinsic rate are competing with each other.

The nuts and bolts of paced ECG interpretation: fusion, pseudofusion and mass confusion

Fusion occurs when both a spike and an intrinsic beat occur together in such a way that both of them contribute to the depolarization. On a paced ECG, a fused beat looks like a cross between a sensed and paced event. Fusion is the result of a timing issue and it actually confirms capture.

Pseudofusion is something else. Pseudofusion occurs when the heart was depolarizing on its own and the pacemaker spike collides with this event in such a way that the depolarization is entirely intrinsic and the spike is just wasted. On a paced ECG, pseudofusion looks like an intrinsic event with a spike. Pseudofusion is also a timing issue. Pseudofusion neither confirms nor contradicts appropriate capture.

Sensing

Ventricular sensing seems appropriate because intrinsic ventricular events reset device timing and inhibit the ventricular output spike.

Underlying rhythm

The patient appears to have sinus bradycardia with intact AV conduction.

What to do next

The loss of ventricular capture should be addressed with a ventricular pacing threshold test and check of the output parameters (pulse amplitude and pulse width).

The nuts and bolts of paced ECG interpretation: how do you actually adjust pacemaker output?

Pacemaker output or the amount of energy actually delivered to the myocardium is governed by two parameters: the pulse amplitude (stated in volts) and the pulse width (stated in milliseconds). Increasing either one will increase device energy, but it is much more energy efficient to adjust the pulse amplitude (voltage).

Many pacemaker programmers will help the clinician by suggesting appropriate output settings, but all pacemaker clinicians should understand how this is done. First, the pacing threshold must be determined. This is the lowest amount of energy (stated as pulse amplitude and pulse width) that will reliably capture the heart.

The pacemaker output settings are based on the threshold plus a safety margin which is typically 2:1 or 3:1. For example, if a patient has a pacing threshold of 0.8 V at 0.4 ms, a good output setting would be 2.0 V at 0.4 ms (0.8 V plus a 2:1 safety margin would be 1.6 V, rounded up for good measure).

Why not just maximize all output settings? Output settings affect battery longevity; the higher the output, the faster the battery is used up, at least in theory. Thus, clinicians try to strike the right balance to assure patient safety but still conserve battery life.

Restoring appropriate ventricular capture will likely address the pseudofusion events this patient has been experiencing. Most pacemaker patients will occasionally experience both fusion and pseudofusion. Should such events be frequent and persistent, this is likely because the patient's intrinsic rate is competing with the programmed base.

Programming hysteresis or lowering the base rate slightly is the most common troubleshooting tactic for frequent fusion and pseudofusion. In this particular case, no such steps are necessary since the patient's native rate is clearly too slow to compete consistently with the programmed base rate.

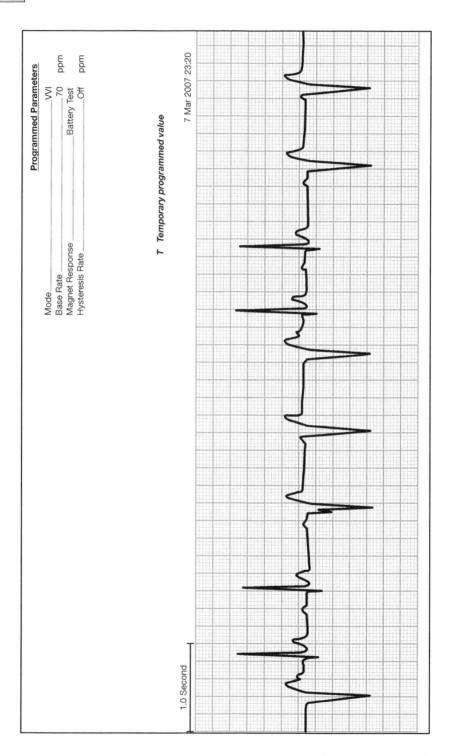

Programmed Parameters

Mode VVI
Base Rate .... 70 ppm
Magnet Response .... Battery Test
Hysteresis Rate .... Off ppm

T Temporary programmed value

7 Mar 2007 23:20

1.0 Second

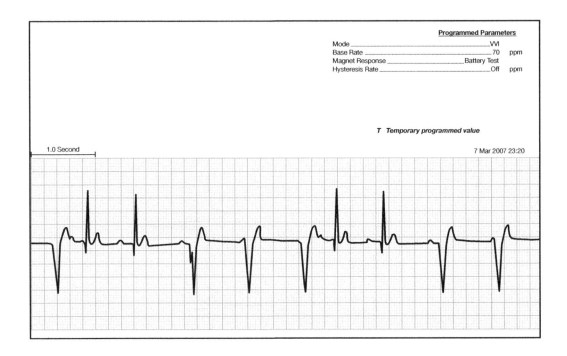

Programmed Parameters

Mode _____VVI
Base Rate _____70   ppm
Magnet Response _____Battery Test
Hysteresis Rate _____Off   ppm

T   Temporary programmed value

1.0 Second   7 Mar 2007 23:20

Mode

Although the pacing spike is not prominent, it is evident in the second downward-deflecting ventricular depolarization. These wide downward ventricular depolarizations are paced events. There is also some apparent intrinsic atrial activity but no atrial pacing. If the pacemaker could sense atrial activity, then the sensed AV delay (AS-VP) would be consistent in the strip; it is not. Further, if this pacemaker were a dual-chamber device, it would have tried to pace the atrium after the third and before the fourth paced ventricular event. In the absence of both sensed and paced atrial activity, this pacemaker has to be a VVI system.

Rate

The ventricular pacing interval (VP-VP) can be measured with calipers from the onset of the second paced ventricular event to the onset of the third ventricular pacing event (or from third to fourth ventricular paced events or using the last two paced ventricular events). They all measure about 880 ms (68 ppm). The printout states that the rate is 70 ppm and that "matches" the caliper reading of 68 ppm in that calipers are always an approximation.

The nuts and bolts of paced ECG interpretation: caliper "rounding"

Calipers should not be underestimated. They are a handy tool and when you get adept with them, they can be quick and easy to use. The main drawback to calipers is that they are approximate. For instance, a pacing rate of 70 ppm corresponds to a pacing interval of 857 ms. Since the smallest unit measured by calipers is 40 ms (and it's hard to interpret units less than 40 ms), clinicians with calipers will either measure pacing intervals of 840 or 880 ms and never hit exactly 857 ms. In this example, the calipers looked like 880 ms. Technically that would mean the pacemaker was set to 68 ppm, which is possible. However, we know from the printout information on the top of the tracing that this pacemaker was set to 70 ppm. That means the pacing interval should be 857 ms long. Was our reading wrong? No, it was just approximate. So when using calipers, allow for "rounding" or "approximation" errors.

By the way, pacing rates like 68 ppm are possible to program but are not very common. Most pacemakers are set to rates such as 60, 65, 70, 75, and so on.

Capture

There are six paced ventricular events of the same morphology (widened, downward deflection) on this strip. Ventricular capture is appropriate.

Sensing

There are four intrinsic ventricular events on the strip (they are the narrow, upward-deflecting ventricular events). Each intrinsic ventricular event inhibited a ventricular output spike and reset device timing. If you measure the VS-VP interval (the escape interval), it corresponds to the pacing interval. Sensing is appropriate.

Underlying rhythm

This patient has sinus node dysfunction and slow AV conduction with some intermittent intrinsic ventricular activity.

What to do next

Capture and sensing appear appropriate, but this patient might have a lot more intrinsic activity if the pacing rate could somehow be slowed down to allow more opportunity for the ventricles to depolarize on their own. One approach might be to lower the programmed base rate, but that has an obvious drawback. What if the patient sometimes needs to be paced at the current rate of 70 ppm? A rate of 60 ppm might allow more intrinsic activity but it might not provide adequate pacing support all of the time.

The best solution is to turn on hysteresis. The printout mentions that hysteresis is currently off. Hysteresis programmed to 60 bpm would allow the heart's intrinsic rate to take over as long as it was above 60 bpm but, if pacing is ever required, the pacing rate can remain at 70 ppm. From what we can observe about the patient's underlying rhythm, hysteresis would encourage more intrinsic rhythm.

This patient has some intermittent intrinsic atrial activity. It is possible that when his device needs to be replaced, an upgrade to a dual-chamber pacemaker might provide him with 1:1 AV synchrony and better rate support.

The nuts and bolts of paced ECG interpretation: modes

Arrhythmias are not static conditions. A patient's rhythm disorders can change, even dramatically, over time, with disease progression, because of drug interactions, or other factors. It is quite common for a pacemaker patient to develop new and different arrhythmias over time. For that reason, you may encounter patients in the clinic who are paced in modes or with pacing systems that may seem less than optimal for their condition. Bear in mind that the patient you see today may present with entirely different rhythm strips than the patient who, 5 years ago, first got a pacemaker.

Most pacemaker patients will need frequent adjustment to their pacemakers over the life of the device. This is not unusual or abnormal.

Many physicians opt for dual-chamber systems with special features to be able to upgrade a patient to more advanced settings and modes, if required. That is, even if a patient does not need a full-featured device today, it can make sense to implant one to accommodate future conditions. (After all, pacemakers can last up to 10 years or more!)

All pacemaker patients will require pacemaker revision at some point, and for some patients, this provides a welcome opportunity for a device upgrade to better meet their needs. This tracing is a good example of a patient who would benefit from a dual-chamber device.

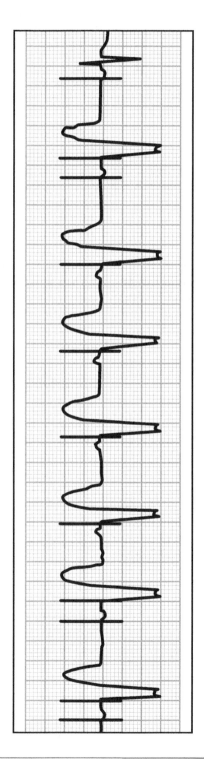

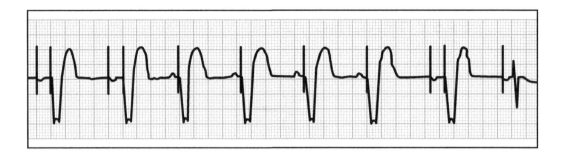

Mode

The presence of atrial and ventricular spikes (for instance, in the first complex) mean that this is a dual-chamber pacemaker.

Rate

To measure the dual-chamber pacing rate, use calipers to measure the atrial pacing interval (AP-AP). On this strip, there are a couple of examples of the atrial pacing interval. They both measure 1000 ms (60 ppm). That is an appropriate and expected rate.

Capture

There are four atrial spikes on this strip and each one is associated with an atrial depolarization that has a different morphology than the intrinsic atrial events. Atrial capture looks appropriate.

Most of the strip shows ventricular pacing. Each ventricular paced event is associated with the ventricular pacing spike and a characteristically "paced look," that is, a widened, bizarre, notched morphology. The next-to-last ventricular event on the strip is intrinsic and has a completely different waveform morphology, which would be typical of an intrinsic event. Ventricular capture seems to be appropriate.

Sensing

There are four intrinsic atrial events in the middle of the strip. When they occur, they inhibit the atrial output spike and reset device timing. Another verification that atrial sensing is appropriate is a consistent sensed AV delay (the timing cycle from the onset of an intrinsic atrial event and the next paced ventricular event). Although it is difficult to measure it too precisely with calipers, it looks to be about 160 ms; at any rate, it is consistent across the strip, even in the last complex on the tracing. Thus, we have good evidence that atrial sensing is functioning appropriately.

There is only one intrinsic ventricular event on this strip (next-to-last complex) but it inhibits the ventricular output spike, resets device timing, and appears appropriate. From what we have to work with, ventricular sensing seems appropriate.

Underlying rhythm

This strip starts with AP-VP pacing (pacing both chambers), then transitions to atrial tracking (AS-VP), and, at the end moves to atrial pacing that conducts (AP-VS). It is rather unusual to see three different pacing states on such a short snippet. The patient has some intrinsic atrial activity and slow AV conduction.

What to do next

This strip shows appropriate atrial sensing and capture and appropriate ventricular sensing and capture, but it would still be prudent to check these functions. In particular, ventricular sensing should be checked since we based our determination on just one single event.

It is almost always good clinical practice in cardiac pacing to encourage intrinsic activity and to try to minimize unnecessary pacing. The AV delay of

160 ms may be too short for this particular patient's intrinsic conduction. That is based on the fact that this strip provides one example of intact AV conduction and that an AV delay of 160 ms is generally considered "short." By extending the AV delay to 200 or even 250 ms, the atrial event (whether sensed or paced) will have more opportunity to conduct via the AV node to the ventricles and cause an intrinsic ventricular depolarization. The best way to evaluate that is to extend the AV delay and observe what happens on the ECG. In my opinion, this patient will likely show more intrinsic conduction, either in the form of AS-VS or AP-VS complexes.

If this particular patient has an advanced pacemaker system with a special feature, such as VIP® technology (Ventricular Intrinsic Preference® technology), that can be activated as well. Such algorithms are designed to help accommodate the patient's rhythm in a way that encourages intrinsic ventricular activity.

The nuts and bolts of paced ECG interpretation: specialty algorithms

Ventricular Intrinsic Preference® technology is just one of many special algorithms that are available in the latest-generation of pacemakers. Even older devices may offer atrial overdrive algorithms, automatic capture features, and algorithms to help manage pacemaker-mediated tachycardia, high-rate intrinsic atrial activity, and premature ventricular contractions. While this book does not go into detail about such features (which vary by manufacturer and even by device model), they are worth getting to know. Many of them automatically adjust to the patient's needs. They are all designed to be easy to set up and program. While we will not delve into them here, I encourage you to learn what you can about these algorithms. The time you spend learning about them will be more than repaid by the time they can save you in the clinic over the long run.

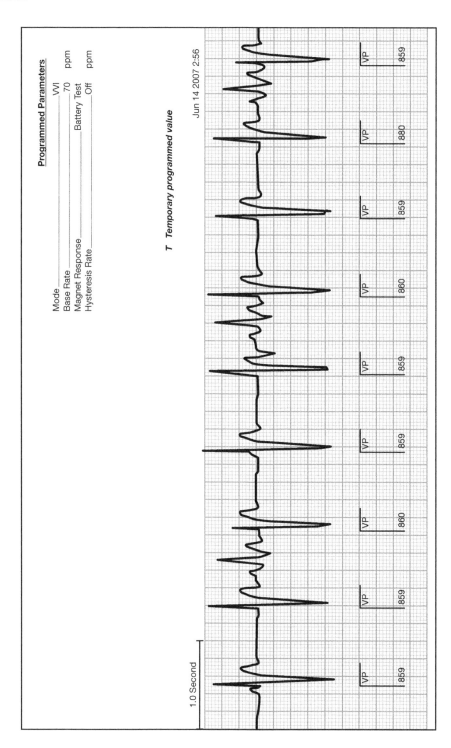

Programmed Parameters

Mode	VVI	
Base Rate	70	ppm
Magnet Response	Battery Test	
Hysteresis Rate	Off	ppm

T Temporary programmed value

Jun 14 2007 2:56

1.0 Second

VP	VP	VP	VP	VP	VP	VP	VP
859	880	859	860	859	859	860	859

The Nuts and Bolts of Paced ECG Interpretation, 1st edition. By Tom Kenny.
Published 2009 by Blackwell Publishing, ISBN: 978-1-4501-8404-5.

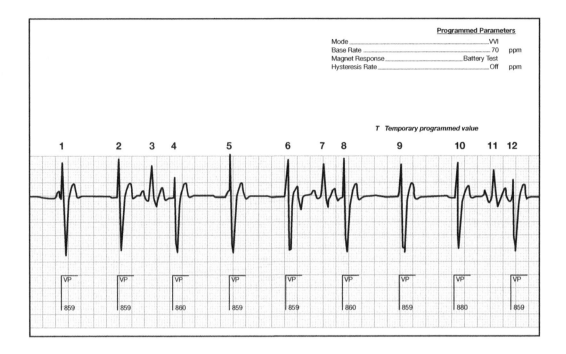

Mode

The strip shows ventricular pacing and there are intrinsic atrial events on this strip, but they appear erratically. There does not seem to be atrial pacing on this strip, because spikes or paced events would have occurred in several places. (A dual-chamber device will try to achieve 1:1 AV synchrony and we see no evidence of that on this strip.)

This is a VVI pacemaker. The printout and the annotations confirm this. Using a systematic approach, you can still confirm this as VVI pacing even in the absence of annotations, printouts, and visible pacing spikes.

Rate

Ventricular pacing is measured by the ventricular pacing interval (VP-VP). With calipers the ventricular pacing interval measures to be about 880 ms but the annotations call it out as 859 ms. Either way, this matches the 70 ppm programmed rate stated on the strip. (Remember, caliper readings are always approximate.) This is an appropriate rate for a single-chamber pacemaker.

The nuts and bolts of paced ECG interpretation: appropriate rate

When we talk about appropriate pacing rates, we need to distinguish that "appropriate" means *appropriate for the patient*. If a patient comes to the clinic and his pacemaker has been programmed to pace at 90 ppm, pacing at this fast rate is the *expected behavior* of the device … but it is probably too fast for the patient and, thus, not appropriate. Whenever unusual rates or rate variations occur, you should try to account for them and then recognize that sometimes the pacing rate is inappropriate *not because something is wrong with the pacemaker*, but rather because the pacemaker was programmed to an inappropriate rate.

While it is relatively rare to see a pacemaker programmed to an inappropriately high or low base rate, it can happen. Always consider it as a possibility if you check out the rate and can find no other explanation.

Capture

Although there are no visible pacing spikes on this strip, the VP annotations serve the same purpose; they tell us when the pacemaker delivered a ventricular output pulse. Every single VP annotation corresponds to a paced ventricular event. While these paced events vary a bit in morphology (some are "taller" than others), they are all examples of ventricular fusion beats. Fusion occurs across a continuum; in other words, some fusion beats can be "more fused" than others.

Since fusion confirms capture, ventricular capture is appropriate across the strip. Every ventricular output is associated with a captured event.

The nuts and bolts of paced ECG interpretation: fusion confirms capture

Fusion beats occur when both an intrinsic depolarization and a pacemaker output combine to depolarize the heart. As such, they actually confirm capture because the fused beat shows that the pacemaker output contributed to the depolarization.

Pseudofusion beats occur when the heart depolarizes on its own and then, at the very last minute, a pacemaker output is delivered right on top of the intrinsic depolarization. Pseudofusion looks like an intrinsic beat with a spike. Pseudofusion neither confirms nor contradicts capture.

Sensing

The third, seventh, and eleventh events are all intrinsic but they did not inhibit the next ventricular output pulse. There is consistent ventricular undersensing.

Underlying rhythm

The patient has sinus node dysfunction and slow AV conduction. The presence of so many fused beats means that the programmed base rate is competing with the patient's own intrinsic rate. The patient's intrinsic ventricular rate has to be quite close to the base rate of 70 ppm.

What to do next

Ventricular undersensing must be addressed by evaluating the sensing threshold and then adjusting ventricular sensitivity. To assess ventricular sensing, lower the base rate in 10-ppm steps until ventricular intrinsic events appears. Since they already appear occasionally on this strip, this should not be difficult.

Although capture looks appropriate, the presence of so many fused events would make me want to test ventricular capture as well. This time, increase the rate (start at about 90 ppm) to get consistent ventricular pacing. It may or may not be necessary to adjust ventricular output parameters (ventricular pulse width and ventricular pulse amplitude).

The string of ventricular fused beats in this strip indicates that the patient's intrinsic ventricular rate is close to 70 bpm. The most efficient and easiest way to address this is to add hysteresis. The printout shows that hysteresis is available but not programmed. The patient's pacing rate could be left at 70 ppm but hysteresis turned on and set to 60 bpm. The programmed base rate could also be lowered, but, in my opinion, the better first step is to add hysteresis and observe how the patient responds. It is probably not necessary to lower the base rate.

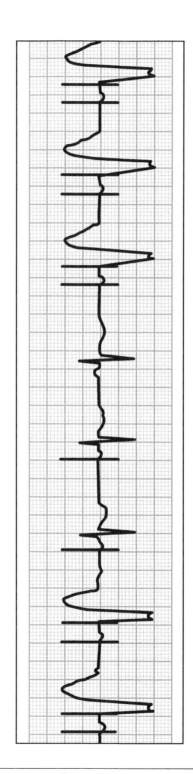

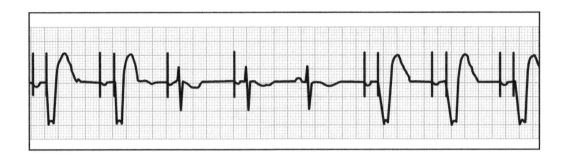

Mode

Atrial and ventricular spikes mean this is a dual-chamber strip.

Rate

In a dual-chamber device, the atrial channel drives the rate. The atrial pacing interval (AP-AP) is 1000 ms (60 ppm), an appropriate rate.

Capture

There are several atrial pacing spikes, all of which are associated with an atrial depolarization of a similar morphology (and this morphology is unlike the morphology of the lone intrinsic atrial event on the strip). Atrial capture is appropriate.

Both intrinsic and paced ventricular events appear on this strip. The first two and last three ventricular events have a widened, bizarre-looking, typical "paced" look to them. However, looking closely at them, the first two events appear smaller and tighter than the last three events. For that reason, the first two events could be ventricular fusion – the collision of an intrinsic event and a pacing spike. Fused waveform morphology usually resembles a hybrid between an intrinsic and a paced beat, and that makes me suspect the first two events are fusion and the last three are "true" paced ventricular events.

However, fusion confirms capture (because the spike contributes to the depolarization). There are five ventricular pacing spikes and five paced events (either five true paced events or three true paced events and two fusion events). In terms of capture analysis, that distinction is not important. Ventricular capture is appropriate.

The nuts and bolts of paced ECG interpretation: when colleagues disagree

It does not take much time in the clinic before you and your colleagues will find rhythm strips that are "subject to interpretation." This strip is a great example of an ECG that two equally competent colleagues could interpret two different ways. The first two ventricular events might be true paced events or they might be fused.

In the clinic, I would probably treat these as ventricular fusion for a couple of reasons. First, they look different than the three ventricular paced beats at the end. The differences may seem very subtle to some, but they look clearly different to me. Second, the patient has intrinsic ventricular activity right after these first two questionable fusion events and that suggests his or her ventricular rate might very well be fast enough to provoke fusion. Thus, I see two beats that are probably fusion in a patient who could definitely support fusion.

However, I am not entirely certain that I am right! With ECG interpretation, you try to "build a case" based on evidence. I think there is good evidence for fusion ... but a strip like this can provoke some discussion in the clinic!

Sensing

There is only one intrinsic atrial event on this strip and it appears to be properly sensed, in that it inhibits the atrial output and resets device timing.

There are three intrinsic ventricular events and they inhibit the ventricular output and reset device timing. Thus, ventricular sensing is appropriate.

Underlying rhythm

This patient has sinus node dysfunction, slow AV conduction, and may have an intrinsic rate that is competing with the paced rate – at least when this strip was recorded.

What to do next

While atrial sensing appears appropriate on this strip, that determination is made from just one atrial event. It would be wise to evaluate atrial sensing. Decrease the base rate in 10-ppm steps until intrinsic atrial activity emerges for testing purposes. Since one intrinsic atrial event appears on the strip, it should be fairly easy to get intrinsic atrial activity by lowering the base rate even slightly. Once the atrial sensing threshold can be measured, atrial sensitivity should be adjusted, if needed.

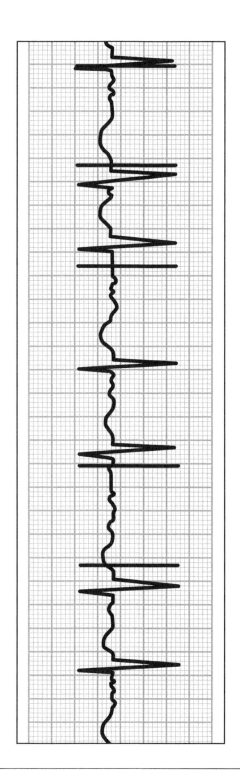

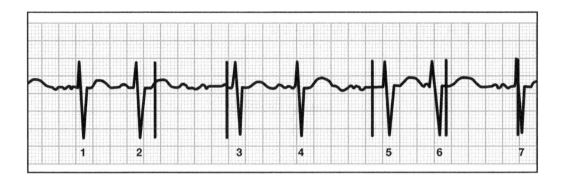

Mode

This is a single-chamber pacemaker. The spikes are associated with the ventricular activity, so this is a VVI pacemaker.

Rate

The ventricular pacing interval (VP-VP) is 840 ms, or about 68 ppm (roughly 70 ppm), an appropriate rate.

Capture

There are seven ventricular events on this strip, which are numbered to make it a bit easier to navigate.

There are five ventricular spikes on this strip (in complexes 2, 3, 5, 6, and 7) and not one of them captures the ventricle. The next logical question: should they have captured the ventricle? Spikes 2 and 6 were delivered during the heart's physiologic ventricular refractory period. These are examples of functional non-capture. The spikes did not capture, but there is no way they could have captured. (Functional non-capture is not really a capture problem; it is likely related to sensing.)

However, spikes in complexes 3 and 5 were delivered to the heart at a time when the ventricular myocardium could have depolarized. Thus, these are true failures to capture. There is a loss of ventricular capture.

The spike in complex 7 is pseudofusion, which neither confirms nor contradicts appropriate capture.

Sensing

The presence of functional non-capture always suggests a sensing problem. There are seven intrinsic ventricular events on this strip. Setting the calipers to the ventricular pacing interval (measure VP-VP on the strip or 840 ms), put one leg of the calipers on the first spike and measure backward to the first intrinsic ventricular event on this strip. The other caliper leg lands on the outset of this first intrinsic ventricular event. This means that first intrinsic ventricular event was properly sensed and reset device timing.

The problem is the pacemaker clearly did not sense the second intrinsic ventricular event. The fourth intrinsic ventricular event is properly sensed and resets device timing, but the sixth ventricular event is not appropriately sensed. There is intermittent ventricular undersensing.

Underlying rhythm

The "bumpy" baseline indicates a lot of high-rate atrial activity. The irregular intrinsic ventricular rate further suggests that the patient may have atrial fibrillation (AF).

What to do next

Ventricular capture and sensing must be restored. For ventricular capture, conduct a capture threshold test and reset device output parameters (ventricular pulse width and ventricular pulse amplitude) to an appropriately high setting.

Ventricular sensing can be checked by the sensing threshold test and reprogramming device sensitivity. Since the pacemaker is undersensing, it should be made more sensitive (lower mV setting).

If changing the output and sensitivity parameter settings of the pacemaker fail to resolve these matters, consider that the problems could relate to a lead problem. The fact that this pacemaker seems to be experiencing simultaneous pacing and sensing problems is a clue that the lead might be involved. Since parameter settings are the more likely reason for what occurs on the strip and they are easy to adjust, make parameter changes first but be prepared that if those changes do not have the desired effect, a chest X-ray should be ordered to evaluate lead integrity.

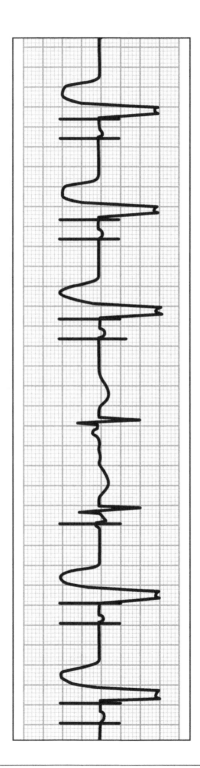

The Nuts and Bolts of Paced ECG Interpretation, 1st edition. By Tom Kenny.
Published 2009 by Blackwell Publishing, ISBN: 978-1-4501-8404-5.

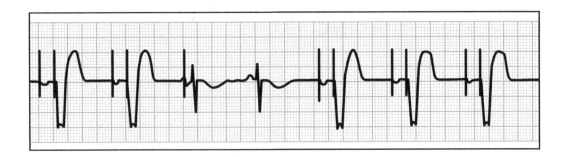

Mode

The atrial and ventricular spikes mean that this is a dual-chamber pacemaker.

Rate

The atrial pacing interval (AP-AP) in this strip – which provides us with the best point to measure the pacing rate in dual-chamber pacing – is 1000 ms or 60 ppm. This is an appropriate rate.

Capture

There are three atrial waveform morphologies on this strip. Atrial spikes occur before downward-deflecting atrial depolarization waveforms. In the middle of the strip is an upward-deflecting intrinsic atrial event. The third atrial spike appears to collide with an intrinsic atrial event in what looks like fusion (a cross between a sensed and paced morphology). Atrial capture appears to be appropriate. (Remember fusion is not a capture problem, it's a timing issue. Fusion actually confirms capture.)

There are two ventricular waveform morphologies on the strip. Ventricular pacing spikes appear before wider, bizarre-looking QRS waveforms (characteristic for paced beats). These waveform morphologies differ from the smaller, tighter, narrower waveforms of intrinsic ventricular depolarizations. Ventricular capture looks appropriate.

Sensing

There is only one intrinsic atrial event on the strip, but when it occurs, it inhibits the atrial output and appears to reset the atrial timing. If you set the cali-

pers to the pacing interval (1000 ms), the intrinsic event is timed to the next atrial paced event. Thus, atrial sensing is appropriate.

There are only two intrinsic ventricular events on this strip and they both inhibit the ventricular pacing spike and reset device timing. Ventricular sensing also seems to be functioning appropriately.

Underlying rhythm

This strip is interesting because in a short span of time, the patient goes from AV pacing (AP-VP) to conduction (AP-VS then AS-VS) and back to AV pacing. This suggests that the patient has both sinus node dysfunction and slow AV conduction, but that these problems are intermittent.

What to do next

At a glance, it seems like everything is functioning appropriately. However, this is just a short snippet of strip and we are basing the decision on appropriate sensing, for instance, on a single event. It is prudent to run pacing and sensing tests anyway, if possible, even when things look like they are functioning appropriately.

The presence of two conducted ventricular depolarizations in the middle of this strip strongly hints that more intrinsic ventricular activity could be encouraged. The paced AV delay appears to be about 200 ms. If that were extended to 250 ms, it would give the atrial event more opportunity to conduct via the AV node down to the ventricles. If an algorithm to encourage intrinsic ventricular activity (such as VIP® or Ventricular Intrinsic Preference® technology) were available, it could also be programmed.

The nuts and bolts of paced ECG interpretation: what about RV pacing?

Right-ventricular or RV pacing has come under scrutiny in the past years. In one landmark clinical trial, the DAVID study, it was found that unnecessary right-ventricular pacing in certain heart failure patients not indicated for bradycardia pacing worsened systolic function.

Based on the DAVID study, many clinicians began to seek out ways to minimize right-ventricular pacing. This becomes a bit of a balancing act between providing adequate pacing support and avoiding unnecessary RV pacing.

The key is not to avoid *all* RV pacing, but to minimize *unnecessary* RV pacing. For that reason, programming longer AV delays, programming appropriately low pacing rates, and taking advantage of algorithms to encourage intrinsic ventricular activity are all excellent strategies that should be considered in patients with some degree of underlying ventricular activity.

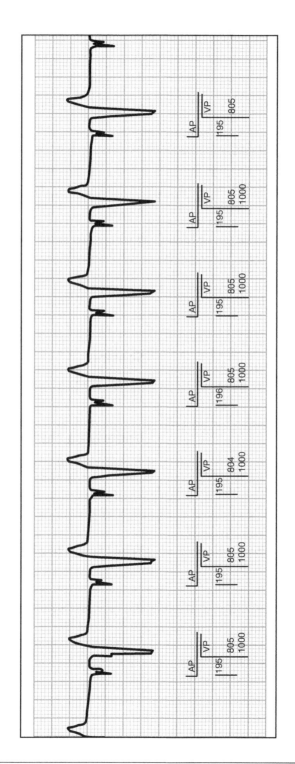

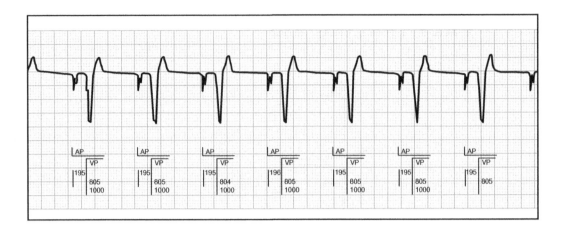

Mode

The atrial spikes are apparent on the tracing, but the ventricular spikes are a bit harder to see (look at the first ventricular event). The annotations can serve as "spikes" and tell where the pacemaker delivered output pulses. This is a dual-chamber pacemaker.

Rate

The atrial pacing interval (AP-AP) provides the rate in a dual-chamber pacing strip; here it is 1000 ms or 60 ppm. This can be measured with calipers, and it is also called out by the bottom numbers on the annotations.

The nuts and bolts of paced ECG interpretation: interval notations on the strip

While calipers will probably never go out of use, intervals noted on the rhythm strip can quickly provide exact measurements in the clinic. In this strip, the pacing interval (AP-AP) is stated in the bottom row (1000). The two upper numbers describe the AV delay (AP-VP), which is 195 ms, and the V-A interval (VP-AP), which is 805 ms. These numbers appear on the annotations with lines to help distinguish the atrial from the ventricular timing segments.

Capture

Every event on this strip is AV pacing (AP-VP). The atrial pacing spikes result in atrial depolarizations, so atrial capture seems to be appropriate. Likewise, ventricular outputs (as seen on the annotations) result in depolarizations and reset device timing. Ventricular capture is appropriate as well.

Sensing

Neither atrial nor ventricular sensing can be evaluated from this strip since every event is paced.

Underlying rhythm

The patient appears to have sinus node dysfunction and slow AV conduction. This strip is 100% paced, so it is unclear what, if any, intrinsic activity this patient might have.

What to do next

Sensing should be evaluated, which means forcing intrinsic events to appear on the ECG. To test atrial sensing, lower the pacing rate in 10-ppm steps until intrinsic atrial activity appears. To avoid patient discomfort, explain to the patient what is going on and lower the rate gradually. Do not go below 30 or 40 ppm, even if intrinsic atrial events do not show up on the tracing. If intrinsic atrial activity cannot be coaxed to appear on the ECG, it may be necessary to forego an atrial sensing test.

To test ventricular sensing, begin by increasing the paced AV delay setting. A gradual stepwise increase is not needed; adjust the paced AV delay temporarily to 300 ms or more and observe if native ventricular activity appears. If no ventricular native activity occurs, an alternate (but less desirable) method of testing ventricular sensing involves temporarily programming the device to VVI mode and lowering the base rate in small 10-ppm steps. In my opinion, the extended AV delay method is by far superior and should always be used first so that you can test this dual-chamber device in a dual-chamber mode.

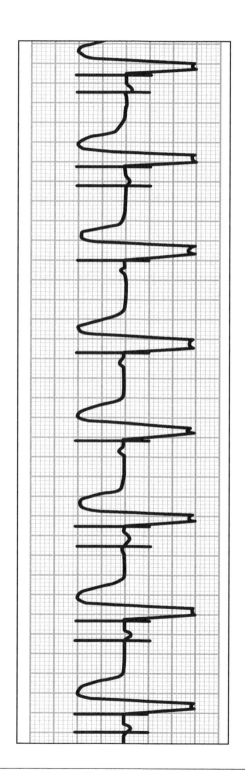

The Nuts and Bolts of Paced ECG Interpretation, 1st edition. By Tom Kenny.
Published 2009 by Blackwell Publishing, ISBN: 978-1-4501-8404-5.

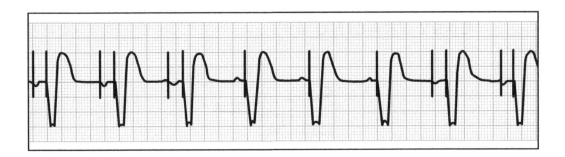

Mode

Clear atrial and ventricular spikes on this strip mean that it is a dual-chamber pacemaker.

Rate

The atrial pacing interval (AP-AP) provides the pacing rate in a dual-chamber pacemaker; it measures 960 ms or about 62 ppm, an appropriate rate.

Capture

The atrial spike appears before several atrial events, all of which share the same distinct morphology. Atrial capture is appropriate.

The ventricular spike appears before ventricular events of the same wide, notched, bizarre look typical of paced events. This suggests that ventricular capture is functioning properly.

Sensing

There are three intrinsic atrial events on this strip, each of which inhibits the atrial output and resets device timing. Measured with calipers, the sensed AV delay appears to be about 160 ms (AP-VS interval). This is further evidence of appropriate atrial sensing.

If you compare the paced AV delay (AP-VP) to the sensed AV delay (AS-VP), it is clear that the paced AV delay in this patient is longer (about 200 ms). It is not unusual for a pacemaker patient to have different sensed and paced AV delay intervals with the paced AV delay typically slightly longer than the sensed AV delay.

Ventricular sensing cannot be assessed from this strip since there are no intrinsic ventricular events.

The nuts and bolts of paced ECG interpretation: sensed and paced AV delays

The AV delay interval is the pacemaker timing cycle between a paced or sensed atrial event and the next paced ventricular event in a dual-chamber pacemaker.

A *sensed AV delay* is the AV delay following an atrial sensed event (AS-VP interval) while a *paced AV delay* is the AV delay following a paced atrial event (AP-VP interval).

These parameter settings are independently programmable and it is actually good clinical practice for the sensed AV delay to be a bit shorter than the paced AV delay in most dual-chamber pacemaker patients. The typical differential is around 25 ms.

The reason for a longer paced than sensed AV delay is that the *paced AV delay interval* timer starts the instant the pacing spike is delivered; the *sensed AV delay interval* timer does not start until the intrinsic atrial event is actually sensed, which means it must occur and be almost done (about 25 ms) before the pacemaker initiates the timing cycle. This particular strip is a good example of how different values for the paced versus the sensed AV delay are used.

Underlying rhythm

The patient has intermittent sinus node dysfunction and consistently slow AV conduction.

What to do next

Ventricular sensing should be evaluated, which means native ventricular activity must appear on the tracing. To force intrinsic ventricular activity to emerge, extend the AV delay temporarily to about 300 ms or even a bit higher. Note that it is not always possible to evaluate sensing in patients who are 100% paced.

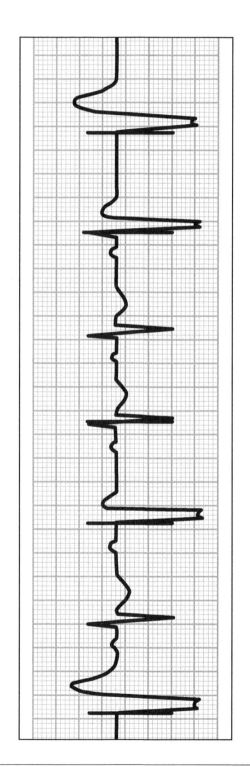

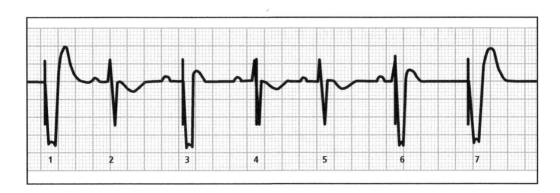

Mode

There are only ventricular pacing spikes on this strip. While there is some atrial activity, there is not an atrial event (paced or sensed) to match every ventricular event, which would have happened in a dual-chamber device. This must be a VVI pacing system.

Rate

The ventricular pacing interval (VP-VP) provides the rate measurement in a VVI device. It measures 840 ms with calipers, approximately, which works out to a pacing rate of around 70 ppm. This rate is expected and appropriate for a VVI patient.

Capture

Although it is tempting to regard single-chamber ventricular rhythm strips as "easy," this particular tracing reveals four distinct ventricular waveform morphologies.

There are intrinsic ventricular events on the strip (second and fifth events). Notice they are small, tight, "sharp-looking" events.

There are true paced ventricular events on the strip, too. They are the first and last complexes.

There are fused ventricular events here: they look like a cross between the paced and sensed events. They are the third and sixth events.

There is also one example of pseudofusion: the fourth event. The spike occurs on top of what otherwise looks like an intrinsic ventricular event.

Appropriate ventricular capture is confirmed, but we have to take into account that we have some ventricular fusion and one pseudofusion event.

Sensing

The intrinsic ventricular events on this strip inhibit the ventricular output and reset device timing. Ventricular sensing looks appropriate.

Underlying rhythm

This patient has sinus node dysfunction and slow AV conduction.

What to do next

Ventricular capture and sensing both seem appropriate, but the presence of two fusion beats and one pseudofusion event is a bit of a concern. Fusion is a timing issue; it occurs when the base rate starts to compete and even collide with the intrinsic rate. The fused beats and the intrinsic beats on the strip offer good evidence that this patient has an intrinsic rate around the programmed base rate (which happens to be 70 ppm).

To allow the patient's intrinsic rate more opportunity to take over, hysteresis should be programmed (for example, leave the base rate at 70 ppm but set up a hysteresis rate of 60 bpm). While it is also possible to program a lower base rate, hysteresis is the better option for most patients because it delivers the best of both worlds – appropriate device inhibition and a sufficiently rapid base rate. Program hysteresis to 60 bpm, leave the base rate at 70 ppm, and observe on the ECG in the clinic how the patient does with this change. If it seems to eliminate fusion and allow intrinsic activity, no further changes would be needed.

The nuts and bolts of paced ECG interpretation: small steps

Your intuition might tell you that if a small change is helpful, a bigger change could be even more beneficial. That's not true when it comes to pacemakers. Even slight changes in pacemaker parameter settings can have significant effects. For that reason, make small, incremental changes in parameter settings and observe the effect on the ECG in the clinic. Since parameters are inter-related and seemingly subtle changes can make a big difference, a big change in a parameter value may solve one problem but introduce several new ones.

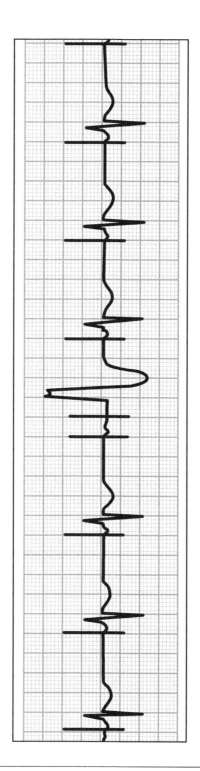

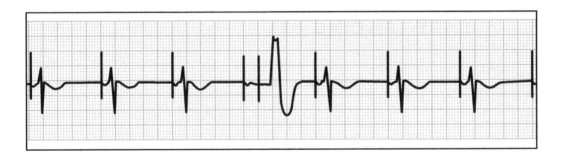

Mode

The presence of atrial and ventricular spikes (even in just one complex) mean that this is a dual-chamber pacemaker.

Rate

The atrial pacing interval (AP-AP) determines the pacing rate. Using calipers, it measures to 1000 ms (60 ppm), an appropriate and expected rate.

Capture

There is consistent atrial pacing in this strip and all of the resulting atrial depolarizations show a similar morphology. This indicates appropriate atrial capture. Atrial capture is also supported by the fact that in the several AP-VS events in the strip, there is a consistent AP-VS interval.

There is only one ventricular pacing spike on the strip and it fails to capture, although it is followed (after a pause of about 200 ms) by an intrinsic ventricular event. Ventricular capture is not appropriate.

Sensing

Atrial sensing cannot be evaluated from this strip since all atrial events are paced.

The first three and last three intrinsic ventricular waveforms all share the same morphology, inhibit the ventricular output, and reset timing. They reflect appropriate ventricular sensing. But what about the fourth event?

This ventricular event is intrinsic but has a different morphology, indicating that it is an escape beat, that is, a beat that originates from a focus within the ventricle.

However, the pacemaker should still sense this ventricular event and use it to reset the timing. That has not happened; the atrial pacing interval remains constant. Had the fourth intrinsic ventricular event been sensed, it should have reset device timing. Whenever something like this is suddenly not properly sensed, the obvious question is: should this event have been sensed? If an intrinsic event occurs during a refractory period, the pacemaker will not sense it or respond to it.

The ventricular spike would have initiated a ventricular refractory period. Did this ventricular event "fall into" the refractory and get missed? Measuring with calipers, it appears that this intrinsic event occurs about 160 ms after the ventricular spike. Since a typical ventricular refractory setting is about 250 ms, this event may well have been missed because it occurred during the refractory period. That would mean ventricular sensing is appropriate.

Underlying rhythm

The patient has sinus node dysfunction but with reasonably good AV conduction.

What to do next

Atrial sensing should be evaluated; reduce the programmed base rate in small steps of 10-ppm to encourage intrinsic atrial activity to appear on the

ECG. Do this gradually, observing the ECG, and checking on the patient that the lower rate is well tolerated. Even if it is well tolerated and no intrinsic atrial events occur, do not drop the rate below 30 or 40 ppm. It may not be possible to test atrial sensing.

Ventricular capture should be restored. To test ventricular capture, ventricular pacing must occur. Temporarily shorten the programmed AV delay to "force" ventricular pacing. It is likely that ventricular output parameters (pulse amplitude and pulse width) will have to be reprogrammed to slightly higher values.

The nuts and bolts of paced ECG interpretation: escape rhythms and PVCs

As far as a pacemaker is concerned, a premature ventricular contraction (PVC) is defined as the presence of two ventricular events without an intervening atrial event. That is not always the same thing as the clinical definition, but it can help you understand pacing annotations.

An escape beat is not annotated as such on the rhythm strip, but it may be defined as an unexpected depolarization with a different morphology from a "typical" intrinsic event. An escape beat has a different waveform morphology because the beat originates from a different focus in the myocardium than a typical intrinsic depolarization. Escape beats originate from the ventricle itself while a classic intrinsic ventricular event originates from an atrial impulse that conducts properly over the AV node and down into the ventricles.

Escape beats and PVCs are not uncommon on ECGs of both paced and non-paced patients. Depending on how frequently they occur, they may be of little concern or they could pose a problem. For a paced patient, the main issue with such beats is not the event itself but the fact that it can sometimes launch a pacemaker-mediated tachycardia (PMT) or might even trigger a potentially lethal ventricular tachyarrhythmia.

Moderate

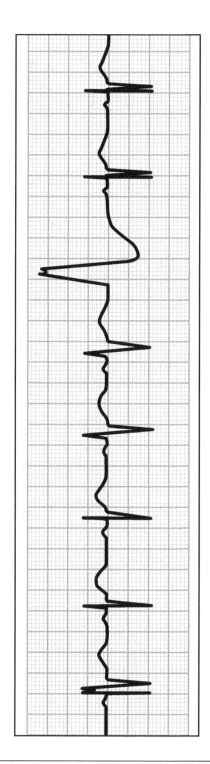

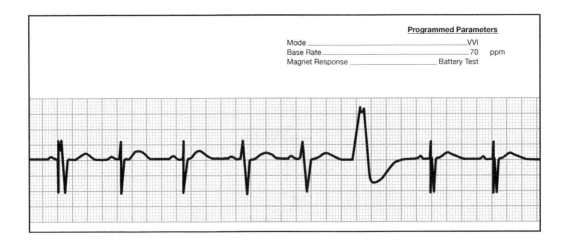

	Programmed Parameters
Mode	VVI
Base Rate	70 ppm
Magnet Response	Battery Test

Mode

There are some ventricular pacing spikes on this pacing strip but it is not clear whether the device is a VVI pacemaker or perhaps a dual-chamber device that is simply sensing atrial activity. If the latter were the case, the intervals in the last two complexes between the intrinsic atrial event and the ventricular pacing spike (the sensed AV delay) would be consistent – which they are. However, we only have two such events. That is really not enough from which to draw a conclusion. If possible, turn on annotations or get printout information about the device. From that, we know that the device is actually a VVI system.

Rate

The pacing rate can be measured on this strip between the last two ventricular spikes. It turns out to be about 840 ms or around 70 ppm, an appropriate rate, particularly for a single-chamber pacemaker.

Capture

Atrial capture cannot be evaluated from this strip since it's a ventricular pacemaker.

The strip has three ventricular pacing spikes, but look at the QRS morphology. These "paced" ventricular events look remarkably similar in morphology to the intrinsic ventricular depolarizations. These events are pseudofusion, which occurs when

the pacing spike happens to land on an intrinsic depolarization; the ventricle depolarizes on its own and the pacing spike makes no contribution to the event. Pseudofusion neither confirms nor refutes capture. Ventricular capture on this strip cannot be assessed.

Pseudofusion events may be controversial. After all, how can we be sure that the event was really intrinsic with a spike and not a fused event, where the spike contributes to the depolarization? A good rule of thumb for evaluating any ventricular morphology is to look not only at the shape of the QRS complex but also at the shape of the resulting T-wave. The T-wave after a pseudofusion event is going to have the same general morphology as a T-wave after an intrinsic event. This is indeed the case.

Sensing

Ventricular sensing appears appropriate in the first four intrinsic ventricular events; each inhibits the ventricular spike and resets device timing. The question is whether the large ventricular escape beat in the middle of the strip is properly sensed.

Using calipers, a distinct sensing problem comes to light. The escape event was sensed in that it inhibits a ventricular output spike. But if you set the calipers to the ventricular pacing interval (840 ms) and use them to measure the outset of the escape beat to the next ventricular pacing spike, a problem appears. The calipers don't reach, in other words, the escape interval (VS-VP) is too long.

The calipers reveal that the pacemaker "sensed" something that coincided with the trailing edge of the ventricular escape beat. This is not a case of undersensing at all, but rather that the pacemaker did not sense this event until the downward slope. While most of the time, pacemakers sense cardiac activity at the outset of the beat, it is sometimes possible for the device to miss a portion of the waveform and sense it on the downslope.

Actually, such sensing peculiarities are particularly common with ventricular escape beats like this. A pacemaker with a bipolar lead senses cardiac activity by the difference in electrical potential of the wavefront energy as it passes by the two electrodes on the distal end of the electrode. Almost all of the time, the pacemaker is on the lookout for "normal" intrinsic activity rather than escape beats, so the pacemaker's sensitivity is programmed specifically for such events. "Normal" intrinsic events travel in a certain direction over the electrodes. An escape beat is a horse of a different color, in that it originates from a different site in the myocardium and its wavefront travels a different path through the heart. The result is that the electrical differentials recorded on the distal electrodes of the bipolar lead may be deceptively small.

It may seem counterintuitive, but an escape beat that appears quite large on the surface ECG may be a barely noticeable electrode differential as far as the pacemaker's sensing circuits are concerned. For that reason, it is not at all unusual for ventricular escape beats to be undersensed. In this case, the ventricular event was not undersensed, just sensed much later in the course of the depolarization than usual. That accounts for the long escape interval.

Ventricular sensing is appropriate.

Underlying rhythm

This patient has sinus node dysfunction but conduction appears to be intact. His intrinsic rate is around 70 bpm, which is why the pseudofusion occurs.

What to do next

Ventricular capture must be assessed. It is likely that the ventricular output parameters (pulse amplitude, pulse width) will have to be increased to deliver more energy to capture the ventricle.

The patient's intrinsic rate is close to the programmed base rate. Hysteresis is a good option for this patient, because it would allow for a hysteresis rate (for example, 60 bpm) to prevail without having to decrease the base rate below 70 ppm for those times when this patient required pacing.

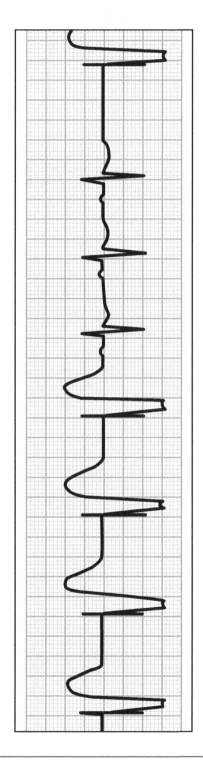

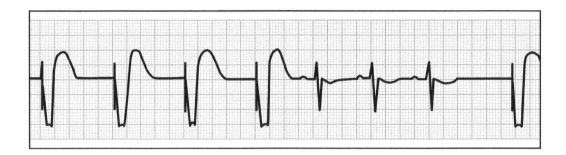

Mode

This pacemaker is a VVI system. While there is some intrinsic atrial activity evident on the tracing, the absence of atrial spikes at the beginning of the strip shows that it is a single-chamber ventricular pacemaker.

Rate

The pacing interval (VP-VP) is 1000 ms (60 ppm), an appropriate rate for a single-chamber system.

Capture

This is a VVI strip, so there is no atrial capture. Ventricular capture appears to be appropriate; ventricular spikes are followed by wider, notched, bizarre QRS complexes. All of the paced events have the same morphology, and there is no sign of fusion or pseudofusion.

Sensing

Ventricular sensing appears to be appropriate in the first three intrinsic ventricular events. Each of them inhibits the ventricular pacing spike. However, there is a long pause between the last intrinsic ventricular event on this tracing and the final pacing spike (VS-VP). The VS-VP interval is also known as the escape interval (sensed event to next paced event in the same chamber). Whenever an escape interval occurs that is longer than the pacing interval … we should consider the possibility of hysteresis. This escape interval measures 1200 ms (50 bpm), a very typical hysteresis rate.

Ventricular sensing is appropriate and hysteresis is programmed to 50 bpm.

The nuts and bolts of paced ECG interpretation: why would you program hysteresis on?

Hysteresis is a very useful feature in pacemakers and other cardiac rhythm management devices, but, in my opinion, it is often not used as much as it ought to be. The purpose of hysteresis is to encourage intrinsic activity to prevail. This might be accomplished by simply programming a low base rate, like "backup pacing" at 30 or 40 ppm.

However, for many patients a lower base rate would not provide adequate rate support during other times of the day when they needed more rapid pacing.

Hysteresis provides the best of both worlds. It allows the normally programmed base rate to prevail when the device starts pacing in the absence of intrinsic activity. Thus, during times when the patient's heart would not be beating very rapidly, the pacing rate takes over and provides appropriate support at rates of 60 or 70 ppm. However, when intrinsic activity occurs, the pacemaker allows it to take control as long as it stays above the programmed hysteresis rate, typically programmed to about 10 ppm less than the base rate.

Use hysteresis for patients with reasonably fast intrinsic activity, even if it is intermittent. There is no harm in programming hysteresis on, even if the patient has little intrinsic activity in that hysteresis remains on standby until some intrinsic events occur.

Underlying rhythm

This patient has sinus node dysfunction and some evidence of intact AV conduction.

What to do next

Ventricular capture and sensing are working properly and hysteresis is programmed on and functioning as expected. Since this patient appears to have intermittent intrinsic atrial activity and intact conduction, he should be a candidate for an upgrade to a dual-chamber system at the next revision.

MODERATE TRACING #3

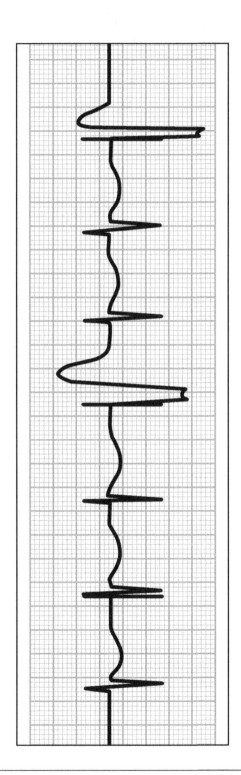

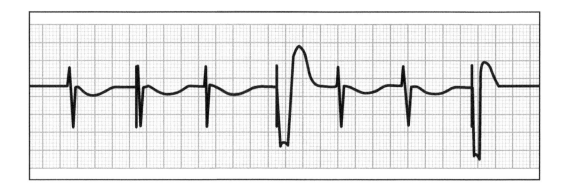

Mode

This is a single-chamber ventricular pacemaker (VVI).

Rate

Normally, the rate could be measured from the pacing interval (VP-VP) but there is no such interval on this rhythm strip. The next best thing to measure is the escape interval (VS-VP) which occurs between the third and fourth complexes and again between the sixth and seventh complexes. The escape interval is 800 ms (75 ppm). That rate would be appropriate.

Capture

There are several different types of ventricular events on this strip. The first, third, fifth, and sixth complexes are intrinsic ventricular depolarizations.

The second complex has the same morphology but with a pacing spike added. This is an example of pseudofusion; pseudofusion has intrinsic morphology but with a spike.

The fourth complex has the typical widened bizarre look of a paced event.

The last event on the strip looks like a blend of intrinsic morphology and paced morphology. This is an example of fusion, where an intrinsic depolarization occurs at the same time as a pacing spike and both contribute to the resulting event.

Both the paced ventricular event and the fused event confirm appropriate ventricular capture.

The nuts and bolts of paced ECG interpretation: when rates compete

Fusion and pseudofusion are timing issues. They occur because the pacemaker is delivering output pulses almost on top of intrinsic events. This occurs when the patient's own intrinsic rate "competes" with the programmed base rate.

Occasional fusion or pseudofusion is nearly unavoidable, in that patients may have rates that approach or even exceed the base rate from time to time. However, lots of fusion and pseudofusion events indicate rates are competing. The best approach is to program hysteresis, lower the base rate, or both.

Technically, fusion and pseudofusion do not "harm" the patient. The heart still depolarizes. The patient will not experience symptoms. At most, fusion and pseudofusion waste battery energy by sending output pulses where none are needed. Nevertheless, they are indications that the intrinsic rate is "bumping into" the base rate.

Sensing

Ventricular sensing is appropriate in that intrinsic ventricular events inhibit the pacing spike and reset device timing.

Underlying rhythm

This patient has sinus node dysfunction; in fact, in this snippet of ECG there is no intrinsic atrial activity at all.

What to do next

Since fusion and pseudofusion are likely frequent events for this patient, it means that the pacemaker timing should be adjusted. Fusion and pseudofusion occur when the patient's intrinsic heart rate starts to compete or "bump" into the programmed base rate. Typically, I recommend using the hysteresis algorithm in cases of a competing intrinsic rhythm, but remember this patient's programmed base rate is set to 75 ppm. Most of the time, base rates are set to 60 to 70 ppm. While 75 ppm is not exceedingly high, the fact that it is a bit above "normal" would make me want to drop the base rate to 70 ppm first. After making that programming change, I would observe the paced ECG and decide whether or not to activate the hysteresis algorithm, programming a hysteresis rate of 60 bpm.

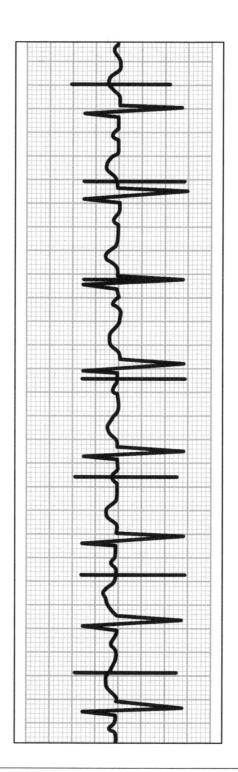

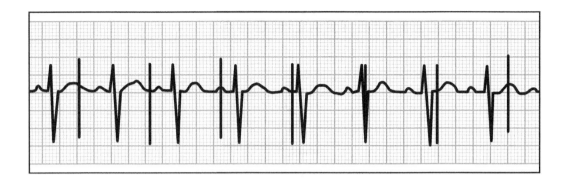

Mode

Normally, pacing mode is easy to determine, but this strip presents some challenges. There are spikes that "march through" this strip at a consistent rate. This is clearly a single-chamber pacemaker operating asynchronously – but is it ventricular or atrial? At first glance, it is very tough to know if the spikes are connected to the atrial or ventricular channel!

Rate

The pacing interval (spike-to-spike) is approximately 840 ms (70 ppm), which is appropriate for a single-chamber system.

Capture

The spikes run through the strip without any relationship to intrinsic activity. But before we can assess capture, we need to ask: should the spikes have captured? The first spike occurs toward the latter portion of a T-wave. If this is a VVI device, it should have captured. The second, third, and fourth spikes should have captured if this was a ventricular system. Thus, there is evidence of non-capture if the device is a ventricular single-chamber pacemaker.

But what if this was an atrial pacemaker? In that case, the first and second spikes also should have captured. Thus, no matter what type of pacemaker (atrial or ventricular) we're dealing with, there is a failure to capture.

Since VVI pacemakers are more common in practice than atrial pacemakers, I am going to make a leap and assume this is a single-chamber ventricular device. If my assumption is true, then the fifth spike is an example of pseudofusion (spike on top of an intrinsic depolarization). If this is a VVI device, the sixth spike could not have captured the heart because it occurs too soon after the intrinsic ventricular depolarization; in fact, the spike occurs during the heart's physiological refractory period. This is an example of functional non-capture, that is, there is no capture but it is a sensing problem rather than an energy problem.

However, no matter how you look at it, this strip shows non-capture.

Sensing

The automatic interval (spike-to-spike) is consistent and appears unrelated to intrinsic events. This is a good indication that there is no sensing going on! The intrinsic events do not appear to ever inhibit the spikes and reset timing. If this was an AAI pacemaker, the fourth intrinsic atrial event should have reset timing and inhibited the pacing spike. If this was a VVI pacemaker, the first intrinsic ventricular event should have inhibited the first pacing spike. Thus, sensing is inappropriate as well or the device is programmed to an asynchronous (non-sensing mode), such as VOO or AOO. Since permanent programming to an asynchronous mode is very rare, it is much more likely that this represents inappropriate sensing.

Underlying rhythm

This patient is fortunate in that his underlying rhythm is reasonably good; there is good sinus node function and what appears to be intact AV conduction. It would be interesting to find out if this patient even had symptoms, despite the troublesome-looking rhythm strip!

What to do next

In many cases when the mode is questionable, I recommend trying to use annotations or finding the programmed parameters to verify the mode. It would also be interesting to check how the device is programmed. Magnet application can induce asynchronous pacing; however, magnet mode often involves higher-than-base-rate pacing which is not the case here. Devices can sometimes enter into a reset or backup mode in the presence of interference; that would force the device to pace asynchronously.

While I would investigate those possibilities first, the total lack of proper capture and sensing (regardless of what kind of device this is) strongly suggests that there is a problem with the pacing lead. Capture and sensing problems that show up simultaneously are a good indicator that there is something more profoundly amiss in the pacing system than just improperly programmed parameters. Once you can rule out magnet mode, noise reversion (backup mode in the presence of interference), or a permanently programmed asynchronous mode, a chest X-ray should be ordered to see if there is some observable problem with lead integrity. Further testing of the device may also be conducted. While I would try to rule out other causes of the asynchronous pacing with failure to capture, this rhythm strip is almost a classic example of how a compromised pacing lead shows up on a paced ECG.

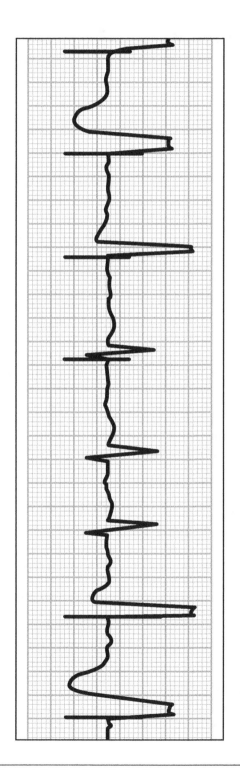

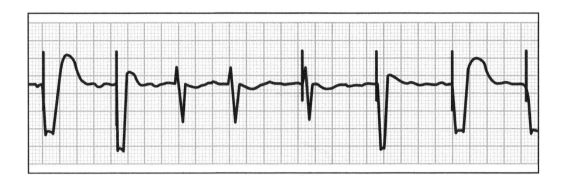

Mode

This strip comes from a VVI pacemaker.

Rate

The pacing interval (spike-to-spike) is around 880 ms (68 ppm), which is appropriate for a single-chamber system.

Capture

The first ventricular pacing spike results in a "classic" example of ventricular capture; notice the widened, notched, bizarre QRS morphology right after the spike. The third and fourth ventricular events are intrinsic. The second ventricular spike looks like a cross between a paced and intrinsic event. This is ventricular fusion. The first and second ventricular spikes both confirm appropriate capture.

The third spike on the strip (fifth complex) is pseudofusion, in that the spike does not change QRS morphology; this is an intrinsic depolarization and the spike simply occurred on top of it. This neither confirms nor refutes capture.

The fourth ventricular spike is another example of ventricular fusion, the fifth is another example of ventricular capture. Although there are three distinct QRS morphologies on this short rhythm strip, capture appears to be appropriate.

Sensing

Ventricular sensing appears to be functioning properly in that the third and fourth events inhibit the ventricular output spike and reset timing. You can verify this by measuring the escape interval from the onset of the fourth event (a sensed ventricular event) to the next pacing spike (VS-VP): it's exactly the same as the pacing interval (880 ms).

Underlying rhythm

This patient has atrial fibrillation (AF). The biggest "clue" to AF is not the bumpy baseline, but rather *the erratic ventricular rate in response to the atrial activity*. Although this is a short strip (just a few seconds of time), the ventricular rate ranges from slow enough to require pacing (less than 68 bpm) to as fast as 94 bpm (640 ms, the interval between the third and fourth ventricular intrinsic events). Irregular ventricular response to AF is often the most visible sign of AF on the ECG. Further evidence of AF appears in the bumpy baseline, which attempts to represent the presence of a lot of low-amplitude intrinsic atrial activity. This patient also has slow AV conduction.

What to do next

This patient should be treated for atrial fibrillation, which should first be done by pharmacological therapy. More severe cases of AF may require electrical or chemical cardioversion. Some dual-chamber pacemakers offer atrial overdrive algorithms or other device-based features to help suppress rapid atrial activity before it can develop.

However, a VVI pacemaker is quite appropriate in a patient like this. AF and fusion go hand-in-hand; an erratic ventricular rate can result in occasional fused beats.

The nuts and bolts of paced ECG interpretation: managing AF in a pacemaker patient

Atrial fibrillation (AF) is a common arrhythmia and one that presents special challenges to the paced population.

Atrial tracking (such as occurs in DDD or DDDR modes) is inappropriate in the presence of AF, since the device will try to force the ventricle to keep up with the rapid intrinsic atrial rate, at least up to the maximum tracking rate. Patients with known AF should be programmed to non-tracking modes; VVI pacing is often used.

Patients with suspected AF or at risk of AF may benefit from mode switching algorithms which temporarily turn off atrial tracking ("mode switches") in the presence of intrinsic high-rate atrial activity.

Some pacemakers offer an AF Suppression™ algorithm or other features to suppress AF before it can develop. While these are very useful algorithms in certain patients, not all pacemaker patients with AF will have devices that offer such algorithms.

The treatment of AF is outside the scope of this book, but the first line of defense is typically pharmacological therapy, followed by cardioversion (chemical or electrical) and possibly surgery or catheter ablation. AF is a progressive disorder, that is, it gets worse over time, so AF patients must be closely followed so that therapy can be adjusted as their condition changes.

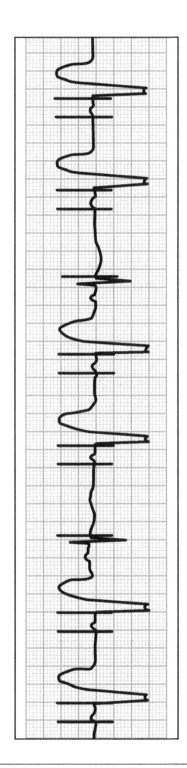

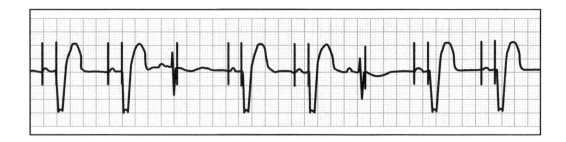

Mode

This strip comes from a dual-chamber pacemaker.

Rate

In a dual-chamber system, the rate is measured using the atrial pacing interval (AP-AP). Here the atrial pacing interval is 1000 ms (60 ppm), an appropriate rate for dual-chamber pacing.

Capture

Six times on this strip, an atrial pacing spike occurs right before an atrial depolarization. In my opinion, they all show appropriate atrial capture. The might be a bit controversial in that there is no obvious difference on this strip between intrinsic and captured atrial event morphology; intrinsic atrial events in this strip look a lot like paced events! The third atrial spike (fourth complex) also occurs slightly "apart" or away from the atrial depolarization, but, in my opinion, atrial capture is appropriate. I say that cautiously – but I think the spikes and depolarizations provide sufficient evidence of proper atrial capture.

There are six ventricular paced events on this strip with the same morphology, and this time the morphology differs from that of an intrinsic ventricular depolarization. There is appropriate ventricular capture.

The third and sixth complex on this strip are a bit puzzling. There is a pacing spike right *after* an intrinsic ventricular event. In my opinion, these are not examples of pseudofusion which occurs when an intrinsic depolarization occurs and a spike lands, ineffectively, right on top of it. Pseudofusion is a simultaneous event. The spikes, in these two examples, occur slightly after the intrinsic ventricular event.

In both instances, the spike fails to capture the heart. But the question whenever there is such an obvious failure to capture must be this: should that spike have captured the heart? The answer, in this case, is no. The ventricular myocardium had just depolarized and was physiologically refractory. The third and sixth ventricular spikes could not have captured the heart, no matter how powerful the pulses were. These are two examples of functional non-capture (which suggests a sensing problem).

Therefore, ventricular capture appears to be appropriate.

Sensing

Any time functional non-capture occurs, we should be on the lookout for undersensing. But before we look at the ventricular channel, let's verify appropriate atrial sensing. There are two intrinsic atrial events on this strip (in the third and sixth complexes). If these intrinsic atrial events were properly sensed, they would have inhibited the atrial output pulse and reset device timing. But in order to determine if that was what happened, we have to double-check the spike that occurs right after the intrinsic ventricular depolarization in the third and sixth beat. Was it an *atrial spike* or a *ventricular spike*?

There are several ways to investigate this.

- If the spike was atrial, it would time itself to the previous atrial event. That means a 1000 ms atrial pacing interval. If you use calipers on the strip, it is clear the third and sixth spikes are not timed to the previous atrial event. That means these spikes were not on the atrial channel.
- We should also check the sensed AV delay interval (AS-VP). In the third event, it measures out to be around 280 ms. That same measurement applies to the sixth event. The presence of a consistent and appropriate sensed AV delay is evidence that the

spike is sensing the atrial event and timing itself to that.

- While we're looking at AV delay intervals, measure the paced AV delay interval (AP-VP), too. It is around 200 ms. The fact that the paced AV delay is shorter than the sensed AV delay is also appropriate.

Thus, we can be confident the third and sixth spikes are ventricular. The intrinsic atrial event did, indeed, inhibit the atrial output pulse. Atrial sensing is appropriate.

Ventricular sensing is another matter. There are just two intrinsic ventricular events on this strip and both are followed almost at once by a ventricular pacing spike. This is ventricular undersensing.

Underlying rhythm

The patient has sinus node dysfunction and slow AV conduction.

What to do next

The most urgent need is to correct ventricular sensing which would require a ventricular sensing test and then appropriate reprogramming of ventricular sensitivity.

The nuts and bolts of paced ECG interpretation: functional non-capture and undersensing

As a general rule of thumb, whenever you see a spike that fails to capture, you should first ask whether or not that spike could have captured the myocardium. If the spike occurs during the physiological refractory period of the myocardium, the pulse could never capture the heart, no matter how powerful it was. That's functional non-capture.

Despite its name, functional non-capture is not actually a capture problem. Nearly always it relates to a *sensing problem*. Functional non-capture occurs during the physiological refractory period of the heart, that is, after an intrinsic beat. However, if sensing were working appropriately, the beat would have been sensed and the pacing output spike would have been withheld. Whenever you have functional non-capture, look for undersensing!

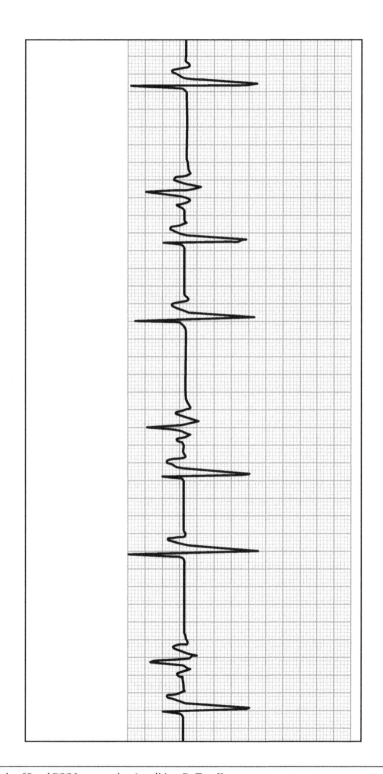

The Nuts and Bolts of Paced ECG Interpretation, 1st edition. By Tom Kenny.
Published 2009 by Blackwell Publishing, ISBN: 978-1-4501-8404-5.

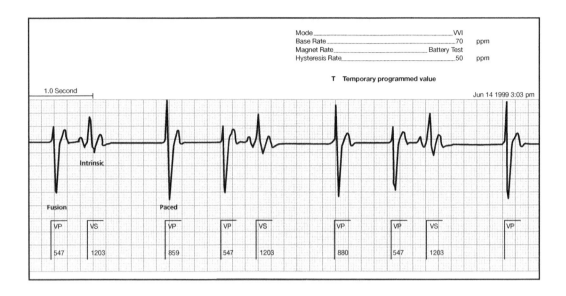

Mode

Look carefully at this strip and you'll see it's from a VVI pacemaker; the complexes on the strip are mostly ventricular with only some sporadic intrinsic atrial events.

Rate

The ventricular pacing interval (VP-VP) may be a bit challenging to find. Since we do not have pacing spikes to go by, a good idea is to turn on annotations, if possible, and use them like spikes. We did that here, but a skilled reader of paced ECGs could actually interpret this strip pretty accurately without benefit of annotations. Here is how it would be done.

Notice that there are three distinct ventricular morphologies on this strip. The first complex shows a large downward-deflecting morphology; the second complex is a smaller upward-deflecting complex; the third complex is a very large, pointed ventricular complex. Every ventricular event on this strip is one of those three distinct morphologies.

That means there are three types of ventricular events going on. The smaller upward-deflecting complexes are intrinsic. The very large, very pointed ventricular events are paced; these are the "tallest" waveforms on the strip. The ones that look like hy-

brids between intrinsic and paced events are fused beats, which count as capture.

When confronting various different morphologies on a single strip, first identify the type of event that is most obvious to you. For me, the smaller, upward-deflecting events (the second, fifth, and eighth complexes) are clearly intrinsic. (This is confirmed by the annotations.) The other two morphologies on this strip look similar but are distinct. One is a "true" paced event and the other one has to be fusion, a combination of intrinsic and paced beat. The "true" paced event is the event less like the intrinsic beat, while the fusion beat has to be the beat that looks more like the intrinsic beat. The third, sixth, and ninth complexes are "true" paced ventricular events, while the first, fourth, and seventh events are fused.

Knowing the types of events, measure the interval between the onset of the third and fourth complexes (or also the sixth and seventh) to get the ventricular pacing interval (VP-VP). It measures to be about 880 ms (70 ppm) with calipers. That rate is confirmed by the annotations (859) and on the printout at the top.

Capture

The ventricular pacemaker spikes do not appear as spikes, but we can see them as annotations. Every spike results in a ventricular depolarization but there are two distinct morphologies. The larger complexes are paced events, the smaller but similar-looking complexes are fused events. Both confirm capture. Ventricular capture is actually appropriate.

Sensing

Ventricular sensing looks appropriate in that sensed ventricular events (the upward complexes) inhibit the output spike. But look what happens with timing! The ventricular escape interval (VS-VP) is longer than the ventricular pacing interval of 880 ms. Measure it from the onset of the QRS to the next pacing spike; it turns out to be about 1200 ms (50 ppm).

Whenever the escape interval (sensed event to paced event in the same chamber) is longer than the pacing interval (paced event to paced event in the same chamber), it is very likely that hysteresis is in force. Hysteresis automatically prolongs the escape interval in the presence of intrinsic activity. Evidence of hysteresis includes:

- An escape interval that is longer than the paced interval
- An escape interval that times out to be a "likely" hysteresis rate (here the pacing rate is 70 ppm and the escape interval works out to be a hysteresis rate of 50 bpm)
- Confirmation on the printout that hysteresis is on!

Underlying rhythm

This patient has sinus node dysfunction and an intrinsic ventricular rate that is competing with the programmed base rate.

What to do next

Hysteresis is definitely appropriate for this patient, but it might be a good idea to lower the programmed base rate as well. The device is programmed to a base rate of 70 and a hysteresis rate of 50 bpm. A gap of 20 bpm between hysteresis and base rate is actually quite large; a 10 bpm differential is typical. For that reason, I would lower the base rate to 60 ppm or at least 65 ppm and leave hysteresis at 50 bpm.

The nuts and bolts of paced ECG interpretation: difference between ppm and bpm

Pacemakers measure rates in intervals, but clinicians like to talk about rates in terms of pulses per minute or ppm. However, sometimes, in particular with hysteresis, it is typical to see the abbreviation bpm, which stands for beats per minute.

Although not everyone does this rigorously, there is actually a method for deciding when to use ppm versus bpm. Pulses per minute refers to what the pacemaker does – it delivers so many spikes or pulses per minute. The base rate of a pacemaker is typically stated as 60 or 70 ppm. Beats per minute refers to the patient's intrinsic rate. A person with an intrinsic cardiac rate of 30 bpm should get a pacemaker.

Since the hysteresis kicks in when the patient's intrinsic rate hits a cutoff, hysteresis rates are rightly stated in bpm – the patient's intrinsic rate. A 50 bpm hysteresis rate means that hysteresis goes into effect when the patient's own native heart rate hits 50 bpm.

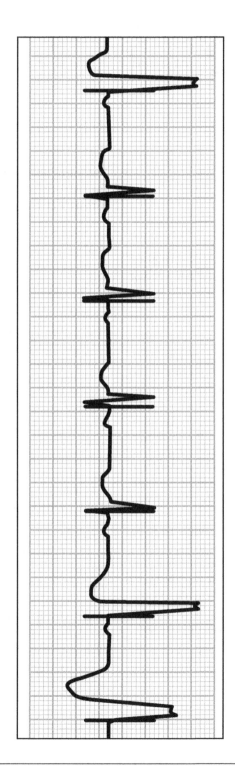

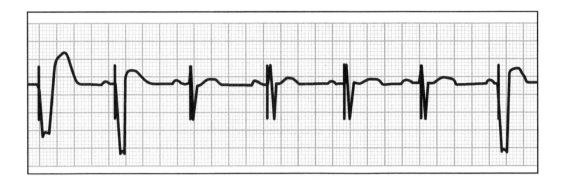

Mode

This comes from a VVI pacemaker.

Rate

The pacing interval (VP-VP) measures out with calipers to around 880 ms, which translates to a pacing rate of 70 ppm.

Capture

There are three distinct ventricular morphologies on this strip. Even without annotations, they can be identified. The first beat is the most obvious to me; it is a "true" ventricular paced event.

The third through sixth events on this strip look like intrinsic events but there is a pacing spike in the middle; these are pseudofusion events. These four pseudofusion events neither confirm nor deny capture, they merely indicate that the patient's intrinsic ventricular rate is competing with the programmed base rate.

The second and last ventricular events are fused ventricular beats, in that they look like a cross between the intrinsic and the paced morphologies. The first "true" paced event and the two fused ventricular events confirm capture. Pseudofusion neither confirms nor denies capture. Thus, from what we have to work with, ventricular capture is appropriate.

Sensing

Sensing cannot be evaluated from this strip.

The nuts and bolts of paced ECG interpretation: don't you forget about T (T-waves, that is)

Evaluating QRS complexes in terms of morphology is somewhat of an inexact science, particularly when it is practiced by rookies or those who don't have a lot of experience with paced ECGs.

On this strip, it might appear to some clinicians that the third ventricular spike distorted the third ventricular complex more than the fourth, fifth, and sixth spikes distorted their resulting QRS complexes. Someone else might notice that the fourth ventricular spike resulted in a kind of notch on top, which didn't happen on some of the other beats. In other words, maybe these four consecutive "pseudofusion events" aren't really the same event at all. There are some subtle morphology differences.

I think all four of these complexes (third through sixth on the strip) are pseudofusion, and here is why. You should always include the T-wave when comparing morphologies. Just as this strip has three different events, there are three different types of T-waves. The first T-wave in the first complex (true paced event) is quite large and rounded; the second and last T-waves (fused events) are rounded but lower. The T-waves associated with what I am calling pseudofusion are all similar: very wide, low, and flat.

Based on that, I would say that the third through sixth events are all the same type of event and that type of event has to be pseudofusion. However, that is subject to "interpretation" and I suspect some colleagues might disagree.

Underlying rhythm

This patient has what appears to be good sinus node function and slow AV conduction. His intrinsic ventricular rate is competing with the programmed base rate.

What to do next

Despite some evidence of appropriate capture, capture should be verified by increasing the base rate to force pacing. To me, this is prudent because there is just not enough evidence on this strip to give me confidence that capture is reliably appropriate.

Ventricular sensing should be evaluated. To do this, decrease the base rate gradually, in 10-ppm increments, to allow intrinsic activity to occur. This patient will likely exhibit intrinsic ventricular activity readily. If necessary, ventricular sensitivity may have to be adjusted.

Since this patient's intrinsic rate competes with the base rate, program hysteresis on. With a programmed base rate of 70 ppm, a good starting place for hysteresis is 60 bpm. That should clear up the persistent pseudofusion.

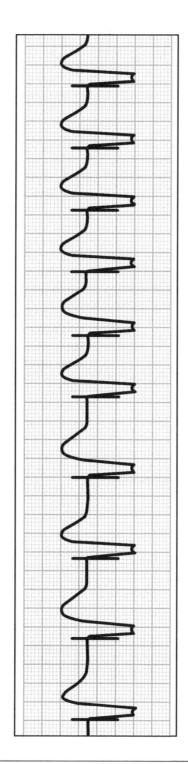

The Nuts and Bolts of Paced ECG Interpretation, 1st edition. By Tom Kenny.
Published 2009 by Blackwell Publishing, ISBN: 978-1-4501-8404-5.

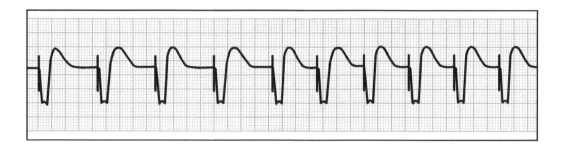

Mode

This is single-chamber ventricular pacing. It might look like atrial tracking, but there are no intrinsic atrial events to track!

Rate

The ventricular pacing interval (VP-VP) on the left is approximately 840 ms (70 ms), but it changes to 610 ms (98 ppm) to the right. Something is "driving" the ventricular pacing rate to exceed the base rate. The only thing that could accelerate a rhythm in this manner is rate response. This is a VVIR device under sensor drive.

Capture

Ventricular capture is consistently appropriate.

Sensing

Ventricular sensing cannot be evaluated from this strip.

Underlying rhythm

The patient has silent atria and likely has chronotropic incompetence.

What to do next

First, check appropriate ventricular sensing. This will require temporarily disabling rate response, which may be done by temporarily programming the sensor to PASSIVE or OFF. Evaluate ventricular sensing by encouraging intrinsic activity; in order to do that, drop the base rate gradually in 10-ppm steps until intrinsic events occur. Monitor the patient's response to the lower rate and do not go below 30 or 40 ppm.

Ask the patient if he feels that the pacemaker's rate is appropriate for his activities. You may also want to download diagnostic reports about rate response that can tell you how much time the sensor drove the pacing rate and at what rates.

The nuts and bolts of paced ECG interpretation: chronotropic incompetence

The healthy human heart has the ability to adjust its rate according to the body's need for cardiac output. During periods of exertion or physical exercise, the heart automatically speeds up its rate to meet the metabolic burden placed on the body under stress. When the exertion is over, the heart gradually resumes its resting rate.

Chronotropic incompetence occurs in patients whose heart has lost the ability to self-regulate its rate. Rate-responsive pacemakers help compensate for chronotropic incompetence by allowing a sensor to help determine when and how much the heart rate should increase.

The main types of sensors are accelerometers, which sense motion or activity, and minute ventilation which senses respiration.

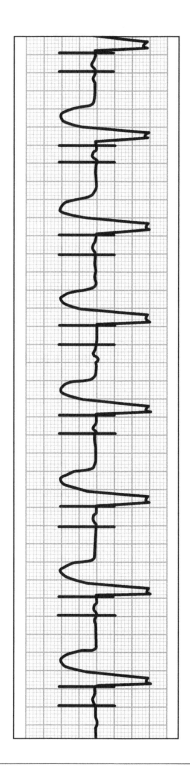

The Nuts and Bolts of Paced ECG Interpretation, 1st edition. By Tom Kenny.
Published 2009 by Blackwell Publishing, ISBN: 978-1-4501-8404-5.

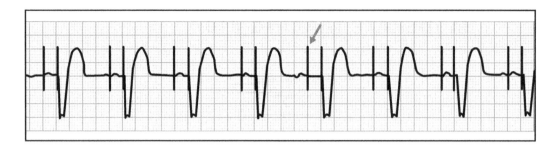

Mode

The presence of atrial and ventricular spikes means that this is a dual-chamber pacing system.

Rate

The atrial pacing interval (AP-AP) is 1000 ms (60 ppm), an appropriate rate for this kind of device.

Capture

This strip shows just AP-VP events, but there are some differences in the complexes.

The fifth atrial pacing spike (see arrow) does not capture. The rest of the atrial spikes all exhibit appropriate atrial capture. With this fifth spike, it is important to ask: could it have captured? Notice that an intrinsic atrial event appears immediately prior to the atrial pacing spike. This means the atria depolarized on their own before the spike and the atrial tissue was physiologically refractory. That fifth atrial spike could not have captured the atrium at that time, no matter how much energy it delivered. This is an example of functional non-capture, which is not actually a capture problem – it's a sensing problem. Thus, atrial capture seems appropriate, but we'll have a sensing issue to tackle.

Ventricular capture seems appropriate. Every ventricular spike is followed by a ventricular depolarization with a characteristic widened, bizarre "paced" look. Even more compelling evidence is the fact that all ventricular morphologies are identical.

Sensing

The atrial functional non-capture (as indicated by the arrow) occurred right after an intrinsic atrial event. The pacemaker did not "see" this intrinsic atrial event and tried to pace right after it occurred. This indicates atrial undersensing.

Ventricular sensing cannot be evaluated from this strip since all of the ventricular events here are paced.

Underlying rhythm

This patient has sinus node dysfunction and slow AV conduction. In the whole strip, there is only one lone intrinsic event – this is a patient who is paced much of the time.

What to do next

Atrial sensing should be evaluated by reducing the programmed base rate in 10-ppm increments to encourage intrinsic atrial activity. It is likely that atrial sensitivity will have to be adjusted (the pacemaker should be made more sensitive, that is, the mV setting should be decreased). Since the patient has some intrinsic atrial activity, there is a very good chance this can be done in the clinic. Even if no intrinsic atrial events occur, do not drop the rate below 30 or 40 ppm and make sure the patient can tolerate the stepwise reduction in pacing rate. Frequently paced patients, like this one, may find lowering the rate uncomfortable.

Ventricular sensing should also be evaluated. The preferred method for assessing ventricular sensitivity in a dual-chamber pacemaker is to extend the AV delay to allow more "lag time" for an intrinsic event to occur. As a rule of thumb, an AV delay of 300 ms or higher should be temporarily programmed.

The nuts and bolts of paced ECG interpretation: is 1 mV more or less sensitive than 2 mV?

A pacemaker set to a ventricular sensitivity setting of 1 mV means that an intrinsic ventricular event has to be at least 1 mV before the pacemaker will "see" it. If the ventricular sensitivity is changed to 2 mV, the intrinsic waveform now has to be at least 2 mV high before the pacemaker can see it. Thus, *the higher the mV setting, the less sensitive the pacemaker.*

As a rule of thumb, when the pacemaker is undersensing, it should be made more sensitive and the mV setting should be decreased. Conversely, when the pacemaker is oversensing, it should be made less sensitive and the mV setting increased.

MODERATE TRACING #11

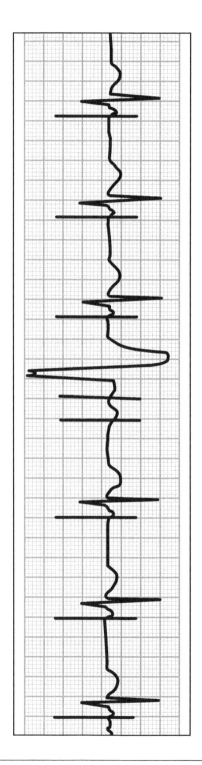

The Nuts and Bolts of Paced ECG Interpretation, 1st edition. By Tom Kenny.
Published 2009 by Blackwell Publishing, ISBN: 978-1-4501-8404-5.

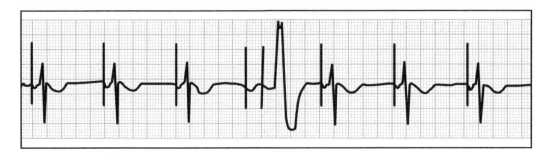

Mode

This is dual-chamber pacing.

Rate

For dual-chamber pacing, measure the atrial pacing interval (AP-AP) to assess the pacing rate. In this case, the atrial pacing interval (AP-AP) is 1000 ms (60 ppm), an appropriate rate.

Capture

At first glance, atrial capture appears to be appropriate. Every atrial output spike results in a depolarization, inhibits the atrial output, and resets device timing. But there is an even better way to confirm appropriate atrial capture in this strip. The AP-VS intervals will be consistent across the strip when there is true atrial capture. That's the case here, so atrial capture is definitely appropriate.

There is only one ventricular spike on this strip and it does not capture. However, it is followed by a ventricular escape beat. Was that beat the result of the spike or an independent event? Actually, this is a case of a *loss of ventricular capture followed by a ventricular escape beat*. Here is how I reached my conclusion:

- The interval between the spike and the event is quite long. With calipers, it looks like just a bit under 200 ms. While I cannot tell you a specific number for how many milliseconds might elapse between a spike and a resulting captured beat, the timing should be virtually immediate. The 200-ms "gap" between pacemaker spike and ventricular event is far too long for capture.
- The morphology of the event looks more typical of an escape beat (very large, very tall, wide,

notched) than a paced event (which is also large and wide, but looks more bizarre).
- The timing of the event would be typical for an escape beat. The pacemaker has just tried to pace the ventricle but did not capture; in the absence of ventricular activity, the heart attempts to beat on its own. This is an escape beat which typically has a very large, widened, and unusual-looking morphology. Looking at the waveform, this is not a beat that conducted down over the AV node to the ventricles; this is a true ventricular escape beat.

Sensing

Atrial sensing cannot be evaluated on this strip since all atrial events are paced.

Ventricular sensing appears appropriate across this strip, if we leave out the escape beat for now. Intrinsic ventricular events cause the ventricular output to be withheld and reset device timing.

Did the pacemaker sense the escape beat? Measuring out the timing cycles, it appears that it did not. This intrinsic event had no effect on timing at all. Of course, it occurred within about 200 ms of the spike, so it is quite likely that it "fell into" the device's ventricular refractory period. If we had annotations on this strip, we would see no VS annotation for this event. The pacemaker failed to "see" it, which is actually appropriate device behavior. Ventricular sensing is appropriate!

Underlying rhythm

The patient has sinus node dysfunction and slow AV conduction. Actually, his underlying rhythm looks pretty good!

What to do next

The most immediate need is to restore ventricular capture. Conduct a ventricular pacing test. It is likely that the ventricular output parameters (pulse amplitude and pulse width) will require some adjustment. Atrial sensing cannot be evaluated from this strip, so atrial sensing should be tested as well and, if necessary, atrial sensitivity might be adjusted.

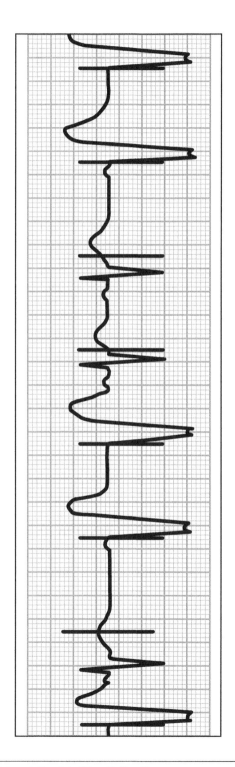

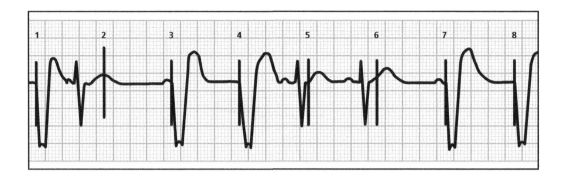

Mode

This comes from a VVI pacemaker.

Rate

The pacing interval (VP-VP) is 800 ms, which works out to be a pacing rate of around 75 ppm. That would be appropriate for a single-chamber system.

Capture

This is a VVI strip, so we will only look at ventricular capture. There are some events on this strip that show appropriate ventricular capture (the first, third, fourth, seventh, and eighth spikes). However, there are three ventricular spikes which do not capture.

Naturally, we have to ask ourselves: should we have expected those ventricular spikes to capture the ventricle? In the fifth and sixth cases, the ventricular spike occurs in such close proximity to the intrinsic ventricular depolarization that the ventricular myocardium was physiologically refractory. Capture was impossible. These are two examples of functional non-capture, which means that we should investigate ventricular undersensing.

However, the second ventricular spike is debatable. The spike occurs during the T-wave but if we measure where the spike appears with respect to the onset of the ventricular depolarization, the interval is about 360 ms. After 360 ms following an intrinsic event, the spike should have captured the ventricular myocardium. While there are no hard and fast rules, in general, the ventricular myocardium is physiologically refractory for about 250 to 300 ms following the onset of the depolarization. This is an example of ventricular non-capture.

Thus, this strip shows several examples of proper capture, a couple of instances of functional non-capture, and one example of failure to capture. It only takes one non-capture event to make us say that overall, capture is not appropriate.

Sensing

There are only three intrinsic ventricular events on this strip, but none of them are properly sensed. They neither inhibit the ventricular output (which occurs right after the intrinsic event) nor do they reset device timing. Ventricular sensing is not appropriate.

Underlying rhythm

The patient has sinus node dysfunction and slow AV conduction. Look closely at the paced rhythm – the pacemaker is probably a VVI device but with a failure to sense properly, this pacemaker is operating in functional VOO mode.

What to do next

Before we move to our next steps, we need to establish why this pacemaker is functioning in VOO mode. Here are the "usual suspects" for asynchronous pacing.

- Asynchronous pacing is typical when a magnet is applied to the device. However, that is very unlikely in this case, because we would expect to see a rate increase with magnet mode.
- Another possibility is that the device might have gone into a reset function or safety pacing. This occurs in the presence of interference; rather than subject the patient to possible device interference,

the pacemaker will revert to asynchronous pacing in such cases to assure that, at a minimum, the patient receives some pacing support even in the presence of interference.

- Inappropriate programming could explain the asynchronous pacing; that is, somebody permanently programmed the pacemaker to VOO. That would be highly unusual but could happen if a test required VOO pacing and the device was never restored to original parameters.
- Another explanation is persistent inappropriate sensing. The device may be programmed to VVI but if sensing is always inappropriate, the pacemaker will operate asynchronously. Although I listed this last, it is actually the most likely cause.

First, use a programmer to determine that the device is set to VVI pacing (not permanently programmed to VOO) and that it is not in magnet mode or some reset or safety mode. If it is, reprogram it to VVI. If the pacemaker is set to VVI pacing already, then we know that the issue is persistent ventricular undersensing.

Evaluate ventricular sensing and adjust sensitivity parameter settings. Ventricular capture should also be evaluated and output parameters adjusted.

The nuts and bolts of paced ECG interpretation: why asynchronous pacing?

Asynchronous pacing is not a desirable choice for pacing except in very specific situations. As a result, whenever you run into VOO, AOO, or DOO pacing in the clinic, you should investigate it thoroughly. While asynchronous pacing can be appropriate in certain instances, it is only appropriate for very short durations. You do not want to leave your patients long-term in asynchronous modes.

Asynchronous pacing occurs during magnet application along with specifically defined other changes (set forth in the pacemaker's technical manual), usually a rate increase.

Asynchronous pacing usually occurs when the device is subject to a lot of interference and goes into a backup or safety mode. In such cases, the device stays in the asynchronous mode until it can be reprogrammed at the clinic.

Asynchronous pacing is also useful in some testing situations but should usually be programmed using the "temporary" parameter settings. When you use "temporary" parameters, the programmer automatically restores the original parameter settings when the test is completed. Many clinicians reprogram devices for tests, which is fine, but it means that the device has to be manually programmed back to the original parameters when the test is over. Although very rare, it has happened that some pacemaker patients leave the clinic with devices still functioning at test parameters. That is why I urge clinicians to rely on "temporary" programming for all tests.

Asynchronous pacing can also occur in the presence of persistent sensing problems, which is the case with this strip.

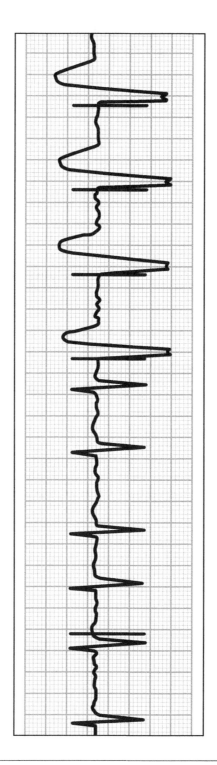

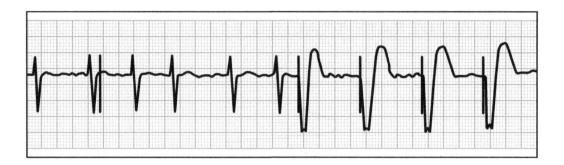

Mode

This comes from a VVI pacemaker.

Rate

The pacing interval (VP-VP) is 800 ms, which works out to be a pacing rate of around 75 ppm. That would be appropriate for a single-chamber system.

Capture

This is a ventricular single-chamber device, so we will only look at ventricular capture. The first ventricular spike fails to capture. However, it occurs immediately following an intrinsic ventricular depolarization, exactly when the ventricular myocardium would be physiologically refractory. This is functional non-capture, which means we are going to have to consider ventricular undersensing. The other ventricular spikes on this strip appear to capture the ventricle appropriately, resulting in immediate ventricular depolarizations with the characteristic paced morphology.

Sensing

The functional non-capture tips us off to ventricular undersensing. The second intrinsic ventricular event is not properly sensed; however, subsequent intrinsic ventricular events inhibit the ventricular output and reset device timing.

Underlying rhythm

This patient has atrial fibrillation (AF) as evidenced by the erratic ventricular rate and the appearance of high-rate intrinsic atrial activity on the strip. The patient has slow AV conduction.

What to do next

Ventricular sensing must be tested and the ventricular sensitivity settings adjusted appropriately. The VVI pacemaker is responding appropriately and as expected to the atrial fibrillation (AF), but the AF should be treated. AF is typically treated with pharmacological therapy, at least in the early stages, although drug therapy is not always effective particularly over the long term.

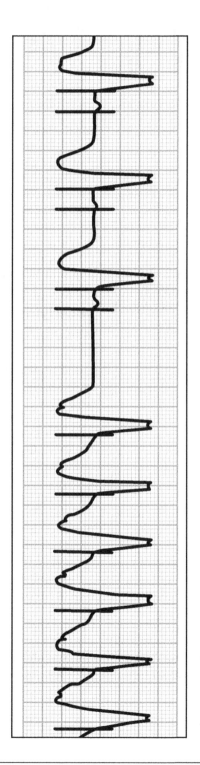

The Nuts and Bolts of Paced ECG Interpretation, 1st edition. By Tom Kenny.
Published 2009 by Blackwell Publishing, ISBN: 978-1-4501-8404-5.

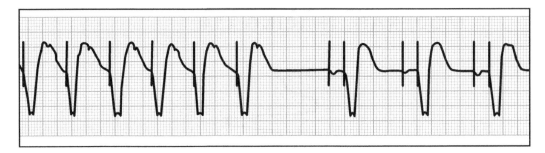

Mode

This comes from a DDD pacemaker.

Rate

The atrial pacing interval (AP-AP) can be measured on the right side of the strip. The interval between atrial spikes there is 1000 ms (60 ppm), which is an appropriate rate. However, the pacemaker was pacing the ventricle very rapidly at the beginning of the strip. The ventricular pacing interval (VP-VP) on the left is just 560 ms (107 ppm). This rapid pacing is followed by a long pause and then base rate pacing. Thus, we have a lot of rate variations to account for.

Capture

Atrial capture is appropriate; so is ventricular capture.

Sensing

The presence of rapid intrinsic atrial events and rapid ventricular pacing indicates atrial tracking. The pacemaker was trying to pace the ventricle in response to high-rate intrinsic atrial events in such a way that 1:1 AV synchrony might be preserved. You may notice that the sensed AV delay interval (AS-VP) is much longer during atrial tracking than during the AP-VP paced events on the right side of the strip. In fact, the AV interval varies during the atrial tracking and at one point appears to be about 320 ms. The paced AV delay at the end of the strip is around 200 ms. The reason the pacemaker violates its own AV delay interval during atrial tracking is because of the maximum tracking rate or Max Track Rate (MTR), an upper rate limit that sets the highest

rate at which the ventricle can be paced in response to intrinsic atrial activity.

Atrial sensing is actually appropriate. The atrial tracking on the left side of the strip and the fact that there is a definite relationship between intrinsic atrial events and the ventricular pacing rate means that the pacemaker is "seeing" and sensing atrial activity properly.

Ventricular sensing cannot be assessed on this strip, since all ventricular events are paced.

Underlying rhythm

The first several events on this strip show pacing at an upper rate limit (MTR). This could occur if the patient's own native atrial rate increased. However, another possibility is that this is pacemaker-mediated tachycardia (PMT).

PMT occurs when a retrograde P-wave "falls into" an endless loop in such a way that the pacemaker actually participates in sustaining a reentry tachycardia. Notice the atrial events on the left side of the strip that the pacemaker was tracking. They occur during the T-wave portion of the preceding ventricular event. Their position suggests that they could be retrograde P-waves. Another hint that that this might have been a PMT is the sudden pause, after which AP-VP pacing at the base rate occurs.

Pacemakers today have algorithms to try to prevent PMTs and then to terminate them if they should occur. Such algorithms usually go into effect after a specified number of PMT events. In this case, it is likely this run of MTR pacing met the PMT criterion, which caused the pacemaker to force a pause and then resume normal base-rate pacing. The pause occurs because the pacemaker abruptly withholds pacing for a long pause and then resumes with an atrial output pulse. (A PMT pause withholds a ventricular output in response to a sensed atrial event, introduces a pause, and then paces the atrium.)

This is a PMT that was successfully broken by a PMT termination algorithm. It is hard to say what this patient's intrinsic rhythm is, but we know he is susceptible to PMTs.

What to do next

Ventricular sensing should be evaluated. The PMT termination algorithm programmed for this patient worked very well; it should be maintained.

This strip tells us that this patient is susceptible to PMTs so, if possible, diagnostic information in the pacemaker should be downloaded to find out what might have triggered this PMT and if other PMTs have occurred recently. The most frequent causes of PMT are PVCs or an abrupt loss of atrial capture. Although atrial capture looks good on this strip, it would be worthwhile to determine if loss of atrial capture caused this particular PMT. For that reason, I would also evaluate atrial capture for this patient, although there are three examples of appropriate atrial capture on this strip.

The nuts and bolts of paced ECG interpretation: managing PMTs

Pacemaker-mediated tachycardia (PMT) is not as common as it used to be, but clinicians still need to know about it. Not all paced patients are susceptible to PMT. To get a PMT, a patient needs to have a dual-chamber pacemaker, retrograde conduction, and then some kind of triggering event (like a premature ventricular contraction or a sudden loss of atrial capture).

Most pacemakers have algorithms to help prevent PMT, which work well in most patients. Since PMTs can cause symptoms and many patients do not tolerate them well, it is advisable to program PMT termination algorithms to go into effect as soon as the pacemaker detects a PMT. If the patient never has a PMT, the algorithm will never go into effect.

These algorithms break the PMT by withholding pacing and then pacing the atrium; this stops the retrograde P-waves from conducting backward and "feeding" the endless loop.

MODERATE TRACING #15

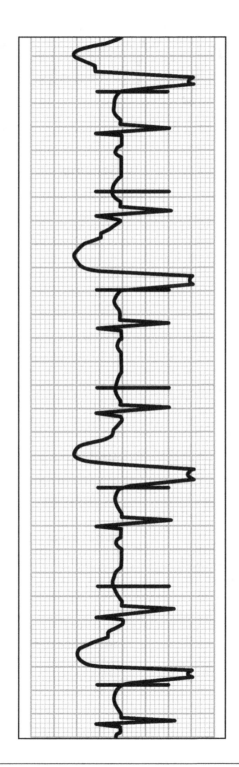

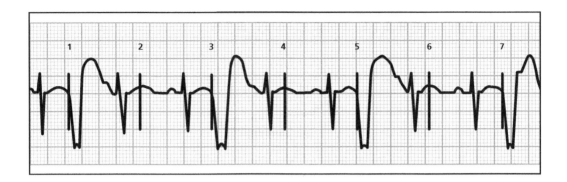

Mode

This comes from a VVI pacemaker.

Rate

The ventricular pacing interval (VP-VP) is around 840 ms (70 ppm), an appropriate rate.

Capture

Every other ventricular spike (first, third, fifth, and seventh) capture the ventricle. Note the immediate ventricular depolarization and the widened, bizarre-looking resulting QRS complex.

There are three other ventricular spikes on this strip that do not capture the ventricle. Before we rule non-capture, we need to determine if they should have captured the ventricle. If the spike occurred during the physiological refractory period following depolarization, there is no way the spike could have captured the heart. To determine this, use calipers to measure the interval between the onset of the intrinsic ventricular depolarization and the spike. As a rule of thumb – and there is some leeway here – the ventricle will be physiologically refractory around 250 ms. The second, fourth, and sixth pacing spikes all occur close enough to the onset of the intrinsic event (around 240 ms) to be ruled functional non-capture. This means that ventricular undersensing must be evaluated.

Sensing

The strip shows several intrinsic ventricular events, none of which are properly sensed. In fact, this strip shows functional VOO pacing. Whenever this kind of asynchronous single-chamber mode occurs, we should consider the possibility of magnet mode, backup-reset or noise reversion, permanently programmed asynchronous mode, or persistent ventricular undersensing. While the last one is the most likely scenario, rule out the others by going to a programmer and verifying that the pacemaker is not in magnet mode (not likely since magnet mode typically increases the base rate), not programmed to VOO, and not in backup or safety pacing mode. If it is not, the cause of the asynchronous pacing is persistent ventricular undersensing.

Underlying rhythm

This patient has sinus node dysfunction and slow AV conduction.

What to do next

The cause of the asynchronous pacing must be determined; most likely this is a case of persistent ventricular undersensing. If no other cause of asynchronous pacing can be found, evaluate ventricular sensing and adjust ventricular sensitivity. Observe the paced ECG after these changes are made. It should resolve the undersensing and functional non-capture.

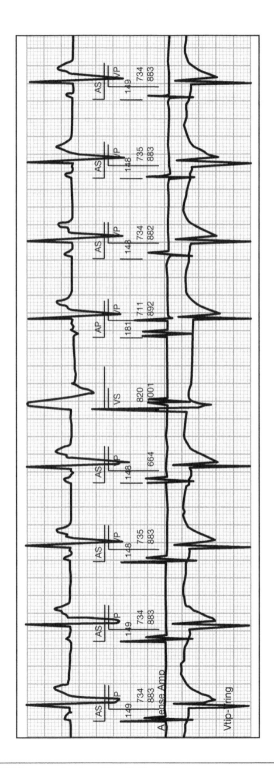

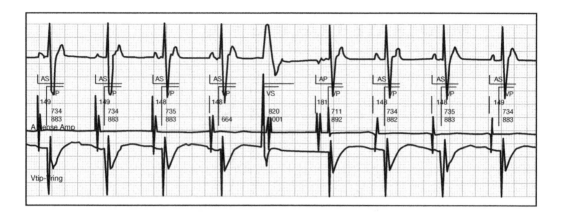

Mode

This is a dual-chamber strip. The pacing spikes are not prominent but the annotations can serve that function here. Note that this strip also contains an atrial and ventricular electrogram, which are the bottom tracings.

Rate

Normally, the atrial pacing interval (AP-AP) would be used to measure the rate of a dual-chamber strip, but this strip provides no such intervals. The ventricular pacing interval (VP-VP) is around 880 ms (70 ppm), an appropriate rate. The rate is consistent except for a long pause after the premature ventricular contraction (PVC). There is one escape interval (VS-VP) and it is 1040 ms (58 bpm). This rate variation must be accounted for in our analysis.

The fact that the long escape interval occurred after the PVC is a clue. This pacemaker is relying on a special algorithm to prevent the PVC from triggering a pacemaker-mediated tachycardia (PMT). The presence of a PVC (which the pacemaker defines as a sensed ventricular event without a preceding paced or sensed atrial event) caused the device to automatically extend the PVARP interval for one cycle. This extension can be seen clearly on the horizontal bar above the VS annotation, which illustrates the duration of the refractory period. This prolonged PVARP affects the timing cycles of the pacemaker and creates this long escape interval.

This particular algorithm extended the refractory period in order to be sure that any retrograde atrial activity would "fall into" the refractory period; that means the pacemaker would not respond to it. This extended PVARP interval is followed by an atrial alert interval which, in this case, times out and results in a paced atrial event. Once the atrium is paced, the device resumes its previous pattern of activity (AS-VP pacing at the base rate).

Capture

There is only one atrial pacing spike on this strip and it appears to capture appropriately. Notice that the paced atrial event has a different morphology from the intrinsic atrial events on the rest of the strip.

Ventricular capture likewise seems to be appropriate.

Sensing

Atrial sensing is functioning properly in that the intrinsic atrial events inhibit the atrial output pulse and reset device timing. The sensed AV delay is consistent at around 150 ms, another indication of appropriate atrial sensing. Last but not least, proper atrial sensing is confirmed by the fact that the annotations (AS) match the strip, meaning the pacemaker is "seeing" things correctly.

There is only one intrinsic ventricular event on this strip, the large premature ventricular contraction (PVC) in the center of the strip. The pacemaker senses it, as confirmed by the fact that the ventricular output pulse is withheld, the event resets device timing, and the pacemaker annotates it as a VS event.

Underlying rhythm

This patient has relatively good sinus node function but slow AV conduction.

What to do next

Atrial capture seems appropriate but should be evaluated since there is only one event on the strip on which we can base our assessment.

Ventricular sensing should also be tested, although what shows up here seems appropriate. This patient experienced a PVC, which launched a PMT-termination algorithm. The success of that algorithm in preventing PMT and restoring normal operation to the pacemaker suggests that it should be left as is, since it seems to be protecting the patient from PMT. If diagnostic reports were accessible, it would be prudent to see how frequently this patient experiences PVCs and PMTs.

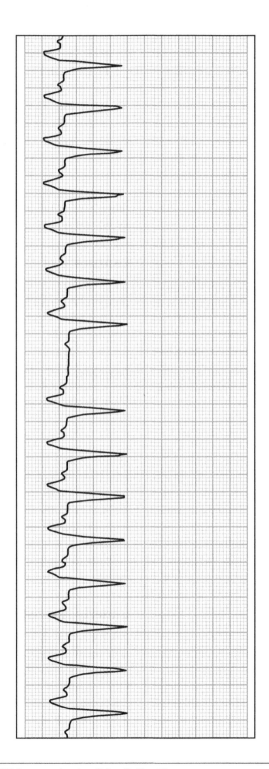

The Nuts and Bolts of Paced ECG Interpretation, 1st edition. By Tom Kenny.
Published 2009 by Blackwell Publishing, ISBN: 978-1-4501-8404-5.

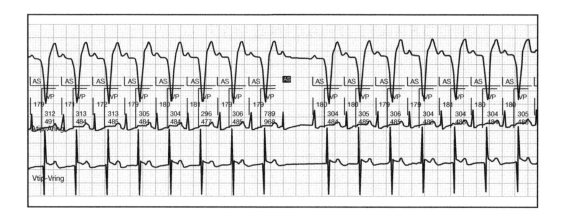

Mode

This is a dual-chamber strip. While the annotations confirm it, the strip alone provides some important clues. Notice the sensed AV delay (AS-VP) is consistent at around 180 ms across the strip. A consistent AV interval suggests proper atrial sensing. The appearance of the strip looks like a run of atrial tracking, followed by a pause, and then the resumption of atrial tracking. That would only occur with a DDD device.

Rate

There is no atrial pacing interval to measure, but the ventricular pacing interval (VP-VP) is quite short: 480 ms (125 ppm). This is much too fast for a programmed base rate, further indicating that the pacemaker is tracking intrinsic atrial activity. In fact, 125 ppm would be a typical value for the Maximum Tracking Rate or MTR.

Notice there is a long pause in the middle of the strip of about 1000 ms (60 ppm). This pause was likely caused by the pacemaker itself in an effort to break what it thought was a pacemaker-mediated tachycardia (PMT). The pacemaker extended the PVARP interval (notice the long horizontal line showing the refractory period); an intrinsic atrial event (shown in the annotations as an AS in a black box) "fell into" the prolonged refractory period. However, after the extended PVARP, atrial tracking at the MTR resumed. There are two possible explanations for this: either the PMT termination algo-

rithm failed or this patient did not have a PMT in the first place.

Capture

Atrial capture cannot be evaluated from this strip, since all of the atrial events are sensed.

Ventricular capture, on the other hand, appears to be appropriate.

Sensing

Atrial sensing is appropriate. Atrial events inhibit the atrial output and reset device timing, not to mention the fact that they appear properly in the annotations. The AS event in the black box occurred during the extended refractory period. Although the pacemaker did actually "see" this intrinsic atrial event (that's why it's annotated in the black box), the fact that it occurred during the refractory period means that the pacemaker will ignore it.

Ventricular sensing cannot be evaluated in this tracing.

Underlying rhythm

This patient has slow AV conduction. However, the rapid atrial tracking is of concern. The pacemaker thought this was PMT, which is why it activated a PMT-termination algorithm that automatically prolonged the PVARP. Just looking at the first half of the strip, it does look a lot like a classic PMT.

However, the fact that it immediately starts up again after the pause means that it probably was not a true PMT. In fact, it may be sinus tachycardia.

To confirm this suspicion, look at the VP-AS interval. In a PMT, the VP-AS interval is consistent because the AS is supported by the pacemaker's timing circuits and thus the VP "drives" the PMT pacing. In a sinus tachycardia, there is a bit more variation in VP-AS intervals, since the AS activity (the heart's own intrinsic atrial rhythm) drives the pacing. In this strip the variation in VP-AS is slight, but notice that the VP-AS intervals on the right side of the strip are slightly shorter than those at the far left. This confirms that this is sinus tachycardia rather than a PMT.

What to do next

Atrial capture and ventricular sensing should be evaluated. If necessary, atrial output settings and ventricular sensitivity settings may have to be adjusted.

If diagnostic reports are available, it would be valuable to look at the patient's history of intrinsic atrial rates to see if sinus tachycardia is a common occurrence. Furthermore, it would also be wise to review prior episodes of PMT (both real and alleged). If the events on this strip are typical for this patient, the PMT termination algorithm could be turned off to prevent it from interrupting physiologically useful atrial tracking.

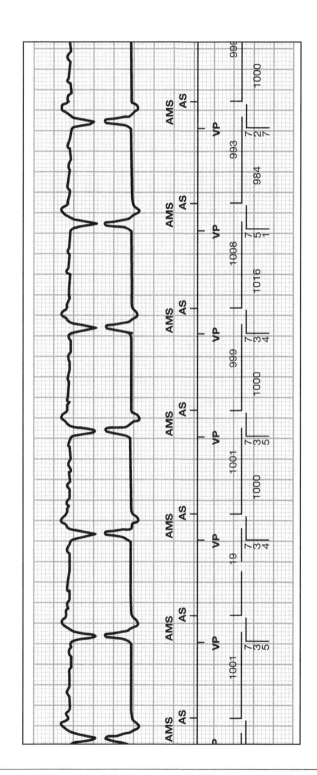

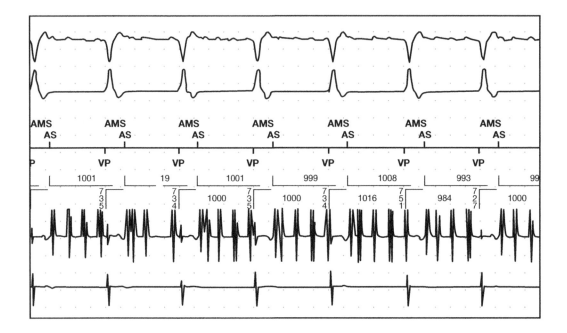

Mode

The annotations show that this is a dual-chamber strip. But the annotations also show that AMS or automatic mode switching is going on! Notice that while the pacemaker is sensing intrinsic atrial activity (AS), the sensed AV delay interval (AS-VP) is not being applied; the sensed AV delay interval (AS-VP) is quite long, over 600 ms! Although the pacemaker is sensing intrinsic atrial activity, the device is pacing the ventricle without any regard to it. Thus, this is a dual-chamber device that is not tracking the atrium. That would be consistent with AMS.

Rate

Since there is no atrial pacing interval (AP-AP) on this strip, the ventricular pacing interval (VP-VP) will have to be used to assess the rate. The annotations show that it measures about 1000 ms (60 ppm), which is an appropriate rate.

Capture

Atrial capture cannot be evaluated from this strip. Ventricular capture appears to be appropriate.

The nuts and bolts of paced ECG interpretation: ECGs and EGMs

The programmer for most pacemakers will often present the clinician with several tracings plus annotations and intervals; it can be confusing to orient oneself. This example was taken from a device programmer. The top two tracings are surface ECGs; the two different leads offered show different "views" of the same cardiac activity.

The annotations indicate how the pacemaker "interpreted" what it saw. Intervals are handy tools and replace old-fashioned calipers (which I still use, by the way).

The two bottom tracings are intracardiac electrograms, giving an "inside view" of the heart. The upper EGM is atrial and the lower one is ventricular. All events are aligned so that you can evaluate at any point in time what the two surface ECG perspectives recorded, how the pacemaker interpreted the event, and finally what the intracardiac electrograms reveal from inside the heart. While these things should all tell the same story, sometimes clues emerge on the intracardiac EGM that are not apparent on the surface ECG.

Sensing

Whenever the AMS algorithm goes into effect, it is crucial to evaluate whether or not it was launched appropriately. Appropriate mode switching occurs in the presence of intrinsic high-rate atrial activity. Looking just at the surface ECG, only a few intrinsic atrial events are annotated. Based strictly on the annotations, AMS is inappropriate. However, it may occur that not every event the pacemaker interpreted will be annotated on the strip.

That's where the atrial intracardiac electrogram (next-to-last tracing) comes in handy. Here it is apparent that there is a great deal of rapid intrinsic atrial activity. While a lot of this intrinsic atrial activity appears on the uppermost surface ECG, many of these events are not evident on the second ECG and they are not fully annotated. From the atrial electrogram, it is clear that mode switching is appropriate. This is a good example why clinicians should make use of all of the information available (including annotations, intervals, surface ECGs, and EGMs).

What about atrial sensing? Since the device is currently operating in AMS, appropriate atrial sensing cannot be evaluated in this interim mode. A pacemaker in AMS mode will not track intrinsic atrial activity.

Ventricular sensing cannot be evaluated from this strip.

Underlying rhythm

This patient has rapid intrinsic atrial activity and slow AV conduction.

What to do next

Atrial and ventricular sensing should be evaluated, which requires the pacemaker to revert back to a "normal" dual-chamber mode. This may not be readily possible because of the high-rate intrinsic atrial activity going on.

While AMS is appropriate, it may not be the best solution if the patient has chronic atrial tachycardia. If diagnostic reports can be accessed, evaluate the frequency of mode switch episodes and the patient's intrinsic atrial rates. For occasional episodes of atrial tachycardia, AMS is a great solution; for chronic atrial tachycardia, the patient may be better served by permanently programming the pacemaker to a non-tracking mode.

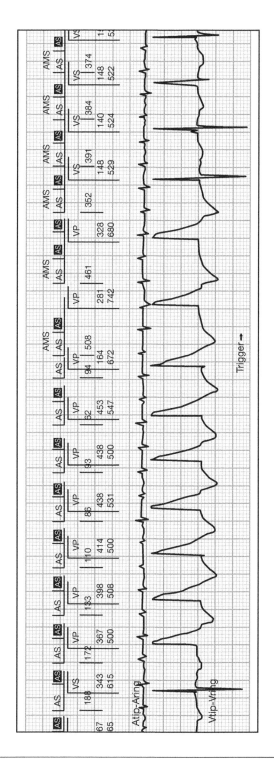

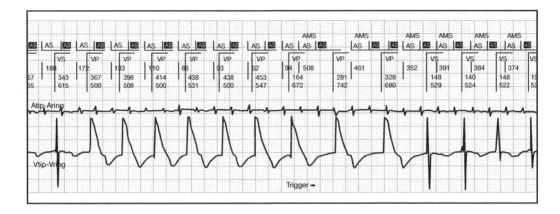

Mode

This is a stored annotated intracardiac electrogram from a dual-chamber device. The AMS annotations show that this strip was stored in memory because the pacemaker initiated mode switching. The main question is whether AMS is appropriate.

Rate

The AMS algorithm is governed by the intrinsic atrial rate. It is quite rapid at the left of the strip (the intrinsic atrial intervals are around 280 ms (214 bpm) but the rate is erratic. Measuring with calipers on the atrial electrogram (next-to-bottom tracing), there are intrinsic atrial intervals ranging from 220 ms to 560 ms (107 to 273 bpm). This kind of seemingly chaotic atrial rhythm is consistent with atrial fibrillation (AF). Considering these rates and the nature of the rhythm, AMS was definitely appropriate.

Before the device began to mode switch, ventricular pacing was quite rapid because the pacemaker was tracking the atrial rate. Ventricular pacing intervals on the left of the strip are around 500 ms (120 ppm). The fact that ventricular pacing only occurred up to 120 ppm suggests that the maximum tracking rate or MTR upper rate limit was set to 120 ppm – a very typical parameter setting for the MTR.

When the device enters AMS (as shown by the annotations), the first complete ventricular pacing interval in AMS is about 720 ms, measured by calipers. This works out to be a rate of about 83 ppm. This is too high for a normal base rate, but it is likely this device has a special mode switch base rate. Some AMS algorithms allow the clinician to program an interim base rate for the duration of the

AMS episode; this AMS base rate is higher than the programmed base rate. An AMS base rate of around 80 ppm would be typical.

The nuts and bolts of paced ECG interpretation: smoothing out mode switching with AMS base rates

Some AMS algorithms allow the programming of a special interim base rate during the AMS episode. This AMS base rate is typically higher than the regular base rate but not as high as the maximum tracking rate. The purpose of this interim AMS base rate is to help smooth out the sometimes abrupt rate transitions that can occur during AMS.

Consider, for a second, the heart rate before and during AMS. Right before AMS goes into effect, the patient will be tracking a high intrinsic atrial rate right up to the maximum tracking rate. This is typically programmed to a value of around 100 to 120 ppm.

When AMS goes into effect, in just one beat, the device stops tracking the atrium but continues to pace the ventricle. This can take a patient from MTR pacing (100 or 120 ppm) to base rate pacing (60 or 70 ppm) in one beat!

Many AMS patients report feeling these "rate bumps" and find them unpleasant. The use of an AMS base rate allows the device to transition to faster-than-base rate pacing during AMS. For example, if the AMS base rate had been programmed to 80 ppm (a typical value), the patient would experience atrial tracking to about 120 ppm, then AMS base rate pacing at around 80 ppm, and finally AMS exit to 60 ppm.

Capture

Atrial capture cannot be evaluated from this strip, since all atrial activity is intrinsic.

The intracardiac ventricular electrogram can help evaluate ventricular capture. Notice the VP annotations all correspond to events on the ventricular electrogram of a particular morphology, while the VS annotations align with ventricular events of a different morphology. This presence of VP annotations and matching ventricular events of a single morphology indicates appropriate ventricular capture.

Sensing

Atrial sensing appears to be appropriate in that the atrial activity is annotated (notice that atrial events on the atrial electrogram can all be accounted for in the annotations), the atrial activity inhibits the atrial output pulse, and the device enters AMS in response to the presence of rapid sensed atrial events. The AS events in the black boxes are atrial events that occur in the refractory period. The pacemaker does not respond to these the same way it would to an AS event in the alert period, but they are still counted to help the pacemaker decide when to activate AMS.

Ventricular sensing appears to be appropriate. There are a few intrinsic ventricular events at the end of this strip that are properly annotated (VS), inhibit the ventricular output pulse, and reset device timing.

Underlying rhythm

This patient has rapid intrinsic atrial activity and slow AV conduction.

What to do next

Everything on this strip seems to be appropriate. The entry into AMS was appropriate, given the rapid intrinsic atrial activity, and capture and sensing seemed to be functioning properly. Atrial pacing could not be evaluated from this strip (and may be difficult to test at all, given the patient's atrial tachyarrhythmia) and should be assessed, if possible. Otherwise, device function looks fine.

The biggest concern in a strip like this is finding a better way to manage the patient's atrial tachyarrhythmia. Check diagnostic reports to see if this patient frequently experiences high-rate intrinsic atrial activity and how often mode switching is activated. If such tachyarrhythmias and rapid ventricular pacing or AMS occur frequently, this patient might be a candidate for anti-arrhythmic drug therapy to better control the atrial tachyarrhythmia.

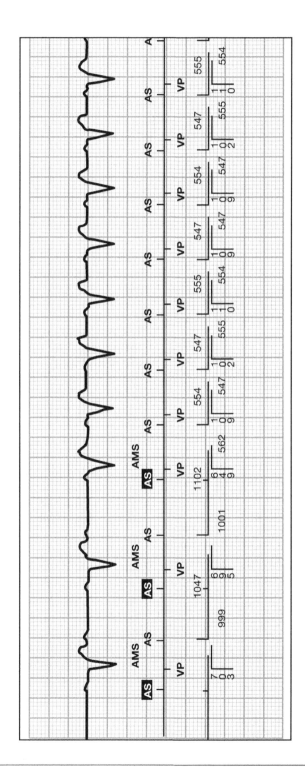

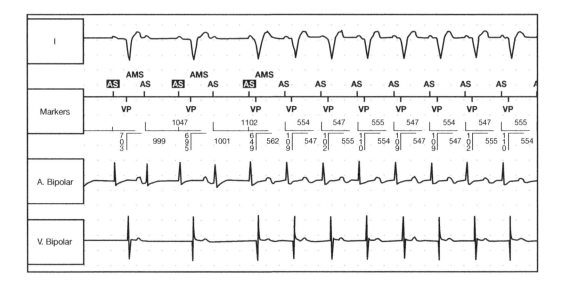

Mode

This is stored data retrieved from the programmer. The annotations show that the pacemaker is exiting AMS (auto mode switch). Whenever the AMS algorithm is in effect, the systematic approach to ECG interpretation will help us decide if the AMS feature was functioning properly and was deployed appropriately.

Rate

Normally, the atrial pacing interval (AP-AP) governs the rate in a dual-chamber pacemaker, but this example shows consistent atrial tracking. The ventricular pacing interval during the AMS algorithm is 1000 ms (60 ppm), an appropriate base rate for a dual-chamber pacemaker. When the pacemaker exits AMS, the device begins tracking the atrium at around 550 ms (109 ppm). This is a reasonable rate for atrial tracking, and it falls within the usual settings of a maximum tracking rate (MTR) upper rate limit, which would typically be programmed somewhere between 100 and 120 ppm. Thus, rate looks appropriate.

This information depicts exit from AMS. AMS ends when the patient's intrinsic atrial rate slows to below the MTR. The intrinsic atrial interval lengthened slightly here and the device exited AMS. Once the intrinsic atrial rate slowed to below 110 ppm

(a likely MTR setting), the pacemaker exited AMS. This is appropriate and the expected behavior of the device.

The nuts and bolts of paced ECG interpretation: appropriate AMS entry and exit

Auto mode switching (AMS) is a very useful feature but whenever it goes into effect, clinicians should evaluate whether it was initiated and ended appropriately. If AMS is programmed on, it should go into effect whenever the patient's intrinsic atrial rate exceeds a certain rate limit. That rate limit is set by the atrial tachycardia detection rate or ATDR. For instance, if the ATDR is programmed to 120 bpm, the pacemaker should mode switch when the intrinsic atrial rate exceeds 120 bpm.

The patient should exit AMS whenever his intrinsic atrial rate falls below the programmed maximum tracking rate or MTR. For example, if the MTR was programmed to 100 ppm, then the patient will not exit AMS until his intrinsic atrial rate is 100 bpm or below.

Inappropriate AMS entry and exit can occur in the presence of atrial oversensing, double-counting, or interference.

Capture

All of the atrial activity shown here is intrinsic, so capture cannot be assessed from this information.

Ventricular capture is functioning properly. Using the VP annotations as surrogates for pacemaker spikes (which are sometimes hard to pick out on a programmer screen), ventricular spikes result in ventricular depolarizations. Every VP "spike" results in a depolarization and all of these paced events share the same morphology.

Sensing

Atrial sensing is appropriate. In this particular configuration, I would look at atrial sensing first on the atrial intracardiac electrogram (next-to-last tracing). There is nothing but intrinsic atrial activity on this strip, and these atrial events are all properly annotated as AS events. Knowing where they are, it is easier to identify them on the programmer's surface ECG (top tracing). Thus, atrial sensing seems to be appropriate.

But notice that there is more than just the tall, pointed intrinsic atrial events on the atrial electrogram! There are also some lower rounded events. This is an example of how the atrial channel is registering the activity on the ventricular channel. If the pacemaker had "seen" these and annotated them, this would be an example of far-field T-wave oversensing. However, they are too small to be sensed by the pacemaker even though they actually do show up on the atrial intracardiac electrogram. It is not at all unusual for the atrial electrogram to pick up the relatively "loud" and large signals from the ventricle. If they do not interfere with proper device function, as is the case here, this is not a problem. You can tell that these far-field signals do not interfere with the pacemaker's function because they do not show up on the surface ECG, they are not annotated, and they don't reset timing intervals.

Ventricular sensing cannot be assessed from these tracings.

Underlying rhythm

This patient has an atrial tachyarrhythmia and slow AV conduction.

What to do next

Atrial capture and ventricular sensing should be tested, if possible. AMS seems to be appropriate, but it would be useful to check diagnostic reports to see how frequently this patient experiences atrial tachyarrhythmias. This atrial tachyarrhythmia is not chaotic and irregular like classic atrial fibrillation (AF); this is good news in that AF is a very challenging and serious condition. On the other hand, the regularity of this particular atrial tachyarrhythmia suggests that it could be a sinus tachycardia.

Sinus tachycardia is often appropriate intrinsic cardiac behavior. For instance, it would be appropriate for a pacemaker patient doing physical exercise to have a sinus tachycardia. During a fever or any periods of exertion, sinus tachycardia is the body's appropriate and expected cardiac rhythm.

Interview the patient. If this patient is active or recently had a fever, this might be a true sinus tachycardia and the body's appropriate (and needed) response. If the pacemaker mode switches during such rhythms, the patient is deprived of the natural rate support he needs.

It can be difficult to distinguish between an exercise sinus tachycardia and a more pathological atrial tachyarrhythmia, particularly when only a few complexes are available for analysis. If the pacemaker is rate responsive, activity should have initiated sensor-driven pacing (rate response) and precluded the AMS episode. This pacemaker is likely not programmed to a rate-responsive mode, but if it is, then the rate-responsive parameters should be checked. If the pacemaker is rate responsive and programmed appropriately, then this episode was not initiated by activity and, therefore, is not an exercise-induced sinus tachycardia. It is likely just an atrial tachyarrhythmia that happens to have regular intrinsic atrial intervals.

If this patient is active but does not have a rate-responsive pacemaker, download diagnostic reports on AMS episodes. This patient may be mode switching during periods when he actually needs more rapid rate support. In that case, AMS should be turned off. Active patients are good candidates for rate-responsive pacemakers when the device is revised.

Tough

TOUGH TRACING #1

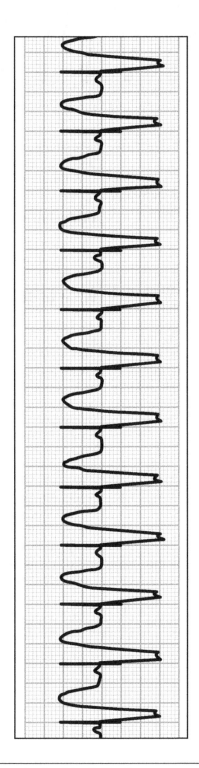

The Nuts and Bolts of Paced ECG Interpretation, 1st edition. By Tom Kenny.
Published 2009 by Blackwell Publishing, ISBN: 978-1-4501-8404-5.

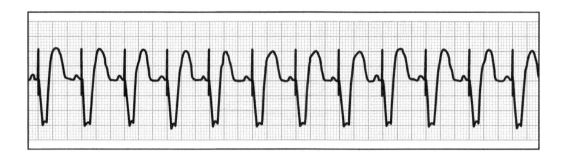

Mode

This rhythm strip comes from a DDD pacemaker. While only ventricular spikes appear on the tracing, the rapid ventricular pacing is being "driven" by the rapid intrinsic atrial rate.

Rate

The ventricular pacing interval (VP-VP) is around 600 ms (100 ppm), which means that the pacemaker is pacing the ventricle above the programmed base rate. Above-base-rate pacing can occur but only in specific instances, such as if the sensor (rate re-sponse) is controlling the rate or if the pacemaker is tracking a rapid intrinsic atrial rate. The presence of high-rate intrinsic atrial activity here means that this is atrial tracking.

Capture

Atrial capture cannot be assessed from this strip.
Ventricular capture is appropriate.

Sensing

Atrial sensing is appropriate, in that the pacemaker not only withholds an atrial output in the presence of an intrinsic atrial event, it also times the ventricular pacing spike to the sensed atrial event.
Ventricular sensing cannot be evaluated here.

Underlying rhythm

The patient has a rapid intrinsic atrial rate and slow AV conduction.

What to do next

If the patient was in the clinic, it would be an excellent first step to ask the patient how he felt and if he had any symptoms. Not every patient tolerates ventricular pacing at 100 ppm. Diagnostic data should be downloaded from the pacemaker to evaluate just how frequently this kind of pacing occurred. If the patient has persistent high intrinsic atrial rates, he is going to experience this kind of pacing for prolonged periods of time. Even if the patient only has atrial tracking with rapid ventricular pacing occasionally and tolerates it without complaint, it should still be minimized.

The first steps would be systematic. Atrial capture and ventricular sensing should be tested and, if necessary, pacemaker parameters adjusted.

A clinical decision must be made in terms of how to manage a patient with intrinsic high-rate atrial activity.

The nuts and bolts of paced ECG interpretation: how to manage high-rate intrinsic activity in the dual-chamber pacemaker patient

There are a few options, each presenting its own advantages and drawbacks.

- If high-rate intrinsic atrial activity is relatively rare and well tolerated, program the maximum tracking rate (MTR) setting to a tolerable rate (such as 100 ppm). This keeps ventricular pacing within reasonable limits. The drawback is that if the patient spends more and more time in high-rate increasing atrial activity, he will be paced at the MTR for longer and longer periods of time.
- Mode switching can be programmed, which will automatically turn off atrial tracking when a cutoff rate is achieved. This prevents rapid ventricular pacing, but can cause some mode switching "rate bumps." If the algorithm allows for a mode switch interim base rate, use that to prevent abrupt changes in pacing rate as the patient enters mode switching. Mode switching deprives the patient of 1:1 AV synchrony, but it prevents rapid ventricular pacing.
- A non-tracking mode can be permanently

programmed, but, as is the case with mode switching, the patient may lose the benefits of AV synchrony. On the other hand, it may be the best solution if high-rate intrinsic atrial activity is frequent and prolonged.

- Many pacemakers offer algorithms to help manage rapid atrial rates, such as overdrive atrial pacing or the AF Suppression™ algorithm from St. Jude Medical. While not all patients are candidates for such algorithms, they work well in patients with certain types of atrial tachyarrhythmias and help "control" the atrium, suppress atrial tachyarrhythmias before they can start, and avoid rapid ventricular pacing.
- Intrinsic high-rate atrial activity can also be addressed with drug therapy. Anti-arrhythmic agents can be highly effective but they do not work equally well in all patients, and they can have serious side effects. Anti-arrhythmic drugs should be monitored closely since adjustments in dosage are frequently required over time.

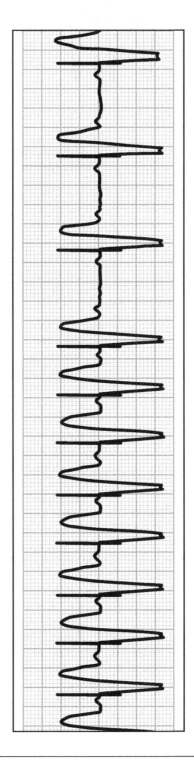

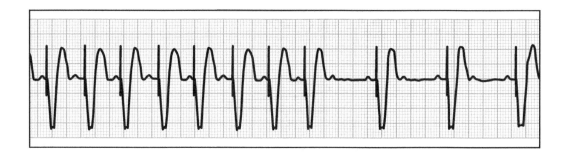

Mode

This strip comes from a DDD pacemaker. Although only ventricular spikes are shown on the tracing, it is clear that the spikes are coordinated to the atrial events.

Rate

On the left side, the ventricular pacing interval (VP-VP) is about 520 ms (115 ppm). The rapid rate then slows abruptly to 1000 ms (60 ppm). The latter rate is an appropriate base rate. Our systematic analysis must account for whatever slowed the rapid ventricular pacing to base rate pacing.

Capture

Atrial capture cannot be assessed from this strip.
    Ventricular capture is appropriate.

Sensing

Atrial sensing is appropriate in that the intrinsic atrial events inhibit the atrial output, and it appears that in both the "slow" and "fast" sections of this tracing, the pacemaker is trying to coordinate some atrial activity to ventricular pacing.

The patient has a rapid intrinsic rate; it is about 115 bpm and is accelerating slightly as you go from left to right on the strip. This is an atrial tachyarrhythmia, although it is at the slower end of the atrial tachycardia spectrum. At first, the pacemaker tracks the atrial rate and paces the ventricle in response. However, right before the ventricular rate slows down, there is an intrinsic atrial event that is not sensed. Had it been sensed, the pacemaker would have tried to track it by delivering a ventricu-

> ### The nuts and bolts of paced ECG interpretation: 1:1 AV synchrony
>
> The healthy heart maintains 1:1 AV synchrony, that is, one atrial depolarization for each and every ventricular depolarization. This allows for the optimal atrial contribution to ventricular filling. Conduction disorders and sinus node dysfunction can disrupt AV synchrony, which, in turn, can quickly lead to less-than-ideal hemodynamics for the patient.
>
> DDD pacemakers strive to maintain 1:1 AV synchrony as much as possible by allowing atrial tracking (pacing the ventricle in response to rapid intrinsic atrial activity, at least within certain rate limits). However, atrial tracking becomes counterproductive at very high rates. In such cases, the DDD pacemaker reverts to a variety of "upper rate behaviors" to help manage the system. These include pacemaker Wenckebach (which actually mimics physiological Wenckebach) and pacemaker block. Pacemaker block is usually described as 2:1 or 3:1 block, etc. In 2:1 pacemaker block, there is a ventricular paced event for every second intrinsic atrial event.

lar output spike. In fact, on the right side of the strip there are several atrial events that are not sensed. They occur right after the T-wave.

Before ruling this a case of atrial undersensing, the question must be asked: should the pacemaker have sensed these atrial events? The answer is no. These atrial events "fell into" the post-ventricular atrial refractory period (PVARP) and, thus, it is appropriate and expected that the pacemaker did not respond to them.

The nuts and bolts of paced ECG interpretation: the world according to TARP

TARP or the total atrial refractory period is not a programmable parameter for a dual-chamber pacemaker, yet it is a very important timing cycle. TARP is calculated by adding the programmed AV delay to the post-ventricular atrial refractory period (PVARP). Taken together, TARP defines the total amount of time that the pacemaker will not respond to events on the atrial channel. For example, if the AV delay is programmed to 250 ms and the PVARP is set to 200 ms, the TARP value is 450 ms (250 + 200 = 450).

TARP defines the point at which the pacemaker will go into 2:1 block (that is, allow two atrial events for every one paced ventricular event). In the above example, a TARP value of 450 ms means that when the intrinsic atrial rate hits 133 bpm (450 ms), the pacemaker will go into 2:1 block.

Many programmers will display the point at which 2:1 block is reached, but you can calculate it yourself if you know the paced AV delay and the PVARP.

In this example, when the intrinsic atrial rate reached a cycle of about 520 ms (115), 2:1 block set in. That means the patient's intrinsic atrial rate exceeded the TARP value. TARP in this case was about 520 ms. Although we cannot determine exactly what the AV delay and PVARP values were, their total was 520.

Ventricular sensing cannot be assessed from this strip.

Underlying rhythm

This patient has an atrial tachyarrhythmia and slow AV conduction. The atrial arrhythmia may be intermittent and in this strip it's around 115 bpm.

What to do next

Atrial capture and ventricular sensing must be assessed and, if necessary, parameter changes made to assure reliable capture and sensing. If the atrial tachyarrhythmia is persistent, it may be difficult or even impossible to evaluate proper atrial capture.

Of special concern is the 2:1 block. If the patient is available, he should be asked about his symptoms. Diagnostic data from the pacemaker should be retrieved to better evaluate the frequency and nature of the atrial tachyarrhythmia.

As a general rule of thumb, it is probably better for the patient to experience atrial tracking with a rapid ventricular response than 2:1 block … at least up to a point. If it seems that the patient could tolerate more rapid ventricular pacing, the TARP value could be shortened to extend the period of time before 2:1 block sets in. This requires good clinical judgment. TARP cannot be programmed directly, but the result could be attained by reducing either the AV delay interval or the PVARP setting or both.

For example, if the clinician decided that 2:1 block should commence only after atrial tracking with ventricular pacing at 120 ppm:
- Calculate the interval (120 ppm = 500 ms)
- Look at the sensed AV delay interval value and the PVARP value and reduce them such that their total equals 500 ms exactly
- Take care to reduce them appropriately: a too-short AV delay virtually assures constant ventricular pacing (not desirable if intrinsic conduction is present, even intermittently)

Using that example, programming combinations that would work include, but are not limited to:
- AV delay 250 ms, PVARP 250 ms
- AV delay 300 ms, PVARP 200 ms
- AV delay 180 ms, PVARP 320 ms

Pacemaker parameters are interrelated and changes you make in one area can affect many others. For that reason, adjusting TARP requires that you still obtain good parameter settings for the AV delay (crucial to avoid unnecessary pacing) and PVARP (crucial to protect against PMT in patient susceptible to PMT).

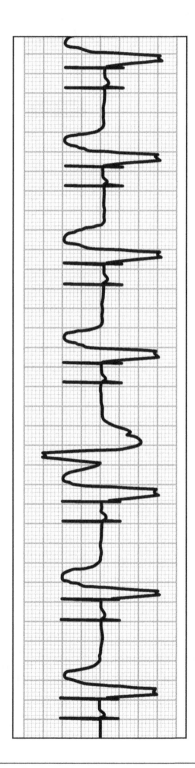

The Nuts and Bolts of Paced ECG Interpretation, 1st edition. By Tom Kenny.
Published 2009 by Blackwell Publishing, ISBN: 978-1-4501-8404-5.

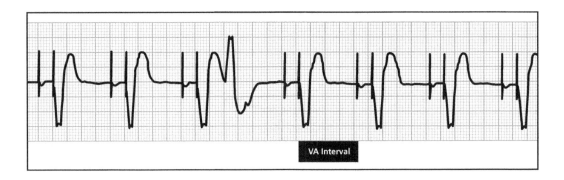

VA Interval

Mode

This is a paced DDD rhythm strip.

Rate

The atrial pacing interval is 1000 ms (60 ppm), which is appropriate.

Capture

Atrial capture is appropriate.

Ventricular capture is appropriate.

Sensing

Almost all of the atrial events on this strip are paced, with one exception. There is one atrial event that occurs within the large intrinsic ventricular event on the strip. Before we tackle this atrial event, let's first go over ventricular activity so we have a better point of reference for this intrinsic atrial event.

There is only one intrinsic ventricular event on this strip, and it is an unusual one. The large ventricular complex in the middle of the strip is a premature ventricular contraction (PVC). The pacemaker defines a PVC a little differently than clinicians do. To a dual-chamber pacemaker, a PVC is an intrinsic ventricular event without a preceding atrial event (either paced or sensed).

This PVC occurs about 400 ms after the onset of the prior paced ventricular event. That means it should have been sensed. To verify appropriate sensing, measure the VP-AP interval (sometimes called the VA interval). It is approximately 800 ms. Still using calipers, now measure the interval from the onset of the PVC to the next atrial pacing spike (VS-

AP). This turns out to be 800 ms. That means that this PVC reset device timing and, therefore, must have been appropriately sensed.

This brings us back to the intrinsic atrial event that occurs right after the PVC. PVCs are associated with pacemaker-mediated tachycardias (PMTs) which are triggered by retrograde P-waves. The presence of a sudden, lone, intrinsic atrial event so tightly associated with a PVC strongly suggests that this is a retrograde P-wave.

The nuts and bolts of paced ECG interpretation: retrograde P-waves

Premature ventricular contractions (PVCs) can be particularly problematic in some pacemaker patients because they are associated with retrograde P-waves which, if sensed, can initiate a pacemaker-mediated tachycardia.

The PVC breaks the synchrony between the atrium and ventricle and allows the patient to conduct retrogradely. That sensed retrograde P-wave initiates the pacemaker-mediated tachycardia. The pacemaker tries to maintain 1:1 AV synchrony, but the intrinsic atrial activity enters an endless loop.

If a dual-chamber pacemaker patient has retrograde conduction (not everyone does) and appears susceptible to PVCs triggering PMTs, the most typical programming strategy is to program an appropriately long PVARP value. A long PVARP will cause any resulting retrograde P-waves to "fall into" the refractory period and not provoke a pacemaker response. That is what happened in this particular strip.

Retrograde P-waves are associated with PVCs, although not all patients with PVCs will have retrograde P-waves.

The pacemaker does not sense this particular atrial event. If this P-wave had been sensed, the pacemaker would have imposed the sensed AV delay and then paced the ventricle in response. Using calipers, it appears that the interval between the onset of this PVC and the appearance of the retrograde P-wave is about 280 ms. Therefore, it is very likely that this retrograde P-wave "fell into" the pacemaker's refractory period and was not sensed. While this atrial event was not sensed, this is the expected and appropriate behavior of the device.

Underlying rhythm

This patient required consistent AP-VP pacing, which means he has both sinus node dysfunction and slow AV conduction. He also has retrograde conduction and is susceptible to PVCs. This kind of patient is vulnerable to pacemaker-mediated tachycardias (PMTs), so the device must be programmed to help prevent them.

What to do next

Atrial sensing should be evaluated, if possible. Reduce the pacing rate in increments of 10 ppm until intrinsic atrial activity occurs to conduct the test. As you reduce the rate, monitor the patient for any signs of discomfort or distress. Even if the patient appears fine and you cannot coax intrinsic atrial activity to appear on the ECG, do not drop the rate below about 30 or 40 ppm.

Although ventricular sensing was appropriate for the PVC, it would be wise to evaluate ventricular sensing as well. To force intrinsic ventricular activity to appear on the strip, extend the AV delay interval to at least 300 ms. The AV interval does not need to be extended incrementally. If intrinsic ventricular activity does not occur, a less desirable option is to temporarily program the dual-chamber pacemaker to VVI pacing and then lower the rate in the same 10-ppm stepwise scheme. However, only use the temporary VVI method if extending the AV delay fails.

Since this patient has retrograde conduction, check the programmed settings of the PVARP. This particular strip is a good example of how PVARP can prevent a PMT, so it is likely the PVARP setting is adequately long.

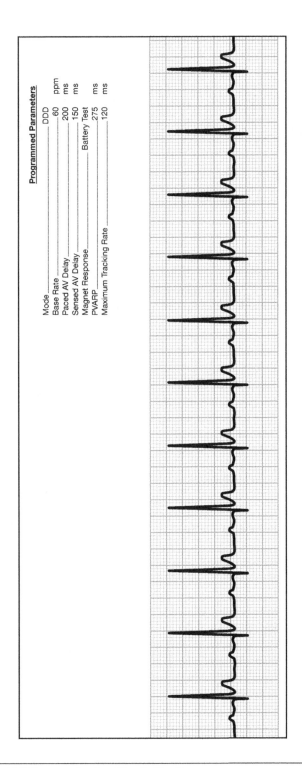

Programmed Parameters

Mode	DDD	
Base Rate	60	ppm
Paced AV Delay	200	ms
Sensed AV Delay	150	ms
Magnet Response	Battery Test	
PVARP	275	ms
Maximum Tracking Rate	120	ms

The Nuts and Bolts of Paced ECG Interpretation, 1st edition. By Tom Kenny.
Published 2009 by Blackwell Publishing, ISBN: 978-1-4501-8404-5.

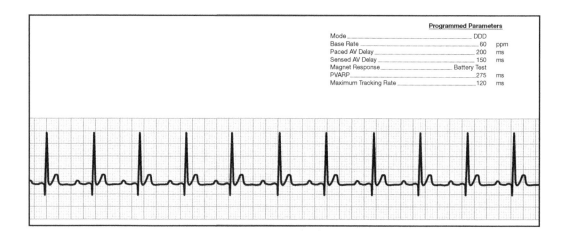

Mode

This strip is an excellent example of how important it can be to know the pacing parameters! If you just saw this strip with no other information, you might think the patient did not even have a pacemaker. That's not the case; the printout reports that the patient has a DDD device.

Rate

You can't determine the base rate from this strip, but it appears on the printout (60 ppm or 1000 ms). If you measure the AS-AS or VS-VS intervals, it shows that intrinsic activity is occurring at approximately 800 ms (75 ppm), which would inhibit the pacemaker spikes.

Capture

Neither atrial nor ventricular capture can be assessed from this strip.

Sensing

There are intrinsic atrial events on this strip and no pacing spikes, but are these native atrial depolarizations being sensed? If they were appropriately sensed, then the sensed AV delay would go into effect, resulting in a ventricular pacing spike after 150 ms elapsed. Using calipers, it appears that the interval between atrial sensed event and ventricular sensed event (AS-VS) is about 240 ms. The sensed AV delay is not imposed. That means the pacemaker did not sense the atrial events appropriately!

If the atrial events were not sensed, you might wonder why the pacemaker withheld atrial pacing. The answer lies in the intrinsic ventricular rate. The intrinsic ventricular rate is about 75 bpm, well above the programmed base rate. Not only did it inhibit the ventricular output pulse, it inhibited AV pacing.

The nuts and bolts of paced ECG interpretation: the V-A interval

This pacemaker is programmed to a pacing rate of 60 ppm, which means we could expect a 1000 ms atrial pacing interval (AP-AP).

For this device as currently programmed, the paced AV delay (interval between AP-VP) is 200 ms. This means that during AV pacing, the timing interval from a ventricular event to an atrial event (VP-AP) would have to be 800 ms. The formula for the VA interval (VP-AP) is the atrial pacing interval minus the paced AV delay (in this case, 1000–200=800).

The pacemaker sensed the intrinsic ventricular event but then waited 800 ms before pacing the atrium. Before the 800 ms could elapse, another intrinsic ventricular event occurred.

In this way, above-base-rate intrinsic ventricular activity can actually inhibit atrial pacing!

Based on the VA interval of 800 ms (base rate minus paced AV delay or 1000 minus 200), the ventricular event is sensed but before the pacemaker can send an atrial output pulse, the next ventricular event is sensed. This effectively prevents atrial pacing – and gives the *appearance* of appropriate atrial sensing. But appearances in paced ECGs can be deceiving!

Underlying rhythm

This patient has good sinus node function and slow AV conduction. However, his intrinsic rhythm has a good rate and provides 1:1 AV synchrony.

What to do next

Atrial sensing is not appropriate, so atrial sensing should be evaluated and suitable atrial sensitivity settings programmed. Both atrial and ventricular capture threshold tests should be performed and output parameters adjusted, if necessary.

Once proper capture is evaluated and proper atrial sensing is restored, the AV delays should be evaluated. This patient apparently has AV conduction, although it is slow (about 280 ms). The current AV delay settings (150 and 200 ms) are so short that once atrial sensing is restored, the patient will experience consistent right-ventricular pacing (AS-VP). It is generally agreed that intrinsic ventricular activity is preferable to paced ventricular activity, as long as it is rapid enough to support the patient's activity. Therefore, long AV delay settings or pacemaker algorithms that encourage intrinsic right-ventricular pacing should be used when possible. The AV delay intervals should be extended to accommodate the patient's intrinsic PR interval and, if available, other algorithms used to encourage more intrinsic ven-tricular activity and minimize unnecessary right-ventricular (RV) pacing.

The nuts and bolts of paced ECG interpretation: RV pacing and the DAVID study

Ever since the DAVID study found that unnecessary and frequent right-ventricular (RV) pacing can exacerbate heart failure in patients with some degree of systolic dysfunction and no standard pacemaker indications, clinicians have tried to limit RV pacing in their patients.

It is generally prudent clinical practice to allow intrinsic activity to emerge in paced patients as much as possible. However, this must be weighed against the patient's intrinsic rates, his or her need for pacemaker support, and symptoms.

Today there are several excellent pacemaker algorithms available, including Ventricular Intrinsic Preference™ technology from St. Jude Medical, that encourage intrinsic ventricular activity without compromising pacing support.

On the other hand, some patients truly require RV pacing. Adequate RV pacing should not be withheld from those who need it.

By the way, the DAVID study results should not be exaggerated; they do not extend to patients with a standard pacemaker indication! Thus, we cannot assume that RV pacing is bad for everyone at all times. The most objective but cautious interpretation of DAVID results is to minimize unnecessary RV pacing, when possible, without compromising adequate pacing support.

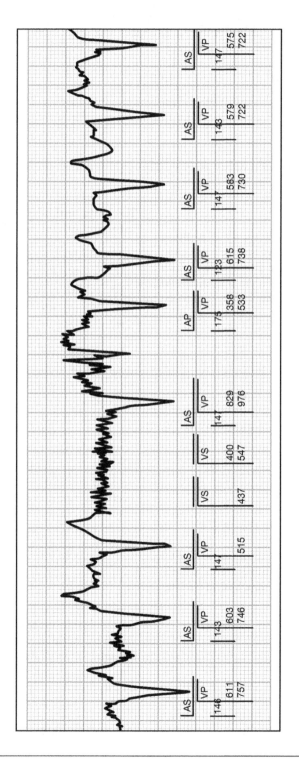

The Nuts and Bolts of Paced ECG Interpretation, 1st edition. By Tom Kenny.
Published 2009 by Blackwell Publishing, ISBN: 978-1-4501-8404-5.

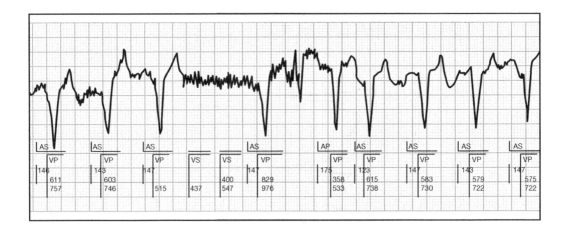

Mode

The annotations show that this is a dual-chamber pacemaker. The appearance of this tracing suggests the presence of some kind of interference. For that reason, we are going to rely on the annotations for this strip more than we usually do. A strip with a lot of interference and no annotations may be impossible to interpret.

Rate

The atrial rate "drives" a dual-chamber pacemaker, but there is no atrial pacing interval (AP-AP) on this strip to measure. The rate cannot be evaluated.

Capture

There is one atrial pacing spike (note the AP event) but it is impossible to ascertain from the strip if this output pulse captured the atrium. There is too much interference going on.

Ventricular pacing looks appropriate in that the VP annotations (which we can interpret as "spikes") result in large, widened QRS complexes of the same morphology.

Sensing

The annotations reveal many atrial sensed (AS) events, but are they all atrial events? Interference can make it difficult to interpret a paced ECG like this, but at least several of the AS annotations align with what appear to be intrinsic atrial events. Atrial sensing seems to be appropriate.

The nuts and bolts of paced ECG interpretation: interference

The pacemaker is designed to sense electrical signals within the body. In order to allow it to selectively pick up electrical signals from the heart and disregard other electrical signals from inside or outside the body, pacemakers today have very sophisticated filtering systems.

However, no system is perfect. Sometimes certain electrical appliances, industrial environments, or myopotential noise within the body can generate electrical signals that the pacemaker not only picks up, but "interprets" (inappropriately) as cardiac activity.

When interference is brief, the pacemaker reverts back to normal operation as soon as the source of interference stops. For example, when a pacemaker patient walks through a metal detector, there may be a moment of interference. Once the patient is clear of the detector, the pacemaker resumes normal operation.

When interference lasts for a longer period of time or is particularly severe, it can cause the pacemaker to automatically switch to asynchronous safety or backup pacing. In such cases, the patient must come back to the clinic for a simple reprogramming step to restore normal operation.

In this example, the interference is intermittent, but that does not make it less serious.

The real issue in this strip is ventricular sensing. The two VS annotations occur during the noisy pause on this strip. The noise is on the ventricular channel and it inhibited ventricular spikes due to ventricular oversensing. While there is clearly a problem with ventricular sensing, this is not the kind of oversensing that is likely due to an inappropriate ventricular sensitivity setting. The root of this problem is the interference.

Underlying rhythm

This patient has some degree of intact sinus node function and slow AV conduction. However, the biggest concern is the interference. In order to manage it, we need to know its source.

What to do next

The source of the interference must be determined. The usual suspects for interference are myopotential or muscle noise within the body, outside sources of interference, or a problem with the pacing lead. To find the source of the problem, we have to start ruling out what we can.

First, the patient should be asked about any symptoms. In talking to the patient, it is important to find out where the patient is when interference occurs. In this particular case, the interference occurred at the clinic which means the source of the interference has to be within the patient himself.

If the problem is muscle noise, then it will be exacerbated when the patient does isometric upper-body exercises. Have the patient do some isometric arm exercises while observing the ECG. If this worsens the interference, the problem is likely myopotential oversensing. This can often be effectively addressed by programming sensitivity settings to less sensitive values to cause the pacemaker to filter out electrical signals generated by the muscles. If such isometrics fail to induce interference, the problem has to be the lead.

If you can rule out myopotential oversensing, order a chest X-ray to visually examine pacing lead integrity. Just looking at the paced ECG, this looks like it might be an insulation breach in the ventricular pacing lead. The problem is not severe enough to cause persistent interference, but that sort of noisy baseline is definitely consistent with an insulation problem. While some lead problems (such as loose connections) are more common in acute implants, an insulation problem may occur at any time over the life of the pacing lead.

The nuts and bolts of paced ECG interpretation: it's a lead problem! What next?

Damaged leads or poor lead connections can manifest on the paced ECG as interference (like this case) or in capture and sensing problems (typically both together). Although not evident on the paced ECG, sudden or very large changes in pacing lead impedance values, as seen from the programmer or diagnostic data, can also suggest lead problems, sometimes before the patient develops symptoms.

Lead problems may be immediate and severe or they may manifest gradually and get progressively worse. When a lead problem is suspected and other likely causes can be ruled out, a chest X-ray should be ordered. Sometimes, faulty connections or damage to the lead can be evident on film.

If there is a lead problem, it usually requires lead replacement. This may or may not involve the extraction of the indwelling lead. While lead extraction is not a procedure to be undertaken lightly, recent advances in this surgical approach and technological developments in lead extraction tools have made it safer and faster than ever. It is beyond the scope of this book to discuss lead extraction, but there will be cases in dealing with pacemaker patients when it is the best and wisest course of action. Lead problems do not self-heal and they compromise device function.

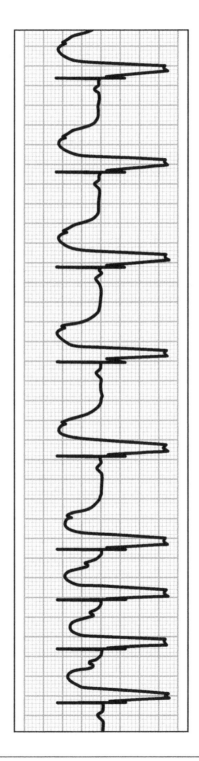

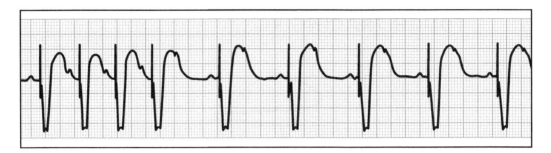

Mode

Although there are no atrial pacing spikes, the atrial tracking behavior in this strip makes it clear that it's a dual-chamber pacemaker.

Rate

The rate cannot be accurately measured here, which would require an atrial pacing interval (AP-AP). However, the ventricular pacing interval (VP-VP) is about 520 ms (115 ppm) at the outset of this strip, then it drops in a single beat by almost half to 1000 ms (60 ppm). A pacing rate of 60 ppm would be appropriate for this system.

Capture

Atrial capture cannot be assessed from this strip.

On the other hand, ventricular capture appears to be appropriate. Note that all ventricular events share the same morphology.

Sensing

In the slower section of the strip, atrial sensing appears appropriate in that the intrinsic atrial event inhibits the atrial output and the ensuing ventricular pacing spike is consistently timed to the sensed atrial event, with a sensed AV delay that measures with calipers to about 160 ms.

The atrial activity in the faster part of the strip requires a closer look. The ventricular pacing interval (VP-VP) shows pacing at 115 ppm. This is an appropriate value for the maximum tracking rate (MTR), which sets the upper rate limit for ventricular pacing in response to atrial tracking. The pacemaker will do whatever it can to keep ventricular pacing at or under the MTR, even violating the

sensed AV delay. If you measure the sensed AV delay in the rapid activity on the left side of the strip, it is clear that these sensed AV delays (AS-VP) are longer than the sensed AV delays in the slower section of the strip. That is perfectly normal and expected pacemaker behavior.

Notice that the sensed AV delay on the left of the strip gets progressively longer. The longest such AV delay interval occurs right before the pause. There is one more intrinsic atrial event on the T-wave right before the pause. Was this intrinsic atrial event properly sensed? The next logical question has to be: should we expect this intrinsic event to have been sensed? Using calipers, it appears that this intrinsic atrial event occurs about 320 ms after the ventricular pacing spike. If the post-ventricular atrial refractory period (PVARP) was set to 320 ms or longer, this atrial event "fell into" the refractory period and the pacemaker did not respond to it.

That is exactly what happened. This is pacemaker Wenckebach (rapid ventricular response to intrinsic atrial activity with a progressively lengthening PR interval, that is AS-VP interval) transitioning into 2:1 block.

Ventricular sensing cannot be assessed from this strip.

Underlying rhythm

This patient has a high intrinsic atrial rate and a pacemaker that responded with pacemaker Wenckebach (a pacemaker version of physiological Wenckebach behavior with a progressive lengthening of the PR interval) that progressed to 2:1 block (two intrinsic atrial events for every one paced ventricular response). The goal of dual-chamber pacing in patients with high-rate intrinsic atrial activity is to delay the so-called "Wenckebach window" as long as possible, that is, to prolong the time the patient spends in pacemaker Wenckebach and delay the onset of 2:1 block. This cannot be done indefinitely, but it looks like this patient might have slipped into 2:1 block before absolutely necessary.

What to do next

Atrial capture and ventricular sensing should be evaluated.

Following that, the patient should be asked about his symptoms to see how well he tolerates rapid ventricular pacing. Device diagnostics would be useful to see how frequent such high-rate intrinsic atrial activity is. One strategy to help manage high intrinsic atrial rates is to increase the maximum tracking rate (MTR). This provides good upper rate response but only if the patient can tolerate higher-than-base-rate pacing. Increase MTR with caution based on the patient's underlying disease and tolerance for above-base-rate-pacing.

It is also beneficial to delay the onset of 2:1 block a bit, which means reducing the TARP. To have the patient enter 2:1 block at 120 ppm (500 ms), the PVARP and sensed AV delay should total no more than 500 ms. While this will not prevent 2:1 block, it will allow the patient to experience more time in pacemaker Wenckebach, which is probably easier to tolerate.

The nuts and bolts of paced ECG interpretation: opening the Wenckebach window

When a pacemaker tracks the atrium, high-rate intrinsic atrial activity can cause unusual behavior. Up to a certain point, an atrial-tracking dual-chamber pacemaker (such as a DDD or DDDR device) will respond by maintaining 1:1 AV synchrony by pacing the ventricle above the base rate. In order to protect the patient from very high ventricular pacing rates, particularly since such rapid pacing is associated with symptoms, a maximum tracking rate (MTR) imposes a "speed limit" beyond which the ventricle cannot be paced. A typical MTR setting is around 120 ppm, but should be adjusted to meet the needs of the individual patient.

This rapid ventricular pacing in response to high intrinsic atrial rates creates what is known as "pacemaker Wenckebach." It preserves 1:1 AV synchrony and most patients feel better with this sort of pacing than with 2:1 block. However, at a certain point, 2:1 block sets in. It occurs when the intrinsic atrial rate exceeds TARP (total atrial refractory period). TARP is not directly programmable as a parameter setting but it is composed of the sensed AV delay plus the PVARP.

When the patient's intrinsic atrial rate exceeds the programmed base rate, pacemaker Wenckebach sets in. It operates up to the point that the intrinsic rate meets the TARP value. Once the patient's native atrial rate exceeds TARP, the "Wenckebach window" closes and 2:1 sets in. This strip is a great example of how abrupt and dramatic the rate change can be. Not all patients do well with this rate transition or with 2:1 pacing!

If the patient can tolerate rapid ventricular pacing, the best tactic is to open the Wenckebach Window. In fact, the goal of upper rate behavior is to stall the onset of 2:1 block as long as possible!

To open the Wenckebach Window, the TARP value has to be shortened. TARP can be indirectly adjusted by changing the sensed AV delay or the PVARP setting or both. In this case, the patient's TARP value was around 115 ms (520 ms). The settings for the sensed AV delay and/or the PVARP should be changed so that their sum is less than 520 ms. If 2:1 block should occur at an intrinsic atrial rate of 120 ppm (500 ms), this patient's TARP should be reduced by 20 ms. For 2:1 block to occur at an intrinsic atrial rate of 130 ppm (462 ms), the patient's TARP would have to be 462 ms, in other words, it would have to be reduced by 58 ms.

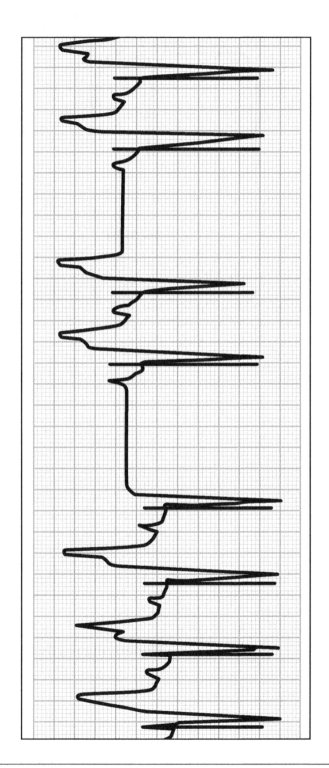

The Nuts and Bolts of Paced ECG Interpretation, 1st edition. By Tom Kenny.
Published 2009 by Blackwell Publishing, ISBN: 978-1-4501-8404-5.

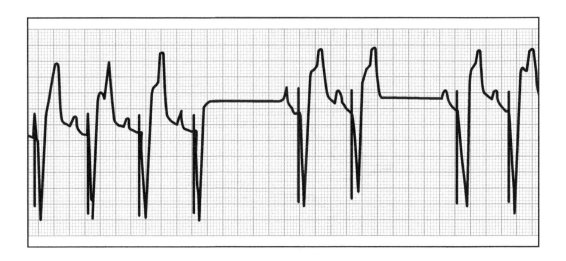

Mode

This is a dual-chamber rhythm strip. Ventricular pacing is tracking intrinsic atrial activity. The strip looks very unusual. Note the squared-off looking pauses and the perfectly straight baselines during pauses. This kind of appearance may be associated with a malfunction of the ECG monitor or some other kind of recording anomaly.

Rate

There are no atrial pacing intervals on the strip to accurately assess the pacing rate, which is erratic. A few of the ventricular pacing intervals (VP-VP) appear to be about 720 ms (around 83 ppm) but that is in response to sensed atrial activity. There are also a couple of long pauses on the strip – the longer one measures 1000 ms (1 second).

Capture

Atrial capture cannot be assessed from this strip.

Ventricular capture appears to be appropriate, with consistent (although unusual-looking) QRS morphologies across the strip. However, there are a couple of pauses. In fact, in the center of the strip the interval between ventricular pacing spikes measures 1400 ms (43 ppm). Unless the base rate was set to 40 ppm or below, the pacemaker should have paced in this period.

Sensing

In much of the strip, atrial sensing appears to be appropriate. Whenever an intrinsic atrial event occurs on the strip, the pacemaker responds with a ventricular pacing spike after an interval of about 200 ms, an appropriate time for a sensed AV delay. However, there are two long pauses in the strip when the absence of intrinsic atrial activity should have caused an atrial pacing spike to be delivered. Such behavior could indicate atrial oversensing.

If those pauses indicate atrial oversensing, they would also indicate ventricular oversensing since no ventricular spike is delivered. In fact, in the first pause, the ventricular pacing interval (VP-VP) is 1400 ms! Is this a case of oversensing?

Not likely! When this alleged "oversensing" occurs, notice that it occurs simultaneously in both chambers: atrial oversensing and ventricular oversensing occur at the same time not once but twice in this short rhythm strip. That alone should cause us to get suspicious but coupled with the squared-off looking tracing, this makes me fairly certain that we are dealing with some kind of ECG monitor malfunction.

Underlying rhythm

This patient has intrinsic atrial activity with slow AV conduction.

What to do next

The overriding concern for any clinician seeing this strip is that the ECG monitor is not working properly. The reasons for this are the appearance of the tracing (particularly the absolutely flat baselines and the odd squared-off look of the complexes) and the fact that inappropriate behavior occurs intermittently but simultaneously on the atrial and ventricular channels. Lead problems often manifest as noisy baselines and often involve simultaneous capture and sensing problems – but on the same lead.

If possible, record another ECG using a different monitor. That should result in a quite different-looking tracing and one that could be confidently evaluated.

TOUGH TRACING #8

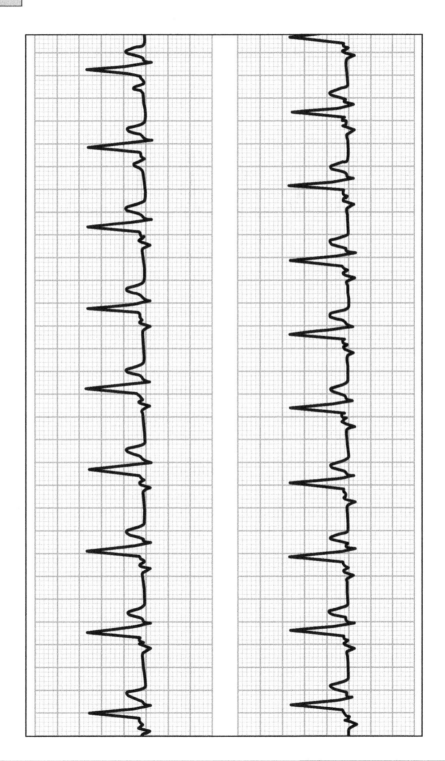

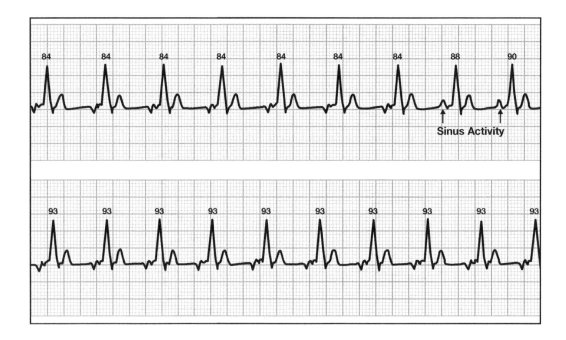

Mode

This is a run of AP-VP complexes, so this is a dual-chamber pacemaker.

Rate

The atrial pacing interval (AP-AP) is about 720 ms if you measure the first two complexes (84 ppm) but it shortens (faster rate) as the strip progresses. It's not unusual to see above-base-rate ventricular pacing when a pacemaker tracks the atrium, but this is a case of above-base-rate *atrial* pacing! This has to involve some kind of specialty pacemaker algorithm. Either it is a rate-responsive pacemaker or atrial overdrive is going on.

The best way to check this is to evaluate programmed settings, if available. But what if the device is both rate-responsive (DDDR) and has an atrial overdrive algorithm? If this strip was obtained in-clinic with the patient seated and at rest, it is unlikely to be rate-responsive pacing! Annotations or diagnostic reports may help. In this case, the patient was at rest at the clinic and the pacing was caused by the AF Suppression™ algorithm, an atrial overdrive feature.

Capture

Atrial capture appears to be appropriate. Ventricular capture also looks appropriate.

Sensing

Atrial sensing is appropriate, but ventricular sensing cannot be assessed from this strip.

Underlying rhythm

The dual-chamber pacemaker with AF Suppression will pace at the base rate and consistently searches for intrinsic P-waves. If it senses two P-waves in a 16-cycle window, it will drive up the atrial pacing rate by approximately 10 bpm. This occurred at the end of the top strip and resulted in above-base-rate atrial pacing.

This rate acceleration will continue for a programmable number of beats and continue to search for intrinsic P-waves. If two more P-waves in a 16-cycle window occur, it will accelerate the rate again by approximately 10 bpm. If intrinsic P-waves do not occur, it will slow the atrial pacing rate back down to the programmed base rate.

The goal is to be pacing the atrium just slightly above the patient's intrinsic rate. This has been proven in clinical studies to suppress atrial fibrillation (AF).

What to do next

Atrial and ventricular sensing should be evaluated, but if the patient is experiencing persistent high-rate atrial activity, this may not be possible. Download device diagnostics to determine how frequently the AF Suppression™ algorithm has been in use and at what rates. If this algorithm has only been recently programmed, it could be interesting to compare "before" and "after" diagnostics. Many times, patients with high-rate intrinsic atrial activity experience lots of pacing at MTR and AMS episodes, which can be reduced with AF Suppression™ or other atrial overdrive features. Interview the patient to find out what symptoms, if any, are associated with overdrive atrial pacing. For many patients, the atrial overdrive algorithm works well. But if the patient does not tolerate it or spends prolonged periods of time at above-base-rate AP-VP pacing or both, it may be appropriate to consider treating the atrial tachyarrhythmia in a different and more aggressive manner. Drug therapy may be appropriate, either new or adjusted from the patient's previous prescription.

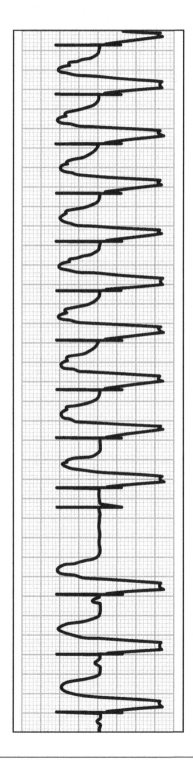

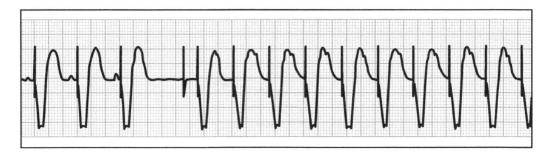

Mode

This is a dual-chamber pacemaker. That is evident from the atrial tracking as well as the presence of one atrial pacing spike and many ventricular spikes.

Rate

The ventricular pacing interval (VP-VP) varies, from about 600 ms (100 ppm) at the outset of this tracing and ending with 520 ms intervals (115 ppm) at the end. The pause in this strip divides it between atrial tracking at around 100 ppm to much more rapid pacing with what appears to be retrograde atrial activity. It looks like after the pause, a pacemaker-mediated tachycardia (PMT) occurred.

Capture

There is one atrial pacing spike in this strip but it fails to capture. Atrial capture is not working properly. Loss of atrial capture is a common trigger of PMT.

Ventricular capture, on the other hand, is appropriate.

Sensing

On this particular strip, we have three areas of investigation for atrial sensing: before, during, and after the pause. Before the pause, it appears that the pacemaker is tracking the atrium at or approaching 100 ppm, which means at or near the maximum tracking rate (MTR). This indicates appropriate atrial sensing. The reason the full sensed AV delay interval does not come into play is that in order to offer 1:1 AV synchrony, the pacemaker has to pace the ventricle too rapidly to allow the full delay interval to be applied.

After the pause, there are what appear to be P-waves on the strip, but these are most likely retrograde P-waves. Tracking these retrograde P-waves causes the PMT.

> ### The nuts and bolts of paced ECG interpretation: which way is retrograde?
>
> The healthy heart has conduction pathways that are all one-way streets, moving more or less from top to bottom. Pacemaker clinicians describe this as antegrade conduction or forward conduction.
>
> Some patients have myocardial tissue that is capable of conducting backward (or upward) through the heart. Not every patient has retrograde conduction.
>
> Being capable of retrograde conduction is not necessarily problematic unless a series of events occur that can cause a cardiac event to "get stuck" and travel around and around in an endless loop tachycardia propelled by both antegrade and retrograde conduction. That's what a pacemaker-mediated tachycardia or PMT is – PMT happens when retrograde conduction that occurs physiologically meets antegrade conduction aided by the pacemaker.
>
> In this case, an atrial event travels faster and faster in a loop, causing rapid pacing. PMTs require three things: a dual-chamber pacemaker patient with retrograde conduction, an adequate "loop" or pathway in the heart, and a triggering event such as the abrupt loss of atrial capture.

The pause occurs when the patient's intrinsic atrial rate abruptly slows. The patient's native atrial rate was rapid, then gave out. When no intrinsic atrial event occurred the pacemaker waited and applied its normal timing intervals. Note that the interval from the preceding intrinsic atrial event to the atrial pacing spike hit 1000 ms (60 ppm), the likely base rate. The problem occurred when this atrial spike failed to capture the heart. In my experience, loss of atrial capture is the most common trigger for PMT.

Atrial sensing appears to be appropriate.

Ventricular sensing cannot be evaluated from this strip.

Underlying rhythm

This patient has sinus node dysfunction and at least intermittent high-rate intrinsic atrial activity along with slow AV conduction. This particular patient also has retrograde conduction and is susceptible to PMTs.

What to do next

If the PMT is ongoing, it must be stopped and appropriate PMT termination algorithms applied. Most dual-chamber pacemakers can be programmed to automatically apply a specific termination algorithm after a run of PMTs. It is possible that this occurred right after this particular PMT started. At any rate, the PMT termination algorithm should be reviewed.

If available, patient diagnostic data should be obtained to see if PMTs were common occurrences and to evaluate the effectiveness of any termination algorithms already in place.

In addition, atrial capture must be restored. A capture test on the atrial channel should be performed and output parameters (atrial pulse width, atrial pulse amplitude) adjusted, as necessary.

Ventricular sensing should be evaluated. If the patient still has high-rate intrinsic atrial activity, ventricular sensing can be tested by temporarily programming the pacemaker to VVI mode and, if necessary, lowering the base rate. If the patient's intrinsic atrial rate is more normal, ventricular sensing can be evaluated by the leaving the device in a dual-chamber mode and temporarily extending the sensed and paced AV delay to 300 ms or more. The latter method is preferred, but not always possible.

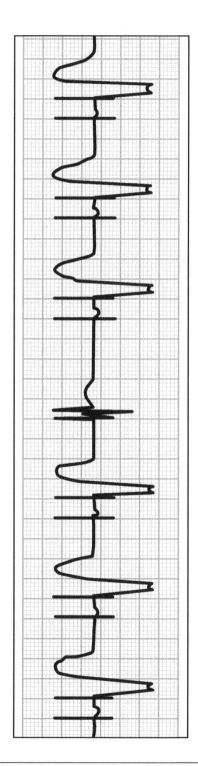

The Nuts and Bolts of Paced ECG Interpretation, 1st edition. By Tom Kenny.
Published 2009 by Blackwell Publishing, ISBN: 978-1-4501-8404-5.

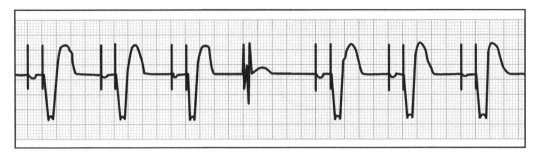

Mode

The pairs of pacing spikes (atrial and ventricular) mean that this is a dual-chamber pacemaker.

Rate

The atrial pacing interval (AP-AP) drives the rate in a dual-chamber system and here that interval measures 1000 ms (60 ppm). The pacing rate is appropriate.

Capture

Overlooking the strange event in the middle of the strip, both atrial and ventricular capture appear appropriate with consistent morphologies.

The unusual looking event appears to be a mixture of an atrial spike, a ventricular spike, and an intrinsic ventricular event. So what could this be? Using calipers, the interval between the atrial and ventricular spikes measures about 120 ms. That is a huge clue. Whenever a ventricular spike follows an atrial spike by 100 to 120 ms (depending on device and manufacturer), safety pacing is involved. This happens to be from a St. Jude Medical device with a 110 ms interval for safety pacing.

Safety pacing involves a few timing cycles. If the ventricular lead senses an atrial pacemaker spike and inappropriately considers it a ventricular event, that phenomenon is called "crosstalk." Crosstalk causes ventricular oversensing, leading to ventricular under-pacing. Thus, after an atrial pacing spike, the pacemaker imposes a very short mandatory blanking period, in order to prevent the pacemaker's ventricular channel from "seeing" the atrial spike and inappropriately sensing it as ventricular activity.

After this brief blanking period following the atrial pacing spike, the pacemaker imposes a second mandatory timing cycle known as the "crosstalk detection window." If any event is sensed during the crosstalk detection window, the pacemaker performs "safety pacing," sometimes called "ventricular safety standby." This means that right after the atrial output pulse (in this device, 110 ms after the atrial spike), the pacemaker will pace the ventricle. It does this *even if the ventricles have depolarized or are depolarizing on their own.*

The nuts and bolts of paced ECG interpretation: crosstalk

Modern pacemakers have done a lot to get rid of the phenomenon known as crosstalk, which occurs when the pacemaker's ventricular sensing circuitry picks up an atrial pacing spike and mistakenly "sees" it as intrinsic ventricular activity.

When crosstalk occurs, it can lead to inappropriate inhibition of the ventricular pacing spike, that is, ventricular under-pacing. It often appears on a paced ECG as a pause on the ventricular channel.

To combat crosstalk, pacemakers routinely impose a very brief blanking period on the ventricular channel whenever an atrial spike is delivered. This blanking period "covers" or conceals the pacemaker spike so that the pacemaker cannot "see" it and therefore will not respond inappropriately. Following the blanking period, a very brief "crosstalk detection window" occurs; during this timing cycle, the ventricular channel can sense activity, but if it does, the pacemaker figures it could be crosstalk and responds with ventricular safety pacing or the automatic delivery of a ventricular spike about 110 ms after the preceding atrial spike.

The idea behind ventricular safety pacing is that if crosstalk is suspected, rather than allow it to interfere with proper pacing and inappropriately inhibit a ventricular output pulse, it triggers a ventricular pacing spike. In this case, the spike falls on top of an intrinsic event (pseudofusion), but it is appropriate pacemaker behavior.

Sensing

Neither atrial nor ventricular sensing can be assessed from this tracing.

Underlying rhythm

This patient has sinus node dysfunction and slow AV conduction.

What to do next

Atrial and ventricular sensing should be evaluated. The presence of one event of safety pacing on this strip is expected device behavior and not necessarily indicative of any problem.

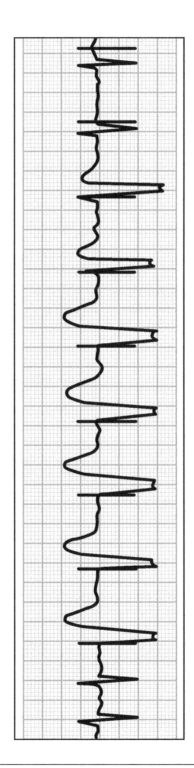

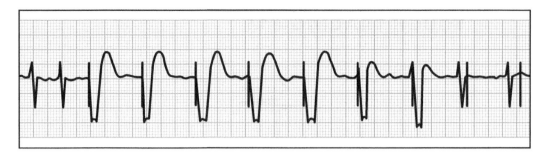

Mode

This is a VVI strip.

Rate

The ventricular pacing interval is about 760 ms (80 ppm). While many clinicians (including me) prefer single-chamber pacemakers be set to rates of 70 ppm, 80 ppm is not particularly alarming or even unusual. For certain patients, depending on symptoms, it may be appropriate. For now, the assumption should be that this rate is high but acceptable.

Capture

There are three distinct ventricular morphologies on this strip. The first two and last two complexes are intrinsic ventricular events; the third through seventh events show appropriate capture.

The eighth and ninth events look like a blend between the intrinsic and captured ventricular depolarizations and are ventricular fusion. Notice the different morphology of the T-wave in the "true" captured events versus the fusion events. Fusion confirms capture. The fused events show that the programmed base rate is competing with the patient's intrinsic rate.

At the end of the strip are two ventricular pacing spikes that fail to capture. This is functional non-capture. They do not capture because they could not possibly capture – they occur right after the ventricles depolarized on their own. Functional non-capture suggests a sensing problem.

Sensing

The first ventricular event is appropriately sensed; it inhibits the ventricular output pulse and resets device timing. Using calipers set to the ventricular

pacing interval (VP-VP), notice that this first intrinsic ventricular event times out to the first ventricular pacing spike (VS-VP). That means the second intrinsic ventricular event on this strip was undersensed.

> ### The nuts and bolts of paced ECG interpretation: intermittent sensing problems
>
> Pacemakers have fixed sensitivity settings but the human heart can exhibit quite a variety in terms of cardiac signal sizes. For that reason, many sensing problems show up on an ECG first as intermittent oversensing or undersensing.
>
> It is good practice for clinicians to check sensitivity settings at every follow-up and to take even the occasional undersensed or oversensed event quite seriously. In this example, the two undersensed ventricular events at the end of the strip were likely "too small" in terms of signal amplitude to be picked up by the device's filters.
>
> The first event was apparently large enough to be properly sensed, but the second was not. Note that waveform appearance on the ECG can be quite misleading; do not assume that because signals look to be the same magnitude that they are the same size to the pacemaker's sensing circuits. PVCs are a great example of this; they can look quite large on the paced ECG but are occasionally undersensed because of the way the wavefront travels through the heart with respect to the pacemaker lead's sensing electrodes.
>
> Intermittent sensing problems can also occur with a lead problem (at least at first before the lead problem becomes severe). However, lead problems are more likely to manifest as a consistent problem with both sensing and capture.

Further sensing problems occur at the end of the strip. Two more intrinsic ventricular events occur which fail to inhibit the ventricular output pulse. Ventricular sensing is clearly not appropriate.

Underlying rhythm

The patient has sinus node dysfunction and slow AV conduction.

What to do next

Ventricular sensing should be checked and the ventricular sensitivity settings adjusted. When ventricular undersensing is corrected, no more functional non-capture events should occur.

The frequent ventricular pacing and the presence of fusion indicates that the patient might have more intrinsic conduction (and less right-ventricular or RV pacing) if pacing was slower. Normally, the best way to achieve this is to activate rate hysteresis and set a hysteresis rate about 10 bpm below the programmed base rate. This patient had a programmed base rate of 80 ppm, which is on the high side. For that reason, in this case, I would first lower the base rate to 70 ppm. Hysteresis could also be programmed to 60 bpm, but just lowering the base rate to 70 ppm is likely to clear up the fusion and encourage more intrinsic activity.

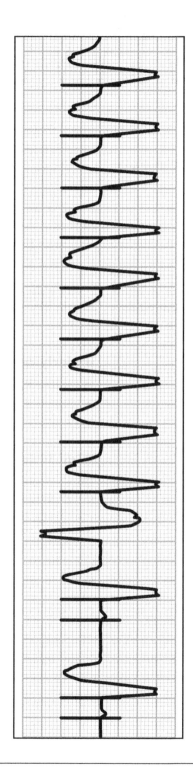

The Nuts and Bolts of Paced ECG Interpretation, 1st edition. By Tom Kenny.
Published 2009 by Blackwell Publishing, ISBN: 978-1-4501-8404-5.

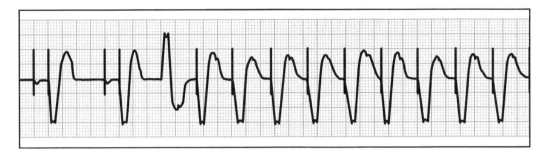

Mode

This is a dual-chamber pacemaker rhythm strip.

Rate

In terms of rate, this strip has two main sections. At the outset, the atrial pacing interval is 1000 ms (60 ppm), an appropriate base rate. The right-hand portion of the strip shows rapid ventricular pacing (520 ms or 115 ppm) in what looks to be a pacemaker-mediated tachycardia (PMT). Between these two "zones" on the strip is a premature ventricular contraction (PVC), a common trigger for PMTs. The PMT is limited by the maximum tracking rate or MTR, which appears to be programmed to 115 ppm, a suitable rate setting for that parameter.

Capture

There are only two atrial spikes on this strip and both exhibit appropriate capture.

Ventricular capture looks appropriate as well. Notice that all ventricular events share the same morphology.

Sensing

The first intrinsic P-wave on this strip occurs in the downward deflection of the PVC and is likely to be a retrograde P-wave. This P-wave then perpetuates the PMT that follows. Notice that the maximum tracking rate (MTR) governs the rate during the PMT, which means that atrial events no longer "drive" the pacing rate. That is why the sensed AV delay interval is no longer imposed; if the sensed AV delay was

used to trigger a ventricular pacing spike, the rate would have exceeded the programmed MTR.

Although this first P-wave was a retrograde event, the pacemaker sensed it – and that is appropriate device behavior. Confirmation of appropriate atrial sensing is that 240 ms following this P-wave the pacemaker delivered a ventricular pacing spike. This means that the pacemaker was programmed to a sensed AV delay of about 240 ms, a reasonable value.

Ventricular sensing also appears appropriate in that the PVC was sensed properly. It reset device timing.

Underlying rhythm

The patient has sinus node dysfunction, slow AV conduction, and retrograde conduction. He is also susceptible to PMTs.

What to do next

This strip reveals a PMT trigger (the PVC), and a spell of PMT but not its termination. Most pacemakers have automatic algorithms to break PMTs, typically by extending the PVARP. Steps should be taken to assure that this patient has normal pacemaker function restored. Furthermore, PMT termination algorithms for this patient should be scrutinized to be sure they are adequate. Clinically, there is little we can do to stop PVCs and retrograde conduction, but we can make sure appropriate PMT termination algorithms are activated.

Although there is some slight evidence (one event) of appropriate atrial and ventricular sensing, sensing tests in both channels are recommended.

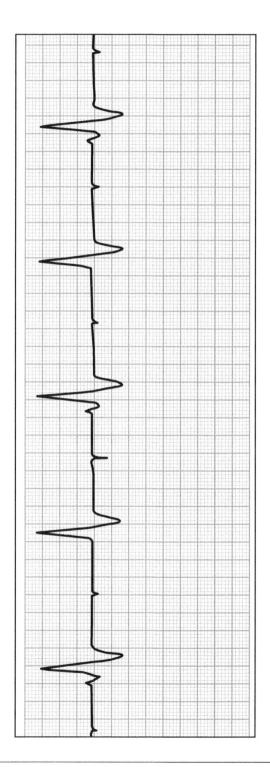

The Nuts and Bolts of Paced ECG Interpretation, 1st edition. By Tom Kenny.
Published 2009 by Blackwell Publishing, ISBN: 978-1-4501-8404-5.

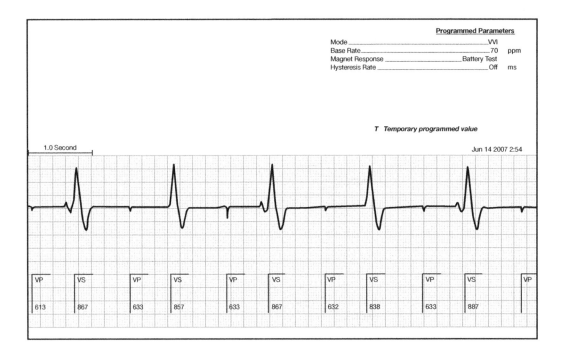

Mode

The printout and annotations make it clear: this is a VVI strip. Even without annotations, there are clues that point to single-chamber pacing. In a dual-chamber system, the pacemaker would have paced the atrium in the prolonged absence of intrinsic atrial activity; yet there are neither spikes nor intrinsic atrial events evident. Even if you thought the small downward-deflecting tick marks were atrial events, that should have initiated the AV delay interval, resulting in a ventricular pacemaker spike in about 200 ms. Thus, the annotations confirm what the strip essentially told us: VVI pacing.

Rate

There is no classic ventricular pacing interval on this strip (VP-VP), but ventricular escape intervals (VS-VP) can be measured. They measure about 880 ms with calipers (around 68 ppm) and a bit less on the annotations, all of which fits with the programmed (and appropriate) pacing base rate of 70 ppm.

This strip looks slow, and, in fact, if you measure the intervals between the large sensed ventricular events, it is about 1560 ms or around 38 ppm. How-ever, it is not "slow" to the pacemaker, because of the presence of the VP events, the little pacemaker spikes between the large intrinsic events. This is a case where the pacemaker "thinks" it is pacing around 70 ppm, but the patient is only getting rate support at around 38 ppm!

Capture

The ventricular pacemaker spikes on this strip are really just small downstrokes, but not one of them captures the ventricle. There is a complete loss of ventricular capture.

Sensing

The large ventricular events on this strip are intrinsic events and they appear to be properly sensed, in that they reset device timing and are annotated as VS events.

Underlying rhythm

This patient has sinus node dysfunction, a junctional rhythm, and slow AV conduction.

What to do next

The most urgent concern is to restore appropriate ventricular capture by performing a ventricular pacing threshold test and adjusting the pacemaker output parameters (ventricular pulse width and pulse amplitude) appropriately. It is unlikely this loss of ventricular capture is due to a faulty lead, since ventricular sensing is working well.

Ask the patient about any symptoms or problems. The patient may notice a change in how he feels right in the clinic as proper pacing support is restored. If the patient experienced particularly debilitating symptoms, it should be noted in the chart so that a generous safety margin is always maintained. In this instance, it would be worth checking to see if a new drug might have altered this patient's pacing threshold.

The nuts and bolts of paced ECG interpretation: hey! Don't forget the patient!

Paced ECGs can become every bit as addictive as crossword puzzles or sudoku, and many scientific sessions among cardiologists and electrophysiologists include some meetings where "lively debate" occurs as experts go over paced rhythm strips to debate what they might mean.

However, in the clinical setting, the patient must always be the focal point. The patient's history, updated drug information, and symptoms are vitally important to any final pacing prescription decisions.

Drugs, in particular, should be monitored closely. Most pacemaker patients take at least one prescription drug and polypharmacy is not unusual. Drugs can affect arrhythmias, pacing

thresholds, and provoke symptoms. For example, a long-time pacemaker patient on a new prescription for beta-blockers may be experiencing fatigue … but that fatigue is more likely attributable to beta blockade than the pacemaker.

Likewise, drugs are sometimes tolerated better by the patient than the pacemaker. Certain drugs are known to increase pacing thresholds, which may result in loss of capture at the previous output parameter settings. The patient's response to drugs, in particular with regard to pacing thresholds, is highly individual; drugs that increase pacing thresholds in one patient will not necessarily have that same effect in another patient.

Treat the patient, not the rhythm strip.

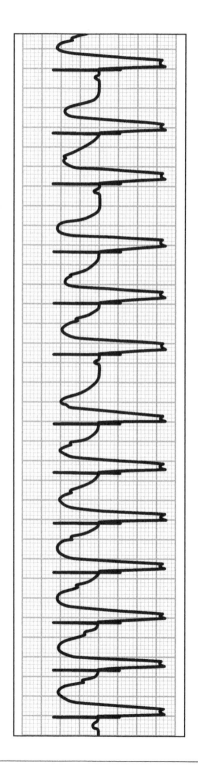

The Nuts and Bolts of Paced ECG Interpretation, 1st edition. By Tom Kenny.
Published 2009 by Blackwell Publishing, ISBN: 978-1-4501-8404-5.

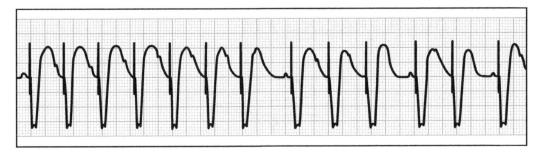

Mode

This is dual-chamber pacing.

Rate

The ventricular pacing rate in this strip is rapid, but it is trying to track rapid intrinsic atrial activity. This is an example of pacemaker Wenckebach; note the sensed AV delay interval (AS-VP) lengthens until an atrial event "falls into" the refractory period and is ignored.

The ventricular pacing interval gets as fast as 520 ms (115 ppm), most likely the maximum tracking rate (MTR).

Capture

Atrial capture cannot be assessed from this strip, but ventricular capture appears to be functioning properly.

Sensing

Atrial sensing is appropriate, in that the pacemaker is tracking rapid atrial activity and inhibiting atrial output spikes. Ventricular sensing cannot be evaluated from this strip.

Underlying rhythm

This patient has an accelerating atrial tachyarrhythmia.

What to do next

The most pressing concern for this patient is managing the atrial tachyarrhythmia. This is not atrial fibrillation (AF) but it can be equally challenging. Appropriately programming the MTR and pro-

longing the "Wenckebach window" by extending TARP as long as reasonably possible to avoid going into 2:1 block too soon are great strategies. But ultimately, this patient is dealing with an intrinsic atrial rate that is fast and getting faster.

If available, use device diagnostics to evaluate how frequently such rapid native atrial activity occurs. If this is not an isolated or unusual occurrence, it becomes important to better manage the atrial rhythm. This might be accomplished through drug therapy (beta-blockers are a good choice). Meanwhile, the device can be programmed in ways to minimize the impact of high-rate intrinsic atrial activity:

- Program an appropriate MTR that the patient can tolerate (this kind of patient is likely going to be paced at the MTR often); the higher it is, the longer the patient retains 1:1 AV synchrony. But don't make it too high or the patient will become symptomatic with the rapid ventricular pacing.
- Shorten TARP (total atrial refractory period or the combined duration of the PVARP and the AV delay interval) as much as reasonably appropriate; this will prolong the time the patient spends in Wenckebach before going to 2:1 block.
- Activate algorithms like mode switching or AF Suppression algorithm (or other atrial overdrive algorithm), if they are available. Many patients benefit from such features, but use them cautiously.
- Some patients with this type of rhythm wind up programmed to a nontracking mode; this is not the best "first choice" option since it sacrifices 1:1 AV synchrony. However, it could be preferable to near-constant above-base-rate pacing.
- Set up pacemaker diagnostics to monitor intrinsic high-rate atrial activity, mode switch episodes, AT/AF burden, and so on, since it can give you valuable insight into the patient's condition (and can help tell you if drug therapy is working).

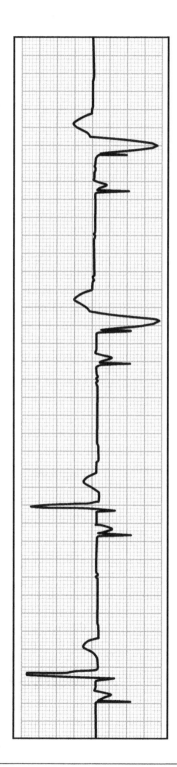

The Nuts and Bolts of Paced ECG Interpretation, 1st edition. By Tom Kenny.
Published 2009 by Blackwell Publishing, ISBN: 978-1-4501-8404-5.

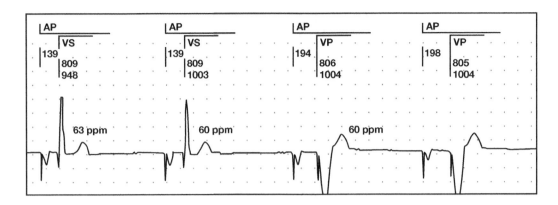

Mode

This is a dual-chamber pacemaker. The sweep speed of this particular tracing makes it look a bit "longer" than some of the other ones in this book, but it's pacing at around 60 ppm. The previous page showed the surface ECG. This image comes from the programmer.

Rate

There is a very interesting rate variation going on in this strip that warrants some explanation. Measure the atrial pacing interval on this strip (AP-AP) and everything looks fine (1000 ms or 60 ppm). But measure the ventricular interval between the first two AP-VS complexes and it indicates above-base-rate pacing at 63 ppm.

This is not rate response (that would have accelerated the atrial pacing interval). This ECG comes from an older device with *ventricular-based timing*. As such, it is set up to allow variations like this to occur in order to preserve the fixed atrial pacing interval. Although ventricular-based timing in pacemakers is getting rarer all of the time, Holter monitors still rely on ventricular-based timing.

A ventricular-based device uses this formula for its timing:

Base rate = AV interval + VA interval

This is easiest to see in AP-VP pacing. If the base rate (determined by the atrial pacing interval or AP-AP) is 60 ppm or 1000 ms and the programmed paced AV delay is 200 ms, then the formula would be:

1000 ms = 200 + 800 ms

When pacing AP-VP, the ventricular-based device preserves the programmed base rate. However, the pacemaker has to make some adjustments to the base rate when intrinsic ventricular activity occurs. Thus, in AP-VS pacing, a ventricular-based system has to make some adjustments to preserve the AV and VA intervals. In the "fast" interval on the strip above, the atrial pacing spike was followed in just 139 seconds by a ventricular intrinsic event. That formula is now:

X = 139 + 809 ms

This means the base rate now has to be 948 ms (139 + 809) or 63 ppm.

Capture

Atrial and ventricular capture appear to be appropriate.

Sensing

Atrial sensing cannot be evaluated from this strip, since all of the atrial events are paced.

Ventricular sensing appears appropriate in that the presence of intrinsic ventricular activity inhibited the ventricular output and reset device timing.

Underlying rhythm

This patient suffers from sinus node dysfunction and slow AV conduction.

What to do next

Atrial sensing must be evaluated, if possible. Lower the base rate of the device in 10-ppm steps down to no lower than 30 or 40 ppm. Monitor the patient as you lower the base rate incrementally. It may not always be possible to get intrinsic atrial activity to occur.

The rate variation apparent here is not a device malfunction; it's the normal and expected behavior of a device with ventricular-based timing. Most modern pacemakers rely on atrial-based timing, but there are older devices and Holter monitors that still use ventricular timing. Note that ventricular-based devices will only show such rate accelerations in AP-VS pacing, not AP-VP pacing.

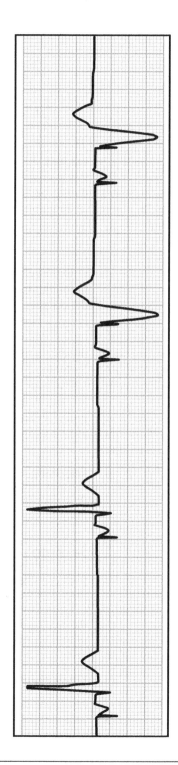

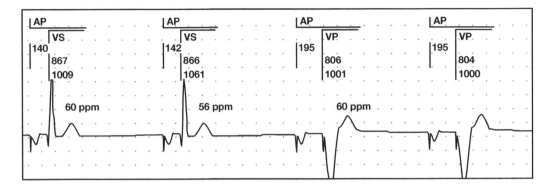

Mode

The presence of atrial and ventricular pacing spikes indicate that this is a dual-chamber strip. The sweep speed of this tracing makes it seem a little "airier" than some of the other ones in this book; that's just a function of how the programmer was set. Pacing is going on at around 60 ppm.

Rate

The atrial pacing interval (AP-AP) drives the dual-chamber pacing rate. In this case the atrial pacing interval is 1000 ms or 60 ppm, an appropriate rate. (As long as we measure the atrial pacing intervals, the rate is constant and appropriate.)

But notice that the ventricular escape interval on this strip (VS-VP) is 1061 ms long according to the interval notation. That converts to a rate of 56 ppm, or lower-than-base-rate pacing. Why does it appear that the pacemaker is violating the base rate?

The answer is that this is not at all unusual. This strip comes from a pacemaker using *atrial-based timing*. That means that the pacemaker regulates its timing such that it tries to maintain a constant atrial pacing interval (AP-AP). When other events occur, such as an intrinsic ventricular event, the pacemaker will adjust the ventricular escape interval or VS-VP (if it has to) in order to preserve a constant atrial pacing interval.

In this case, in order to maintain a constant atrial pacing interval, the pacemaker had to make adjustments and it did this by lengthening the ventricular escape interval (VS-VP). This caused slower-than-base rate pacing if you measure the ventricular pacing intervals; if you measure the atrial pacing inter-

vals only, it is not noticeable. You will not observe this phenomenon during AP-VP pacing or even during consistent AP-VS pacing but when ventricular escape intervals occur (VS followed by a VP), an atrial-based device may vary the ventricular pacing interval to preserve a constant atrial pacing interval.

To the best of my knowledge, all pacemakers on the market today use atrial-based timing and most devices you will see in the clinic are atrial-based systems. However, ventricular-based timing was once in widespread use and it will also turn up at the clinic in older devices and is commonly used in Holter monitors.

The important thing to recognize is that this seeming "rate variation" is actually the normal and proper behavior of a dual-chamber device with atrial-based timing.

Capture

Atrial and ventricular capture appear to be appropriate.

Sensing

Atrial sensing cannot be evaluated from this strip, since all of the atrial events are paced.

Ventricular sensing appears appropriate in that the presence of intrinsic ventricular activity inhibited the ventricular output and reset device timing.

Underlying rhythm

This patient has sinus node dysfunction and slow AV conduction

The nuts and bolts of paced ECG interpretation: atrial- versus ventricular-based timing

While most of the time you'll encounter atrial-based pacemakers in the clinic, it is important to understand that there are two types of timing systems employed by pacemakers and both have their own unique (and sometimes very confusing) eccentricities.

A dual-chamber pacemaker with atrial-based timing will maintain a consistent atrial pacing interval (AP-AP), adjusting the ventricular pacing interval if it has to in order to keep a constant atrial pacing interval. This shows up in slower-than-base-rate ventricular escape intervals (VS-VP).

When dealing with an atrial-based system, measure the atrial pacing interval to get the rate and do not be surprised if you occasionally encounter a slightly "too long" ventricular escape rate.

What to do next

Atrial sensing should be evaluated; lower the base rate by 10-ppm increments to encourage intrinsic atrial activity. Even if no intrinsic atrial activity occurs, do not drop the rate lower than 30 or 40 ppm or below what the patient can tolerate comfortably. It may not be possible to see intrinsic atrial activity.

Otherwise, this pacemaker is functioning appropriately.

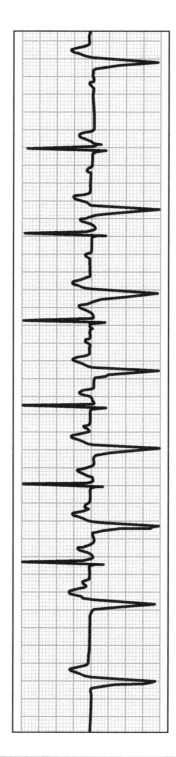

The Nuts and Bolts of Paced ECG Interpretation, 1st edition. By Tom Kenny.
Published 2009 by Blackwell Publishing, ISBN: 978-1-4501-8404-5.

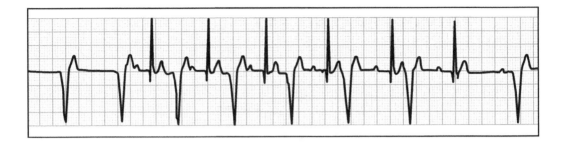

Mode

Although intrinsic atrial activity is present on the strip, it has no influence on the pacemaker's behavior. This is a single-chamber ventricular pacemaker.

Rate

There are two types of ventricular events on this strip. The wider, downward events are paced ventricular events, while the narrower, upward events are intrinsic ventricular events. The ventricular pacing interval (VP-VP) measures to be about 880 ms or 68 ppm. The rate marches through the strip without regard to the intrinsic activity – that is functional VOO pacing. However, there is a normal escape interval (VS-VP) at the end of the strip. Thus, this pacemaker was pacing asynchronously (VOO) but ends by pacing in VVI mode.

Capture

The downward ventricular events are paced events; the morphology is consistent. There do not appear to be any ventricular spikes on the strip that do not cause a paced event. Ventricular capture seems to be appropriate.

Sensing

Most of this strip reveals consistent ventricular undersensing. The intrinsic ventricular events are ignored by the pacemaker as the ventricular pacing interval marches through. The last intrinsic ventricular event is properly sensed; it inhibits the ventricular spike and resets device timing. Notice the last paced complex is timed to that last intrinsic ventricular event.

It is possible that this strip just shows an extended period of ventricular undersensing with a sudden resumption of proper ventricular sensing. But since the device is performing in VOO mode for so many beats, it is very appropriate to ask: what's going on? Why is this VVI pacemaker pacing consistently in VOO mode?

One possible answer is that this is some sort of magnet mode behavior. Pacemakers are designed to revert to specific behaviors when they come near a magnet. While magnet mode varies by device and manufacturer, it generally involves asynchronous pacing at a fixed rate. However, magnet mode pacing rates are often higher than normal base rates.

VOO mode is sometimes used as a temporarily programmed parameter for testing purposes. It is possible that VOO was temporarily programmed and then turned off.

Another explanation for this strip is intermittent ventricular undersensing. Rule out magnet mode and temporary VOO, if need be, by checking programmed device settings.

The nuts and bolts of paced ECG interpretation: magnet mode

Magnet mode behavior can vary by device and manufacturer, but, in general, look for pacing at a fixed and often somewhat high rate without any sensing. Magnet mode disables features like rate response or other parameters that might affect pacing rate, so you should see a constant rate as well as asynchronous pacing. Magnet mode essentially forces pacing and is typically used for specific tests. It can validate to the clinician that the pacemaker has sufficient output to capture the heart and that hardware (generator and leads) is working properly.

Most of the time, magnet mode strips are marked or obtained while you yourself are conducting the test. However, if you are assessing strips in a patient chart, you may run into magnet strips that are maintained on file.

Appropriate ventricular sensing is restored at the end of the strip, indicating that the device is capable of VVI pacing and capable of properly sensing the ventricle.

Underlying rhythm

The patient has sinus node dysfunction and slow AV conduction. The intrinsic atrial events seem to conduct down over the AV node to the ventricles but with a long and slightly variable PR interval (about 240 ms).

What to do next

If the patient is available, a longer tracing should be obtained! Without knowing for certain the cause of the asynchronous pacing, ventricular sensing should be evaluated and ventricular sensitivity re-programmed, if necessary.

Since this patient appears to have relatively good underlying cardiac function, he should be considered for a device upgrade to dual-chamber pacing at the next generator revision. It is possible that with a DDD device and a long AV delay interval, this patient might have 1:1 AV conduction and less right-ventricular (RV) pacing.

TOUGH TRACING #18

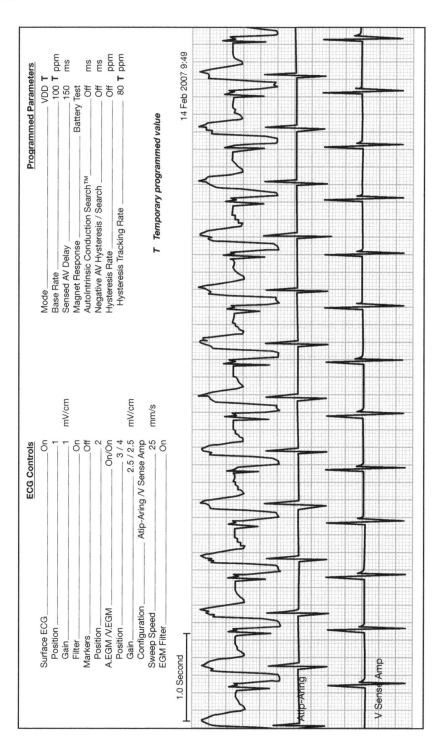

ECG Controls

Surface ECG	On	
Position	1	
Gain	1	mV/cm
Filter	On	
Markers	Off	
Position	2	
A.EGM /V.EGM	On/On	
Position	3 / 4	
Gain	2.5 / 2.5	mV/cm
Configuration	Atip-Aring /V Sense Amp	
Sweep Speed	25	mm/s
EGM Filter	On	

Programmed Parameters

Mode	VDD	**T**
Base Rate	100	**T** ppm
Sensed AV Delay	150	ms
Magnet Response	Battery Test	
AutoIntrinsic Conduction Search™	Off	ms
Negative AV Hysteresis / Search	Off	ms
Hysteresis Rate	Off	ppm
Hysteresis Tracking Rate	80	**T** ppm

T Temporary programmed value

14 Feb 2007 9:49

1.0 Second

Atip-Aring

V Sense Amp

The Nuts and Bolts of Paced ECG Interpretation, 1st edition. By Tom Kenny.
Published 2009 by Blackwell Publishing, ISBN: 978-1-4501-8404-5.

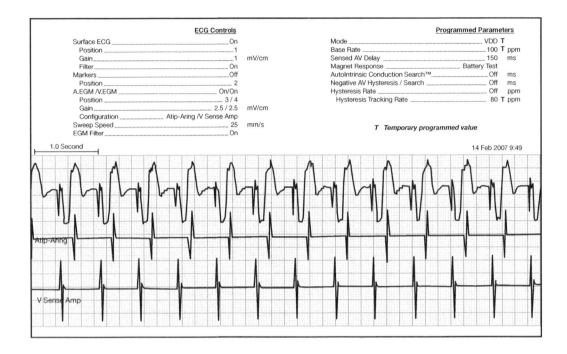

ECG Controls

Surface ECG	On
Position	1
Gain	1 mV/cm
Filter	On
Markers	Off
Position	2
A.EGM /V.EGM	On/On
Position	3 / 4
Gain	2.5 / 2.5 mV/cm
Configuration	Atip-Aring /V Sense Amp
Sweep Speed	25 mm/s
EGM Filter	On

Programmed Parameters

Mode	VDD **T**
Base Rate	100 **T** ppm
Sensed AV Delay	150 ms
Magnet Response	Battery Test
AutoIntrinsic Conduction Search™	Off ms
Negative AV Hysteresis / Search	Off ms
Hysteresis Rate	Off ppm
Hysteresis Tracking Rate	80 **T** ppm

T   Temporary programmed value

1.0 Second   14 Feb 2007 9:49

Atip-Aring

V Sense Amp

The nuts and bolts of paced ECG interpretation: using intracardiac electrograms (EGMs) with a paced ECG

In the clinic, strips like the one shown here are quite common. The upper tracing is a surface ECG; that is what most of us are trained to evaluate. Below that tracing are two intracardiac electrograms or IEGMS (sometimes also called EGMs). These tracings are taken from the electrodes on the pacing leads within the heart and they reveal a somewhat different perspective of the heart's electrical activity.

The middle line on this strip is the atrial EGM and the bottom line is the ventricular EGM. The tracings align so that the surface ECG can be contrasted to what the pacemaker electrodes report is going on within the heart.

Use atrial and ventricular intracardiac information to give you a fuller, more complete picture of what is going on in the heart. Sometimes the EGM can help solve difficult ECG interpretation puzzles.

Mode

Look just at the ECG and you might have trouble identifying the mode. There is consistent ventricular pacing, but it is difficult to see if atrial activity is present (that's where the atrial EGM comes in … there are indeed atrial events present but they are swallowed up in the T-wave of the preceding ventricular event). A glance at the printout reveals that this is VDD pacing! The T annotation after the VDD mode indicates that this is a temporarily programmed setting. Although there are dedicated VDD pacemakers on the market, this is likely a dual-chamber system temporarily operating in VDD mode. (If the device's highest mode was VDD, as would be the case in a dedicated VDD pacemaker, then it's unlikely VDD would be used as a "temporary" setting.)

Rate

The rate in VDD mode is reflected by the ventricular pacing interval (VP-VP), which measures to 600 ms (100 ppm) here. This is a surprisingly high pacing rate. Checking the annotations at the top of this

The nuts and bolts of paced ECG interpretation: VDD mode

VDD mode senses both chambers of the heart but paces only in the ventricle. When you review a VDD strip, you may see ventricular pacing timed to intrinsic atrial events, but you won't ever see atrial pacing.

Dedicated VDD or VDDR pacemakers work with a so-called "single-pass lead." This pacing lead anchors in the ventricle, where it can both pace and sense. But it has ring electrodes in the section of the pacing lead that would be located within the blood pool of the right atrium. A single-pass lead can sense atrial activity through the blood in the atrium using these special electrodes.

A dedicated VDD or VDDR device would be indicated for a patient with reliable sinus node function but poor conduction. The advantages of such a device are less hardware in the body and a slightly lower device cost. The disadvantage of VDD is that if sinus activity quits, the patient is left with a VVI pacemaker. Also if atrial pacing is ever required, a device revision is needed and an additional lead must be implanted.

VDD can also be used as a test mode. It is particularly useful to test for retrograde (VA) conduction.

mode, but is atrial activity present in this strip? The atrial electrogram confirms that intrinsic atrial activity is going on. Using the atrial EGM, it is possible to identify atrial events on the ECG. They are obscured by the large T-wave but once you know where to look, they can be seen as notches or bumps at the top of the QRS complex.

The first problem with the intrinsic atrial activity is that it is clearly not used to drive the device. In a typical VDD system, the intrinsic atrial event would launch a sensed AV delay and be followed by a ventricular pacing spike. The interval between AS and VP measures to be about 400 ms, which is far too long for a sensed AV delay.

However, something interesting shows up. *The intrinsic atrial event appears consistently 200 ms after the ventricular pacing spike.* This is most clearly visible on the two EGMs. Measure the distance from the VP event (lower EGM) to the AS event (upper EGM) and it marches through consistently at 200 ms. A constant VA interval (VP-AS) indicates retrograde conduction. In this case, you can measure the retrograde conduction interval (200 ms).

Underlying rhythm

This is a test strip, so it is not a good idea to misuse it to evaluate normal rhythm. Instead, it was used to assess retrograde conduction, which it found. Not all patients have retrograde conduction, but it is good to know if a patient can conduct in retrograde manner since it can affect how the device is programmed.

What to do next

Although capture and sensing might be evaluated from this strip, I hesitate to use a test strip to evaluate device function or underlying rhythm. For this patient, more ECG should be recorded to assess the basics. This strip does, however, alert us to retrograde conduction and even provides us with a way to measure the retrograde conduction interval (200 ms).

Dual-chamber pacemaker patients with retrograde conduction are at risk of pacemaker-mediated tachycardia (PMT). One of the best defenses against PMT is a long PVARP interval. While retrograde conduction cannot be prevented, the clinician can

strip, it is clear that 100 ppm was deliberately programmed, but on a temporary basis. These temporary settings are clear indications that this rhythm strip reflects some kind of test.

Capture

Atrial capture cannot be assessed on a VDD strip, since there is no atrial pacing. Ventricular capture on this strip looks appropriate. Notice that you can compare the very prominent spikes on the lower tracing (ventricular EGM) against the surface ECG on the top to confirm ventricular paced activity.

Sensing

The pacemaker will sense atrial activity in the VDD

program the pacemaker to prevent it from responding to that retrograde conduction. In order to do that, the pacemaker patient should have a PVARP interval that is *longer than his retrograde conduction interval.*This makes it more likely that any retrograde P-waves will "fall into" the refractory period and not reset device timing.

The PVARP value for this patient is not shown on this strip, but we know that his retrograde conduction interval is 200 ms. A typical PVARP setting is 250 ms and that is probably acceptable for this patient. Since retrograde conduction is a known factor for this patient, I might be inclined to add a bit of a cushion to the PVARP and set it at 280 ms.

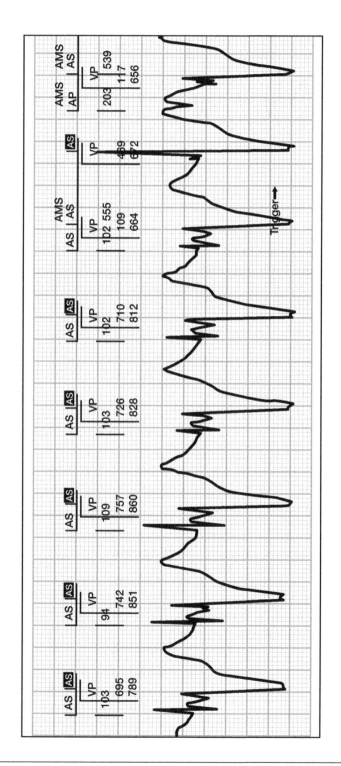

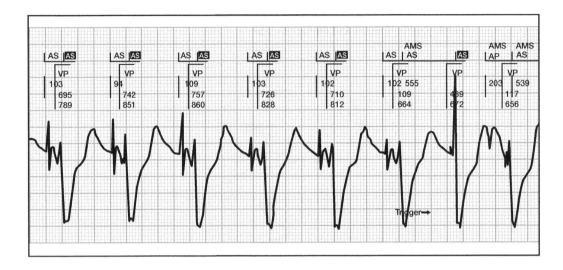

The nuts and bolts of paced ECG interpretation: stored electrograms

This is an intracardiac electrogram (IEGM or EGM) that was retained in the pacemaker's memory and downloaded during a programming session. While this is not truly a paced ECG, pacemaker clinicians must develop skills at retrieving and interpreting these recordings, which offer a snapshot of remarkable cardiac events.

Most EGMS are stored because of some sort of triggering event annotated on the strip. In this case, it is a mode switch (AMS annotations, top right) and notation "Trigger" at the bottom right.

The tracing itself is a dual-channel electrogram. This is an intracardiac electrogram composed of both atrial and ventricular input. It's neither a true atrial nor a true ventricular electrogram – it's somewhere in the middle. Many pacemaker clinicians prefer this kind of electrogram, because it looks more like a surface ECG and it is the most economical kind of stored EGM in terms of pacemaker memory capacity.

Mode

The presence of mode switching (AMS annotations at the top right) means that the device has to be a dual-chamber system. This could be determined even without annotations in that atrial and ventricular activity are clearly timed to each other. Notice an intrinsic atrial event occurs (AS) and then about 100 ms later, a ventricular pacing spike is delivered. This indicates a sensed AV delay is in play, meaning it is a dual-chamber system. Even if it was unclear from the tracing whether these atrial events were sensed or paced, this would have to be a dual-chamber system.

After AMS is activated, there is an AP-VP event. It seems as if this pacemaker has moved from DDD pacing to DDI pacing (dual-chamber, no tracking).

Rate

The rate cannot be determined here because intrinsic atrial activity is in control of pacing.

Capture

There is only one atrial output pulse on this strip and it appears to capture appropriately. Ventricular capture seems consistently appropriate.

Sensing

Events annotated with a plain AS are appropriately sensed. The atrial depolarization shows up on the ECG and the annotation confirms that the pacemaker "saw" it. The pacemaker also "sees" some intrinsic atrial events that are just about impossible to

The nuts and bolts of paced ECG interpretation: AMS concepts

It is the patient's intrinsic atrial rate that drives a DDD pacemaker; the pacemaker will do what it can, within reason, to provide 1:1 AV synchrony even if it means pacing faster than the programmed base rate to keep up with a rapid intrinsic atrial rate. However, there is a point at which the pacemaker will apply the "brakes" to the ventricular pacing rate. For instance, atrial tracking at a rate of 100 ppm is probably beneficial for most patients, but atrial tracking at 200 ppm is never a good idea. The maximum tracking rate (MTR) sets the fastest rate at which the ventricles can be paced in response to intrinsic atrial activity.

One device feature to help dual-chamber devices better manage high intrinsic atrial rates is mode switching, sometimes called auto mode switch (AMS). The concept is simple: when the patient's native atrial rate starts to go faster than a programmed atrial cutoff rate, atrial tracking is simply turned off until the intrinsic atrial rate returns to a lower rate.

This results in a change of pacing mode (for example, from DDD to VVI or even DDD to DDI), which is where the algorithm gets its name. Some pacemakers allow the clinician to select the temporary mode that is used when AMS goes into effect.

In order to be able to enter and exit AMS appropriately, the pacemaker has to recognize and count atrial events, including those that might technically "fall into" the refractory period. The pacemaker does not respond to such events or use them to reset device timing … but the AMS algorithm recognizes them and counts them. They appear on this particular tracing as black boxes with white AS letters. (Other manufacturers may use other conventions to represent this kind of atrial activity.)

read from the tracing; these are shown in the black boxes marked AS. On this particular type of device, an AS annotation in a black box refers to an intrinsic atrial event that "fell into" the atrial refractory period. As such, the pacemaker will not recognize or respond to it. However, the pacemaker has seen it and counts it; it counts toward meeting the criteria to initiate the AMS algorithm.

Whenever AMS is activated, the clinician has to ask: was AMS appropriate? Inappropriate AMS can occur when the pacemaker oversenses atrial activity. For example, if the pacemaker picks up far-field signals from the ventricle and counts them as atrial events, this can result in atrial oversensing leading to inappropriate AMS. This phenomenon has been nicknamed "double counting" or "far-field sensing" (sometimes called "far-R"). Therefore, it is important to determine whether the pacemaker was counting actual atrial events or picking up far-field signals.

On this particular strip, it is unclear. The AS events in the black box might represent where the pacemaker sensed the ventricular pacemaker spike (VP) and inappropriately labeled them atrial sensed events. On the other hand, they could be genuine intrinsic atrial depolarizations that are just obscured by the larger ventricular depolarization. An atrial intracardiac electrogram would come in handy here! Since we do not have access to an atrial EGM, the best evaluation to make is that it is unclear if this is appropriate atrial sensing and an appropriate entry into AMS.

I suspect far-field sensing, in that the AS event in the black box occurs so closely in conjunction with the ventricular pacing spike and creates pairs of two atrial sensed events … with gaps in between. An intrinsic high atrial rate is more likely to show up as AS events in rapid sequence, not in pairs that have an apparent relationship to ventricular pacing.

Ventricular sensing cannot be evaluated from this strip, since it is all ventricular pacing.

Underlying rhythm

This patient has slow AV conduction and may have rapid intrinsic atrial activity.

What to do next

This is a stored EGM to help the clinician determine if AMS entry was appropriate. Unfortunately, it is not completely clear from this strip. If we had an atrial electrogram, we might have been able to determine it, but if the device offers this kind of stored

EGM, it does not offer the option of a simultaneous stored atrial and ventricular EGM, too. Instead, I would get a surface ECG.

Using the surface ECG, I would do a systematic analysis with special attention on possible atrial oversensing of far-field signals. If diagnostic reports are available, I would check how frequently AMS episodes occurred. If frequent AMS occurs, it would make me want to look very hard for possible atrial oversensing.

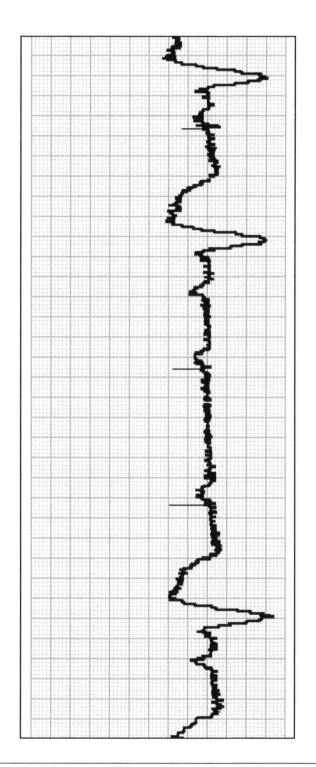

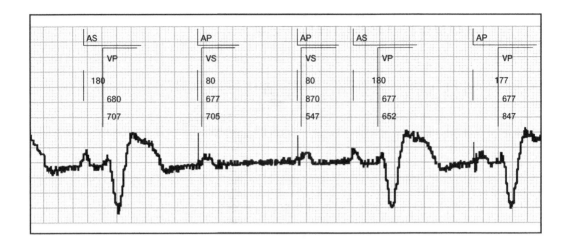

Mode

This is a dual-chamber strip. Note the chart speed on this tracing is faster than usual.

Rate

The atrial pacing interval (AP-AP) is around 700 ms (85 ppm). This is a bit faster than typical, but not inappropriate.

Capture

There are three atrial spikes on the strip and atrial capture appears to be appropriate.

There are three ventricular spikes on the strip; ventricular capture seems to be appropriate.

Sensing

There are two intrinsic atrial events on the strip, both of which inhibited the atrial output pulse, reset device time, and show up on the annotations. Thus, atrial sensing is appropriate.

Ventricular sensing is more problematic. There are no intrinsic ventricular events on the tracing, but the annotations show two VS events. This is ventricular oversensing. While this might be just a simple case of oversensing, we should always ask ourselves why this might have occurred.

Notice that both sensed and paced AV delay intervals (AS-VP or AP-VP) are about 180 ms. But the oversensed ventricular activity occurs almost immediately after the atrial pacing spike (there is just 30 ms offset). This indicates that the pacemaker is suffering from "crosstalk inhibition." The atrial pacing spike is being picked up by the ventricular sensing circuits and inappropriately counted as an intrinsic ventricular event. As a result, the pacemaker withholds the ventricular pacing spike. This manifests itself on the ECG as a pause that looks like ventricular oversensing.

Underlying rhythm

This patient has sinus node dysfunction and slow AV conduction. He also has a case of "crosstalk" which is a device-based condition! Notice that crosstalk occurs for two beats but then the pacemaker resumes normal operation.

What to do next

A number of things can contribute to crosstalk inhibition, whether working in isolation or in combination. The first thing to check out is the atrial output. While atrial capture is appropriate, the atrial output settings may be higher than necessary. If the atrial pulse amplitude and/or atrial pulse width can be safely reduced, this will minimize one of the causes of crosstalk.

Second, ventricular sensing should be evaluated. Not only can it not be assessed from the strip, the presence of crosstalk should make us at least consider the fact that the ventricular sensitivity setting may be too high (the mV setting too low). This would make the ventricular sensing circuits "too alert" to electrical signals.

Finally, the blanking period on the pacemaker should be extended slightly to help "blind" the pacemaker to the atrial output.

These three programming strategies can all help minimize the occurrence of crosstalk.

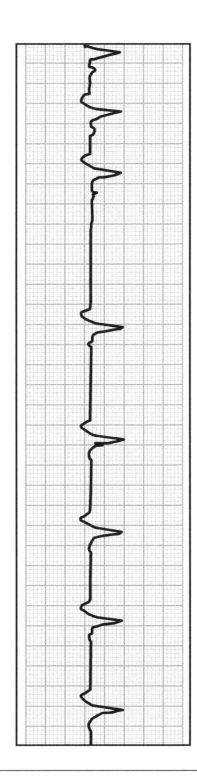

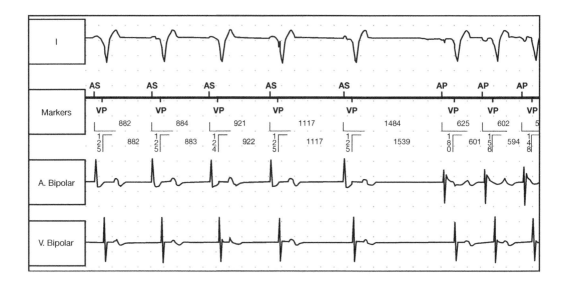

Mode

This is a dual-chamber strip. You can see it in the atrial tracking, the way the ventricular pacing rate changes as the sinus node slows down, and from the presence of paced events in both chambers. The annotations confirm this.

Rate

The atrial rate, whether paced or sensed, typically "drives" dual-chamber pacing. The left side of the tracing shows atrial tracking with a sinus node that is slowing down rapidly (in five beats, the intrinsic atrial interval changes from 882 to 1117 ms, that is, it drops from 68 ppm to 54 ppm). On the right side of the strip, the atrial pacing interval (AP-AP) is 625 ms (96 ppm) and 602 (100 ppm). This relatively slow atrial tracking followed by a pause and then 100 ppm AP-VP pacing indicates something unusual is going on. We should be on the lookout for special algorithms or features that might explain this behavior.

This rhythm strip is an example of an advanced hysteresis function. Ordinarily, hysteresis is a function that prolongs the escape interval periodically to encourage the heart's intrinsic activity to prevail. There are advanced functions of hysteresis which follow hysteresis intervals with periods of above-base-rate pacing. This is particularly useful in patients who experience neurocardiogenic syncope. The idea is that when the heart's intrinsic rhythm slows, rapid pacing can help preserve cardiac output.

If this pacemaker had been programmed to a base rate of 60 ppm, the atrial tracking behavior seen in the first five complexes would be normal and handled appropriately by the pacemaker. After the fifth beat, the escape interval is prolonged as the pacemaker searches for intrinsic ventricular activity. When none occurs, the pacemaker begins AP-VP pacing at 100 ppm. That's caused by the advanced hysteresis algorithm. It's a feature called "rate drop response."

The concept behind "rate drop response" is that if a patient's intrinsic rate starts to slow rapidly and abruptly, the pacemaker comes in with above-base-rate pacing to preserve cardiac output.

Capture

Atrial capture appears to be appropriate, as does ventricular capture which occurs consistently across the tracing.

Sensing

Atrial sensing is appropriate, in that the left side of the strip shows intrinsic atrial events to which the ventricular output timed itself. These intrinsic atrial events inhibited an atrial output spike, too.

Ventricular sensing cannot be assessed from this strip, since it shows consistent ventricular pacing.

The nuts and bolts of paced ECG interpretation: neurocardiogenic syncope

Neurocardiogenic syncope is a broad term used to describe syncope or dizziness up to and including loss of consciousness attributed to neural or cardiac causes.

Syncope can be an extremely difficult symptom to manage, since it has many potential causes and may or may not be indicative of a serious health issue. Patients with neurocardiogenic syncope experience large and abrupt rate drops, that is, their hearts beat at a normal rhythm and can slow down suddenly, even resulting in asystolic pauses. Neurocardiogenic syncope patients are prone to syncope or even passing out from this sudden decline in their heart rate.

If regular base rate pacing were used, that would definitely help. But patients with neurocardiogenic syncope may already be in distress due to a falling rate. That's why advanced hysteresis can be helpful in such patients. It is not a commonly used feature since most patients will never need it. But for those who do, it can be a very important feature to enable!

Advanced hysteresis with rate drop response is not a common way to program a pacemaker, but pacemaker clinicians will encounter it. If a patient has a history of neurocardiogenic syncope or fainting spells, look for this kind of programming of a dual-chamber pacemaker.

Underlying rhythm

The patient has sinus node dysfunction and slow AV conduction. The sudden, abrupt drop in sinus node function strongly suggests that this patient could become syncopal (which would be neurocardiogenic syncope).

What to do next

Ventricular sensing should be evaluated. Temporarily program a long AV delay of 300 ms or higher and see if intrinsic ventricular activity occurs. If it does not, the device can be temporarily programmed to VVI and the base rate lowered in 10-ppm steps down to no lower than 30 or 40 ppm. The extended AV delay is by far the better method.

Advanced hysteresis is working appropriately in that after the sudden rate drop, the pacemaker began above-base-rate pacing. This was appropriate and expected device behavior and likely helped preserve cardiac output in the patient and prevented a dizzy spell or fainting.

While advanced hysteresis with rate drop response is very useful for patients with neurocardiogenic syncope, it is not an appropriate algorithm for all patients.

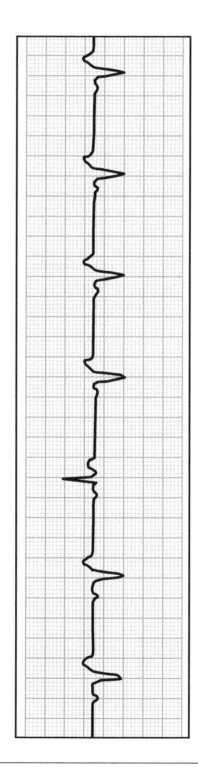

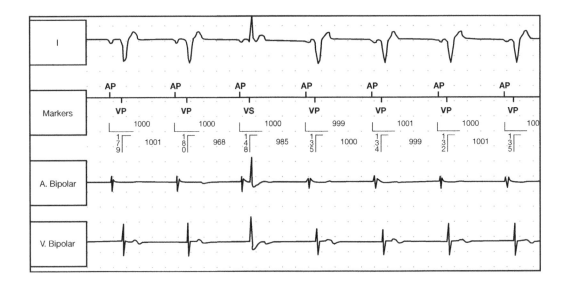

Mode

The clear atrial and ventricular relationship means this is a dual-chamber pacemaker; that is confirmed by the annotations.

Rate

The atrial pacing interval (AP-AP) is 60 ppm (1000 ms), which is appropriate and typical. Notice the AV delay values. The first two complexes show a paced AV delay of about 180 ms. The third complex is an AP-VS event, that is, the atrial output pulse conducts down over the AV node and causes a ventricular depolarization. The intrinsic ventricular event interrupts the paced AV delay before it can time out. But in the remaining four events on the left of the strip, the paced AV delay is considerably shorter (about 133 ms). Whenever we see such changes in AV delay intervals, we have to suspect a specialty algorithm of some sort.

Capture

Atrial and ventricular capture are appropriate.

Sensing

Atrial sensing cannot be assessed from this strip. Ventricular sensing seems to be appropriate, although this strip only provides us with one example of a ventricular sensed event.

Underlying rhythm

This patient is being paced close to 100% of the time in both chambers (AP-VP). The one time that intrinsic ventricular occurred spontaneously, the paced AV delay automatically tightened up to force ventricular pacing again.

This is an example of negative AV hysteresis. Regular hysteresis is an algorithm that promotes intrinsic conduction; negative hysteresis is an algorithm that does the opposite, that is, it tries to pace the patient as much as possible. In this case, the intrinsic ventricular event occurred, was properly sensed, and launched the Negative AV Hysteresis algorithm, which shortened the paced AV delay in a successful attempt to restore consistent AP-VP pacing.

> ### The nuts and bolts of paced ECG interpretation: negative AV hysteresis
>
> Negative hysteresis, which forces pacing, is an algorithm available in many newer devices. Negative hysteresis is useful in patients with hypertrophic obstructive cardiomyopathy or HOCM. These patients have a heart with very thick and inflexible ventricular walls. It is believed that HOCM patients derive better cardiac output and hemodynamics when the heart is artificially paced than when it beats on its own. As a result, negative hysteresis can be used in such patients to force-pace the heart as much as possible.

What to do next

Atrial sensing should be evaluated, if possible, and it may be prudent to test ventricular sensing as well, although the one intrinsic event that occurs on this strip was properly sensed.

The algorithm which intended to force-pace the heart worked well and successfully restored AP-VP pacing. The patient's history and symptoms should be checked to verify the presence of HOCM. If diagnostic reports are available, they should be checked to see how much pacing the patient receives. Unlike a typical bradycardia pacemaker patient, HOCM patients should be paced as close to 100% of the time as possible. If this is not happening, it may be necessary to permanently program a slightly shorter paced AV delay while still maintaining the Negative AV Hysteresis algorithm.

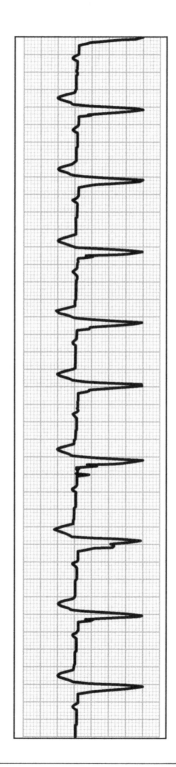

The Nuts and Bolts of Paced ECG Interpretation, 1st edition. By Tom Kenny.
Published 2009 by Blackwell Publishing, ISBN: 978-1-4501-8404-5.

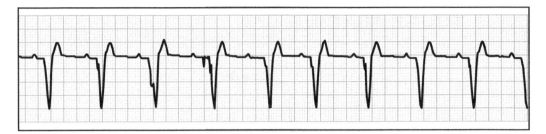

Mode

This is a dual-chamber strip. It might look like a single-chamber strip in that pacing is occurring only in the ventricle, but notice that ventricular pacing appears to be timed to the atrial activity (atrial tracking) with the exception of the fourth and fifth complexes.

Rate

Since atrial tracking is occurring, the programmed base rate cannot be assessed. Notice that the sensed AV delay is consistent in the strip except for the fourth event (which shows an unusual downward output spike) and the fifth event (which has a longer-than-usual sensed AV delay). These variations do not seem random; they most likely indicate the presence of a special algorithm at work.

Capture

Atrial capture cannot be evaluated from this strip since all of the atrial activity is intrinsic.

Most of the strip shows appropriate ventricular capture, except for the fourth complex. Notice an intrinsic atrial event occurs, launching the sensed AV delay. When it times out, a ventricular output pulse is delivered. This output pulse shows up as a little downward notch on the strip, but it fails to capture the ventricle. About 100 ms after the first (failed) ventricular output spike, a second is delivered … and this time it captures the ventricle.

The presence of two ventricular output pulses so close together indicates that a capture algorithm is at work. The first spike was insufficient in energy to capture the ventricle so the device delivered a backup safety pulse, which captured the ventricle.

This backup safety pulse affected the next complex in that the sensed AV delay was prolonged by 100 ms for one cycle only. This temporarily extended AV delay interval is also known as the fusion avoidance feature. It prevents a possible fused beat (intrinsic depolarization colliding with a pacemaker spike) by extending the AV delay slightly for one cycle only.

Ventricular capture in this strip is being controlled by a capture algorithm (in this case, it's the AutoCapture Pacing Systems® algorithm from St. Jude Medical) so that even when capture was lost for a beat, it was restored in a moment (just 100 ms later). The ventricular capture algorithm is working appropriately.

The nuts and bolts of paced ECG interpretation: automatic capture algorithms

Nowadays there are two ways to assure long-term appropriate capture: program a very large safety margin or use a special algorithm to promote capture.

While capture algorithms may not be right for every patient, they can benefit most patients by using lower amounts of energy to pace the heart, monitoring the heart to be sure capture occurred, and delivering a backup safety pulse, as shown in this example, whenever capture is lost. Such algorithms frequently state that they enhance patient safety while simultaneously using less energy.

The energy savings of such an algorithm are considerable; pacemakers equipped with the AutoCapture Pacing Systems® algorithm can last a decade or more. One minor downside of these algorithms is that they can create ECGs which puzzle clinicians not familiar with these features!

Sensing

Atrial sensing appears to be appropriate in that ventricular pacing is being driven by the intrinsic atrial events and atrial activity inhibits atrial output pulses.

Ventricular sensing cannot be evaluated from this strip.

Underlying rhythm

The patient has good sinus node function and slow AV conduction.

What to do next

Atrial pacing and ventricular sensing should be evaluated.

The AutoCapture® algorithm is working well in this strip, but the tests relative to that particular algorithm should be performed as well to assure on-going appropriate operation of this feature. These tests can be conducted semi-automatically from the programmer.

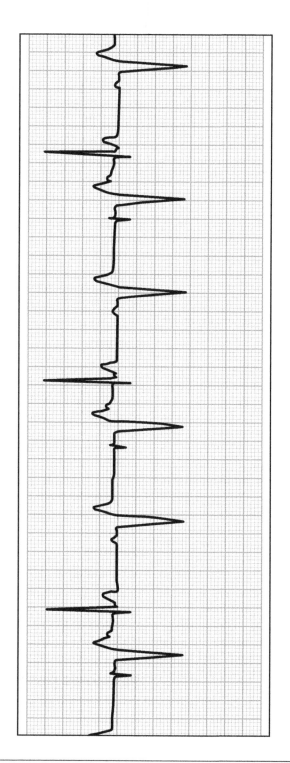

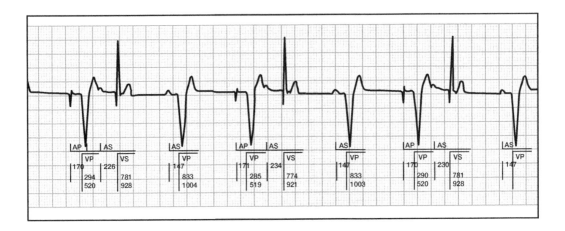

Mode

The presence of atrial and ventricular pacing spikes indicates that this is a dual-chamber strip.

Rate

Normally, one would look for an atrial pacing interval (AP-AP) to confirm the pacing rate, but there is no such interval on this strip. Instead, measure the atrial escape interval (AS-AP), which occurs on this strip. That measures 1000 ms (60 ppm), an appropriate rate.

The great puzzle on this strip is the AV delay interval. The paced AV delay (AP-VP) is 170 ms, which is an appropriate setting. The sensed AV delays (AS-VP), however, are all over the map! The first sensed atrial event results in a pause of 226 ms before an intrinsic ventricular event occurs; that means the first sensed AV delay exceeded 226 ms. The second sensed AV delay interval was 147 ms. What's going on?

Look at the pattern on the strip. The long sensed AV delay intervals only occur in close proximity to a previous paced atrial event. The pacemaker automatically overrode the programmed sensed AV delay in order to preserve the maximum tracking rate or MTR. The first complex on this strip is AP-VP. The next atrial event occurs so close to the previous atrial event that the device would have violated the MTR (even if it was set as low as 100 ppm or 600 ms) if it had imposed the programmed sensed AV delay of 147 ms. The pacemaker will not pace faster than the MTR, so it temporarily suspended

the sensed AV delay and waited to pace. Before it could pace, an intrinsic ventricular event occurred, resulting in the second complex (AS-VS).

This pattern repeats itself on the strip and is the result of the pacemaker's preserving the MTR even at the cost of sacrificing the sensed AV delay. This is actually normal and appropriate device behavior.

Capture

There are three atrial pacing spikes on this strip (AP annotations) but it is unclear to me if they captured the atrium or not. At the very least, they look suspiciously like loss of atrial capture.

On the other hand, ventricular capture looks good. Notice that the strip contains ventricular depolarizations with the typical "paced morphology" following ventricular pacing spikes. The few intrinsic ventricular events on the strip have a distinctly different shape.

Sensing

Atrial sensing is appropriate. The intrinsic atrial events on this strip inhibit the atrial output pulse and reset device timing.

Ventricular sensing is likewise functioning properly.

Underlying rhythm

This patient has sinus node dysfunction and slow AV conduction.

What to do next

Atrial capture should be evaluated; while some colleagues might say that this strip might show appropriate atrial capture, there is some doubt in my mind. When in doubt, test it out! Otherwise, this pacemaker is exhibiting appropriate (if somewhat unusual) behavior.

TOUGH TRACING #25

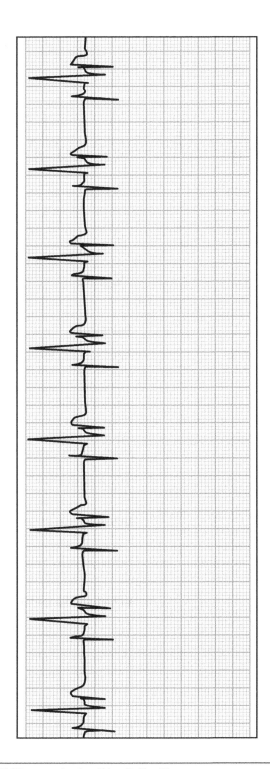

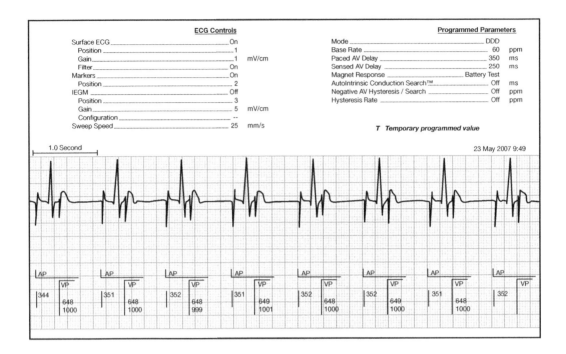

Mode

This is a dual-chamber pacemaker.

Rate

The atrial pacing interval (AP-AP) is 1000 ms or 60 ppm, an expected and appropriate rate.

Capture

Atrial capture is appropriate.

Ventricular capture is another story. After the paced atrial event in each complex, an intrinsic ventricular event occurs followed by a ventricular pacing spike. In each instance, the ventricular spike fails to capture.

In such cases, we need to figure out if the ventricular spike ought to have captured the ventricle. In every complex in this strip, there is no way that ventricular output pulse could have caused a ventricular depolarization, because the ventricular myocardium was physiologically refractory. This is functional non-capture. Functional non-capture goes hand-in-hand with undersensing.

Sensing

Atrial sensing cannot be evaluated from this strip, because every atrial event here is paced.

Functional ventricular non-capture suggests ventricular undersensing. The intrinsic ventricular complexes on the strip are definitely "overlooked" by the pacemaker. They neither inhibit the output pulse, nor reset device timing, nor are they annotated on the tracing. Thus, ventricular sensing is inappropriate.

Underlying rhythm

This patient has sinus node dysfunction, but it looks like he has intact AV conduction.

What to do next

The most pressing need for this patient is to restore proper ventricular sensing. A ventricular sensing test should be conducted and the ventricular sensitivity setting adjusted.

Atrial sensitivity should be tested as well.

Scramble

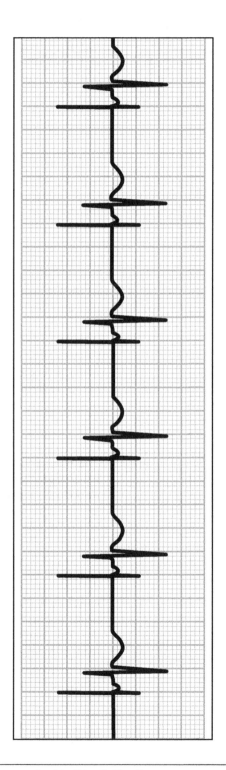

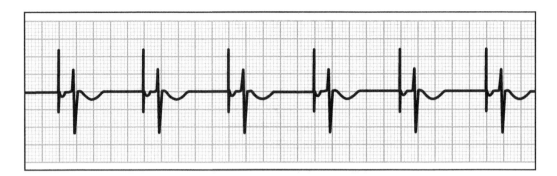

Mode

This strip could be from a single-chamber atrial pacemaker (AAI) or a dual-chamber pacemaker that is pacing in AAI mode. The latter is more likely, since dual-chamber devices are much more common in clinical practice than atrial pacemakers.

Rate

The atrial pacing interval (AP-AP) is 1000 ms or 60 ppm, an appropriate rate.

Capture

Atrial capture appears to be consistently appropriate; the atrial output pulse results in a depolarization and resets device timing. The atrial depolarization conducts via the AV node down to the ventricles. The delay between a paced atrial event and the onset of the intrinsic ventricular depolarization (AP-VS) is consistently about 200 ms, as measured with calipers, which is further evidence of appropriate atrial capture.

Ventricular capture cannot be assessed from this strip since there is no ventricular pacing evident on the tracing.

Sensing

Atrial sensing cannot be evaluated from this strip.

Ventricular sensing is appropriate in that the intrinsic ventricular events inhibit the ventricular output pulse and reset device timing.

Underlying rhythm

The patient has sinus node dysfunction but intact AV conduction.

What to do next

The pacing behavior in this strip is appropriate, but provides an incomplete picture. An atrial sensing test and a ventricular capture test should be conducted.

To test atrial sensing, the base rate should be reduced temporarily in increments of 10-ppm to see if intrinsic atrial events break through. Observe and talk with the patient as you gradually decrease the base rate but even if the rate is tolerated and no intrinsic atrial activity emerges, do not go below 30 or 40 ppm.

Ventricular pacing can be tested by shortening the AV delay interval temporarily. That is the preferred method. In the event that does not work, temporarily program the device to VVI and then lower the base rate in 10-ppm steps (but never below 30 or 40 ppm) to see if intrinsic ventricular activity appears.

The nuts and bolts of paced ECG interpretation: AAI pacing in single- and dual-chamber pacemakers

Single-chamber atrial pacemakers have been around for years, but are not routinely seen in clinical practice. In most instances, AAI pacing observed in the clinical setting comes from a dual-chamber pacemaker. While I would not make an official ruling on whether this particular strip is a single-chamber atrial system or a dual-chamber pacemaker operating in AAI mode, in the absence of other data, I would proceed in my assessment by assuming that this strip comes from a dual-chamber pacemaker. Clinicians trying to evaluate a rhythm strip with incomplete information must always opt for "most likely" situations based on the available data.

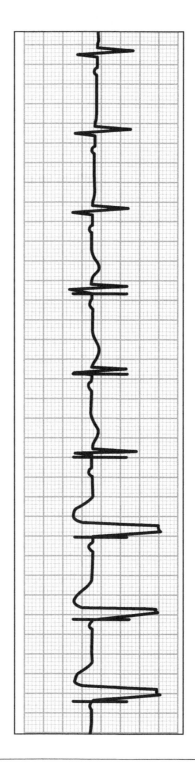

The Nuts and Bolts of Paced ECG Interpretation, 1st edition. By Tom Kenny.
Published 2009 by Blackwell Publishing, ISBN: 978-1-4501-8404-5.

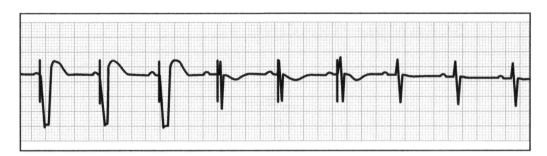

Mode

This is a VVI pacemaker.

Rate

The ventricular pacing interval (VP-VP) is 800 ms (75 ppm), an appropriate rate.

Capture

Ventricular capture is appropriate in the first three complexes: the spike leads to a depolarization that resets device timing. The QRS morphology exhibits the characteristic widened bizarre look of a paced ventricular event.

The next three spikes occur on top of what appear to be intrinsic ventricular events. In fact, if you compare the QRS morphology of the last three complexes (true intrinsic ventricular events) to the preceding three complexes, it is apparent that spikes and intrinsic events occurred "on top of each other." This is pseudofusion. Pseudofusion does not confirm capture, but it does not contradict it, either. Ventricular capture appears appropriate, but pseudofusion suggests that the patient's intrinsic rate is competing with the programmed base rate.

Sensing

Ventricular sensing can only be assessed from the last three complexes on this strip. These events appear to be properly sensed in that the pacemaker withholds a ventricular spike and resets device timing.

Underlying rhythm

The patient has good sinus node function but slow AV conduction. His native rate sometimes approaches the programmed base rate of 75 beats a minute.

What to do next

The presence of several pseudofusion complexes indicates that the pacing rate sometimes "bumps into" the patient's own intrinsic rate. This could be addressed by programming a hysteresis rate of 60 or 65 bpm.

The nuts and bolts of paced ECG interpretation: why program hysteresis when you can lower the base rate?

When a patient's intrinsic rate starts to compete with the programmed base rate, fusion and pseudofusion appear on the paced ECG. The best course of action is to encourage more native activity. Lowering the base rate may seem more straightforward, but many patients have only intermittent periods when their intrinsic rate competes with the base rate. Furthermore, they may need pacing at the currently programmed base rate for most of their daily activities. Exposing them to permanently programmed slower base rates may provoke symptoms.

Hysteresis offers a great solution, in that it goes into effect only in the presence of intrinsic activity and lasts only as long as the patient's intrinsic rate remains above the programmed hysteresis rate. Thus, it adjusts automatically to the patient's changing heart rates. It's a great way to give the patient the best of both worlds – an adequately high base rate and the benefits of intrinsic conduction when possible.

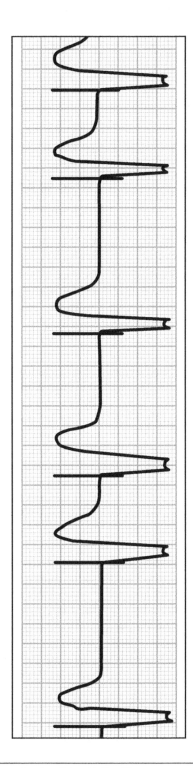

The Nuts and Bolts of Paced ECG Interpretation, 1st edition. By Tom Kenny.
Published 2009 by Blackwell Publishing, ISBN: 978-1-4501-8404-5.

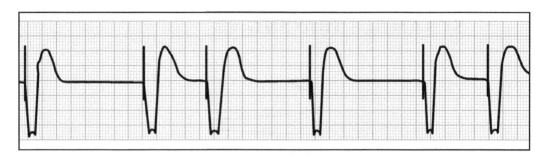

Mode

This is a VVI pacemaker.

Rate

The rate is very confusing! There are two ventricular pacing intervals on the strip (VP-VP) that measure about 880 ms (around 68 ppm), which is likely to be the programmed rate. It is an appropriate rate for single-chamber ventricular pacing. However, there are three longer-than-normal ventricular pacing intervals; two of these long intervals measure about 1600 ms (38 ppm) and one is 1440 ms (42 ppm). The most likely explanation is that the programmed base rate is 70 ppm but we need to account for the pauses on the strip.

Capture

Ventricular capture is appropriate in the strip.

Sensing

Since there are only ventricular paced events on this strip, appropriate ventricular sensing cannot be assessed. However, the pauses suggest ventricular oversensing. Setting the calipers to the ventricular pacing interval (VP-VP) or 880 ms and measuring backward from one spike into the pause, the exact position where something was inappropriately sensed can be determined. Using this method, sometimes the phenomenon that was oversensed can be determined. However, here it is not clear what exactly might have caused the oversensing.

Underlying rhythm

This patient has sinus node dysfunction (maybe even what is called "silent atria") and slow AV conduction. It is possible he is pacemaker dependent.

What to do next

The ventricular oversensing must be corrected. Normally, this would be accomplished by trying to force intrinsic ventricular to emerge and then conducting a sensing test. However, this patient could be pacemaker dependent. The appearance of the tracing suggests to me that intrinsic ventricular activity may never appear at all, even if the base rate were temporarily set very low. For that reason – and for this type of patient only – I would approach the oversensing problem backward.

Instead of finding intrinsic ventricular activity and then adjusting sensitivity, I am going to start off by adjusting the sensitivity.

This device is oversensing, so the goal is to make the pacemaker less sensitive. To make a pacemaker less sensitive, you should increase the mV setting. For example, if this pacemaker had a ventricular sensitivity setting of 2.0 mV, it should be reduced to make the device less sensitive. I would program it to 1.0 mV. Then I would observe how the patient responded. If it solved the problem with oversensing, I would leave the matter at that. If it did not, I would keep making the pacemaker less sensitive until I could resolve the oversensing issue.

The downside of adjusting sensitivity first is that the first change (from 2.0 mV to 1.0 mV) might make the device less sensitive to the point that it could miss intrinsic ventricular events. For most pacemaker patients, that is a risk the clinician does not want to take. But in this kind of patient, intrinsic ventricular activity is not the issue at all. In fact, intrinsic ventricular activity may never occur. The more important concern here is to fix the oversensing.

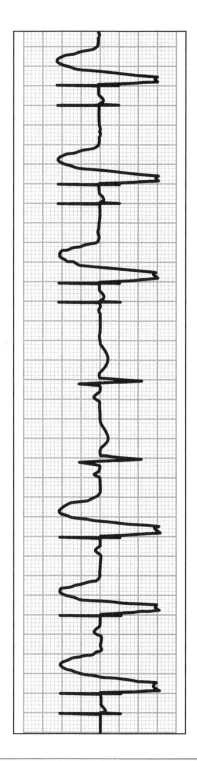

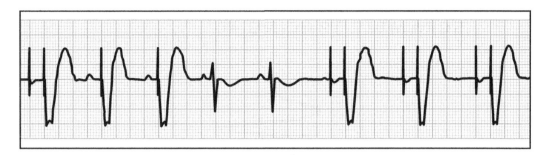

Mode

This is a dual-chamber rhythm strip.

Rate

In a dual-chamber system, the rate is best assessed by measuring the atrial pacing interval (AP-AP). There are two on the strip, both of which measure 1000 ms (60 ppm), an appropriate rate. There is also one atrial escape interval (AS-AP), which also measures 1000 ms.

Capture

Atrial capture is appropriate; there are four atrial pacing spikes on the strip and all of them result in an atrial depolarization. Note, in particular, that paced atrial event morphology differs from intrinsic atrial morphology.

Ventricular capture also looks good. Every ventricular pacing spike is followed by a ventricular depolarization with a characteristic widened, bizarre look. The paced events have a distinct morphology compared to the intrinsic events.

Sensing

Atrial sensing seems to be functioning properly. The intrinsic atrial events inhibit the atrial output pulse and reset device timing. The paced and sensed AV delays are about 200 ms (measured by calipers), an appropriate setting. They are consistent across the strip.

There are only a couple of intrinsic ventricular events on this strip, but they are appropriately sensed in that they cause the pacemaker to withhold ventricular pacing and reset device timing.

Underlying rhythm

This patient has sinus node dysfunction and slow AV conduction.

What to do next

The pacemaker is working appropriately. No changes are needed.

The nuts and bolts of paced ECG interpretation: filling in the missing beats

This strip is a great example of how pacemakers can help "fill in the missing beats" as a patient's heart rhythm changes. The strip begins with one AP-VP event, but the intrinsic atrial rate speeds up, and a couple of atrial tracked events occur (AS-VP). Then intrinsic AV conduction is restored and there are a couple of textbook-perfect intrinsic beats (AS-VS), at which time, the atrial rate and intrinsic conduction are interrupted and AP-VP pacing returns.

While the patient experienced changes in his intrinsic atrial rate and his intrinsic conduction, the pacemaker made sure that he maintained 1:1 AV synchrony on every single beat.

SCRAMBLE TRACING #5

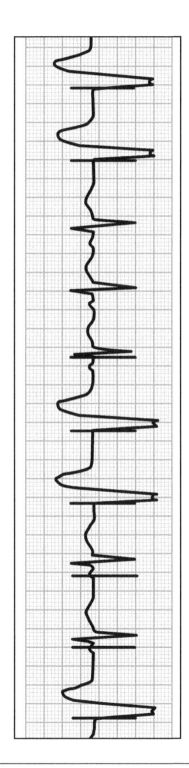

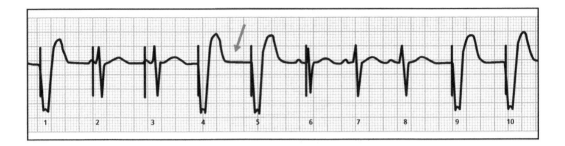

Mode

This comes from a VVI pacemaker. Do not be confused by spikes that seem to appear on the "atrial channel." They just happen to occur simultaneously with an intrinsic atrial event. If this were a dual-chamber pacemaker, there would be an atrial pacing spike in the flatline area indicated by the arrow.

Rate

The ventricular pacing interval is about 800 ms (measured by calipers) which works out to be a pacing rate of 75 ppm. That is appropriate, but not the most usual value (70 ppm is more common).

Capture

Ventricular capture is problematic. The first ventricular pacing spike appears to capture appropriately. Note that that same typical "paced morphology" appears after several other ventricular pacing spikes on the strip. However, the second and third pacing spikes do not capture the ventricle and are followed by intrinsic ventricular events. The sixth pacing spike falls on top of an intrinsic ventricular event. The sixth event is pseudofusion (simultaneous spike on an intrinsic event). The second and third spikes are failure to capture rather than pseudofusion because the spike is clearly distinct from the intrinsic event. Ventricular capture is inappropriate.

With failure to capture, we should ask if the second and third ventricular spikes ought to have captured the ventricle. The answer is yes. The myocardium was not refractory.

Sensing

The second and third complex show two ventricular intrinsic events which are not sensed, but that is actually appropriate in that they occurred in the pacemaker's refractory period. (You can tell they were not sensed because they did not reset device timing; the ventricular spikes are timed to each other, not the intrinsic activity.) A typical ventricular refractory setting is 250 ms and both intrinsic events occurred within 200 ms of the ventricular pacing spike. The intrinsic events on the right side of the strip were appropriately sensed in that they inhibited the output pulse and reset device timing. Thus, ventricular sensing is appropriate.

Underlying rhythm

This patient has some sinus node dysfunction and slow AV conduction.

What to do next

The most pressing concern is to restore appropriate ventricular capture. Run a ventricular pacing threshold test and adjust output parameters (amplitude and pulse width) to assure reliable capture.

The presence of one pseudofusion event and some intrinsic activity strongly suggests that this patient's intrinsic rate is competing with the programmed base rate. When this happens, in general, the best approach to this is to activate the hysteresis algorithm; however, since this patient's base rate is relatively high anyway, in this case, I would bring the base rate down to 70 ppm (from 75 ppm) and turn on hysteresis (60 bpm).

The nuts and bolts of paced ECG interpretation: strategies for generator change-outs

Pacemakers have to be replaced when their batteries run out. This occurs every 5 to 10 years or even longer, depending on the patient and the device. Pacemaker revision not only gives the patient a fresh battery, it offers the patient the opportunity to get a device with the latest features and algorithms.

In some cases, it can make sense to change the type of pacemaker the patient has. While I would hesitate to upgrade this patient from VVI to DDD based on this small section of rhythm strip alone, a VVI patient who appears to have intrinsic atrial activity, no atrial fibrillation (AF), and some degree of native conduction is actually a good candidate for a DDD pacemaker. A DDD device would assure that this patient received more consistent 1:1 AV synchrony.

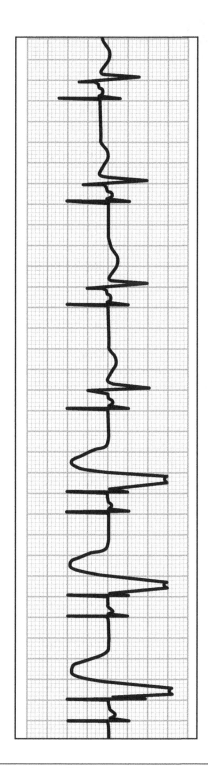

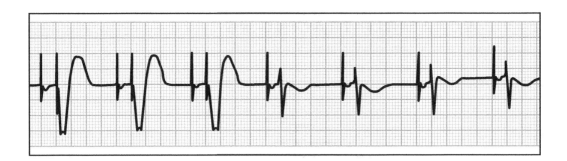

Mode

This is a dual-chamber pacemaker rhythm strip.

Rate

The atrial pacing interval (AP-AP) is 1000 ms or 60 ppm, an appropriate rate.

Capture

Atrial capture looks appropriate.

Ventricular capture also looks to be working properly. Note that paced ventricular events have a different morphology than the intrinsic ventricular events toward the end of the strip.

Sensing

Atrial sensing cannot be assessed from this strip because every atrial event shown is paced.

Ventricular sensing seems to be appropriate in that the intrinsic ventricular events shown inhibit the ventricular output and reset device timing.

Underlying rhythm

This patient has sinus node dysfunction and an AV conduction disorder. However, sometimes a paced atrial event conducts reliably over the AV node to cause an intrinsic ventricular depolarization.

What to do next

Atrial sensing should be evaluated. This requires intrinsic atrial activity to emerge. That can best be accomplished by temporarily reducing the programmed base rate. Do this in 10-ppm steps while observing the patient. Decrease the rate gradually and do not go below the rate at which the patient becomes uncomfortable or 30 or 40 ppm, whichever comes first.

This patient has intrinsic conduction at least intermittently. One way to encourage more intrinsic ventricular activity is to lengthen the programmed AV delay (sensed and paced AV delay). Some pacemakers have special algorithms, such as Ventricular Intrinsic Preference™ technology, which can offer this type of AV delay extension automatically.

SCRAMBLE TRACING #7

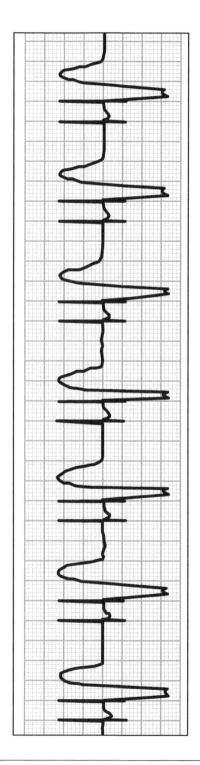

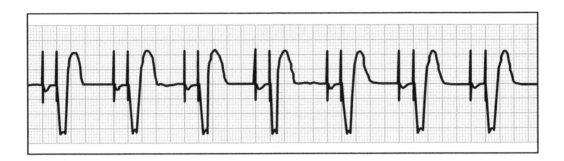

Mode

This is dual-chamber pacing.

Rate

The atrial pacing interval (AP-AP) is 1000 ms or 60 ppm, an appropriate rate. The paced AV delay (AP-VP) is consistent at about 200 ms.

Capture

Atrial and ventricular capture are appropriate.

Sensing

Neither atrial nor ventricular sensing can be evaluated from this strip, since it shows consistent AP-VP pacing.

Underlying rhythm

This patient has sinus node dysfunction and slow AV conduction.

What to do next

This strip shows appropriate AP-VP pacing but atrial and ventricular sensing should be evaluated. Both require intrinsic activity to appear.

For atrial intrinsic activity, lower the programmed base rate gradually, in steps of about 10 ppm. Observe the patient. Stop this process if the patient does not tolerate it or if you have to decrease the base rate lower than 30 or 40 ppm. It is not always possible to get intrinsic atrial activity to appear.

For intrinsic ventricular activity, temporarily program a prolonged AV delay. There is no need to do this gradually; temporarily set the paced AV delay interval to 300 ms or higher. This gives intrinsic ventricular activity good opportunity to appear. If it does, test ventricular sensing and also observe the patient's intrinsic conduction interval. If it is, say, 230 ms, programming the paced and sensed AV delay to greater values (for instance, 250 ms) will encourage more intrinsic ventricular activity and discourage unnecessary pacing.

I do not recommend testing ventricular sensing by lowering the base rate unless all else fails. In that case, temporarily set the device to VVI mode and then lower the base rate in 10-ppm increments. Do this gradually and while observing the patient for distress. Do not drop the base rate below 30 or 40 ppm, even if the patient tolerates it and intrinsic events do not appear.

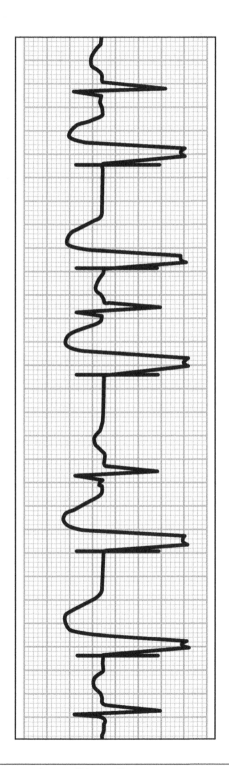

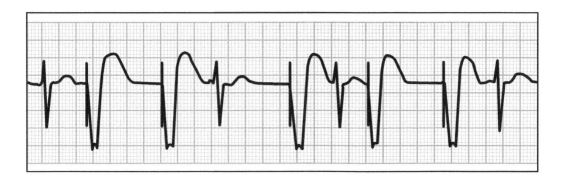

Mode

This is a VVI strip.

Rate

The ventricular pacing interval (VP-VP) is about 880 ms (around 70 ppm), which is appropriate.

Capture

Ventricular capture looks appropriate. The ventricular spike causes a widened, bizarre-looking ventricular morphology that differs markedly from the morphology of intrinsic ventricular depolarizations. Every spike is associated with such a ventricular event.

Sensing

The first intrinsic ventricular event on this strip was undersensed; notice the escape interval (VS-VP) is just 520 ms. If it had been appropriately sensed, the pacing spike would have occurred 880 ms following the onset of the intrinsic ventricular depolarization.

The second intrinsic ventricular event on this strip was properly sensed; the escape interval is 880 ms (VS-VP).

The third intrinsic ventricular event was undersensed. Since it is close to a paced event, we should ask: should the pacemaker have sensed this intrinsic event? Measuring from the pacing spike to the intrinsic event, the interval is about over 500 ms. That is more than enough time for the sensing circuitry to be on alert. Thus, the third intrinsic ventricular event exhibits inappropriate sensing.

The last event on this strip is an intrinsic ventricular event that was properly sensed in that it inhibits the pacemaker output pulse.

Underlying rhythm

This patient has sinus node dysfunction and slow AV conduction.

What to do next

Consistent ventricular sensing must be restored. The pacemaker should be temporarily programmed to a lower base rate to allow intrinsic ventricular activity to emerge. Based on this strip, that will be relatively easy to accomplish. A sensing threshold test can be conducted and the ventricular sensitivity setting adjusted appropriately.

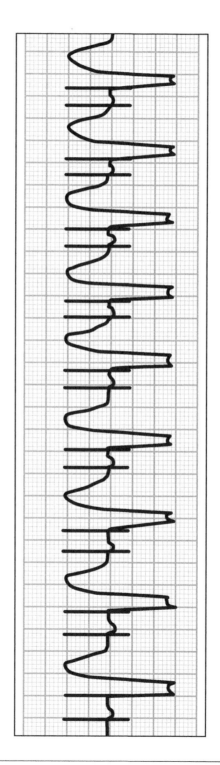

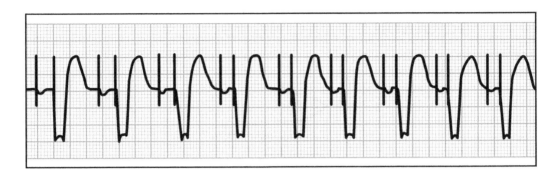

Mode

The atrial and ventricular spikes make this easy to identify as a dual-chamber strip.

Rate

At first glance, this strip seems very straightforward. The atrial pacing interval (AP-AP) drives the dual-chamber rate in a strip of AP-VP events. However, in this strip the atrial pacing interval varies from complex to complex! It progressively shortens, meaning the rate is gradually increasing by a small amount.

This kind of rate variation can be challenging to interpret, but there is a very likely explanation. If this pacemaker had rate response, it is possible that the pacing rate is under sensor control. This means that the device's built-in activity sensor has "decided" that the patient's activity level requires a bit faster pacing support than the base rate. This would increase the rate; this kind of subtle ramping up of the rate is consistent with a rate-responsive device.

Capture

Both atrial and ventricular capture seem to be functioning appropriately.

Sensing

Sensing cannot be evaluated for either chamber from this tracing, since every event is paced.

Underlying rhythm

This patient probably has chronotropic incompetence, which is why the pacemaker came under sensor control to drive up the rate. The patient also exhibits sinus node dysfunction and slow AV conduction.

What to do next

First, verify that the device is a rate-responsive pacemaker. If it is, rate-responsive parameter settings can be checked to be sure that sensor drive is providing adequate rate support. Ask the patient about his activity level and symptoms and download diagnostic reports on how frequently the pacemaker operated in a rate-responsive mode.

Both atrial and ventricular sensing should be evaluated. Conduct sensing tests in both chambers and adjust sensitivity parameters for each channel, if appropriate.

SCRAMBLE TRACING #10

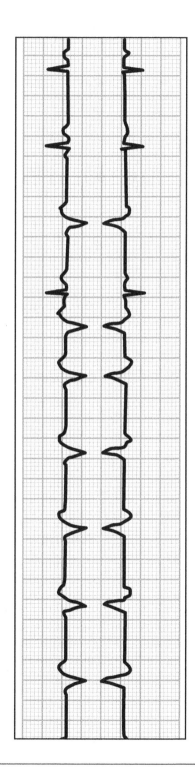

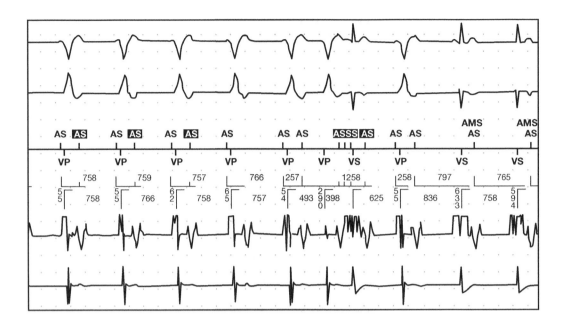

Mode

The first strip was isolated from this programmer screen, and it illustrates just how much faster and simpler programmers have made paced ECG interpretation – however, you can't forget the basics. While it is easy to see from the annotations and the presence of both an atrial and ventricular intracardiac electrogram (bottom two tracings) that this is a dual-chamber strip, the strip alone gives us some clues.

Notice the timing of the sixth event; it occurred more rapidly than the base rate would indicate, suggesting the pacemaker is tracking the atrium.

The last two events look backward: an intrinsic ventricular event followed by an intrinsic atrial event. The atrial event does not seem to invoke the sensed AV delay (which would mean the pacemaker would pace the ventricle).

This is a dual-chamber pacemaker going suddenly from atrial tracking to non-tracking behavior. Whenever the device seems to shift abruptly from atrial tracking behavior to non-atrial-tracking behavior, mode switching should be suspected. The annotations confirm that this was, indeed, the case.

Rate

Atrial tracking governs the first part of this strip, so

the programmed base rate cannot be determined. The ventricular pacing interval (VP-VP) is about 758 ms (80 ppm) which is a likely rate for atrial tracking.

Capture

There are no atrial pacing spikes on this strip, so atrial capture cannot be evaluated.

Ventricular capture appears to be appropriate. Using the second ECG tracing, notice that paced ventricular morphology is positive, while intrinsic ventricular morphology is negative. That helps facilitate strip interpretation.

Sensing

Mode switching occurs when the pacemaker senses rapid intrinsic atrial activity that the pacemaker should avoid tracking. For that reason, atrial sensing is key to understanding any AMS strip. Whenever a pacemaker mode switches, the first question in the mind of the clinician should be: was the mode switch appropriate? In other words, the presence of high-rate intrinsic atrial activity should be confirmed.

The annotations indicate atrial sensed events with the AS annotation; those AS annotations in a dark box indicate a sensed atrial event that "fell into" the refractory period.

The nuts and bolts of paced ECG interpretation: variations in annotations

Annotations have been in widespread use for decades and have greatly facilitated the rapid, clinical interpretation of paced rhythm strips. However, it must be noted that every manufacturer has its own system for annotating specific events. In this example, the manufacturer uses a dark box with white AS lettering to indicate an atrial event that was sensed but to which no response was made because it occurred during the refractory period. This is not a universal symbol; it is particular to this manufacturer. Most annotations are intuitively understandable, but if you need help with a "master key" of annotations, talk to your device company representatives or refer to the programmer manual.

Let's look closely at the first pair of AS events; there is one regular AS and one AS in a dark box. These annotations tell us the pacemaker "saw" two intrinsic atrial events. One of those intrinsic events is visible on the top surface ECG (but not the second ECG); the second AS, the one in the box, is not visible on either ECG. However, it is possible the second intrinsic atrial event might have been obscured by the repolarization represented by the T-wave.

This is where intracardiac electrograms are of great help. The atrial electrogram (next-to-last tracing) indeed shows two distinct events, but they have different morphologies. There is one event with a large, square-looking morphology followed by a second event with a smaller, downward-deflecting, pointier morphology. These are not two identical events; they are two events from different points of origin in the heart.

Moving to the ventricular electrogram (bottom tracing), the ventricular electrodes in the heart detected something on the ventricular channel. The pacemaker annotates this as a VP or ventricular pacing spike. The surface ECG shows this as a ventricular depolarization.

And the atrial electrogram represents this as the squared-off looking event! Thus, the two events that show up on the atrial electrogram are actually one ventricular event (that's the first event with a squared-off morphology that aligns with the VP annotation and the event on the ventricular electrogram) followed by one genuine intrinsic atrial event.

This is an example of far-field sensing, that is, the pacemaker's atrial channel is sensing "far-off" signals from the ventricle and inappropriately interpreting them as atrial events.

But what about the "apparent intrinsic atrial activity" that is seen on the top electrogram? It was likely a true intrinsic atrial depolarization that got obscured on the surface ECG by the ventricular event. Thus, a real intrinsic atrial fell into the pacemaker's refractory period and got missed, but a ventricular pacing spike was inappropriately labeled as an intrinsic atrial event. Moving over to the run of atrial sensed events near the middle of the strip, there is further evidence of far-field oversensing. Atrial sensing is inappropriate and because of the double counting, the AMS algorithm was inappropriately activated.

Ventricular sensing appears to be functioning properly.

Underlying rhythm

This patient has sinus node dysfunction and slow atrial conduction. Despite what the strip, the annotations, and the mode switch suggest, the patient is *not* experiencing high-rate intrinsic atrial activity.

What to do next

The most pressing concern for this patient is to eliminate far-field R-wave sensing and prevent future inappropriate mode switches. The strip shows that the patient was in normal sinus rhythm (a good thing) as the device mode switches. To prevent far-field oversensing, atrial sensing should be evaluated and adjusted to be as insensitive as clinically prudent. Ventricular capture should be tested (although it looks appropriate) because it would be wise to set ventricular output parameters as low as possible without jeopardizing patient safety. Finally, the refractory period after the ventricular event (PVARP setting) should be extended to help prevent the pacemaker from responding to far-field signals.

SCRAMBLE TRACING #11

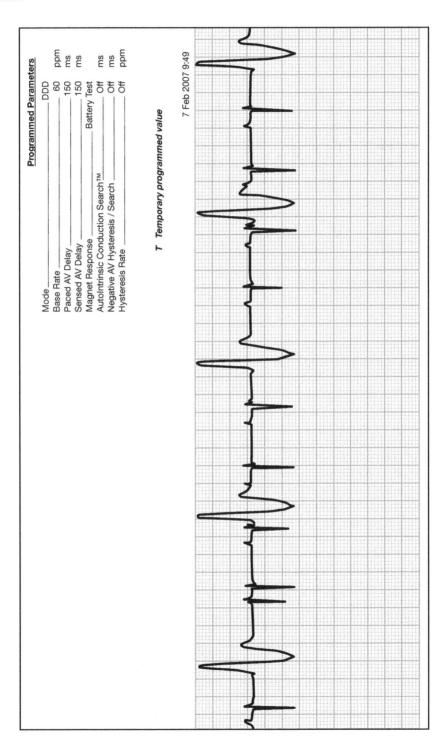

Programmed Parameters

Mode	DDD	
Base Rate	60	ppm
Paced AV Delay	150	ms
Sensed AV Delay	150	ms
Magnet Response	Battery Test	
AutoIntrinsic Conduction Search™	Off	ms
Negative AV Hysteresis / Search	Off	ms
Hysteresis Rate	Off	ppm

T Temporary programmed value

7 Feb 2007 9:49

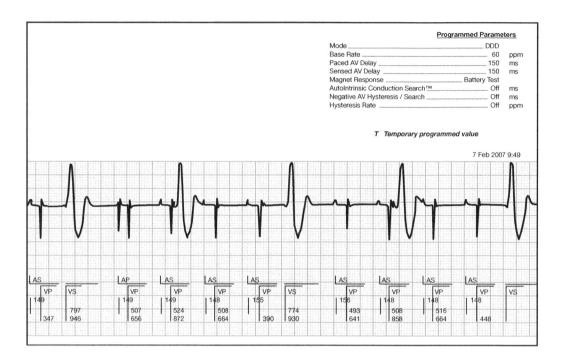

Programmed Parameters						
Mode					DDD	
Base Rate					60	ppm
Paced AV Delay					150	ms
Sensed AV Delay					150	ms
Magnet Response					Battery Test	
AutoIntrinsic Conduction Search™					Off	ms
Negative AV Hysteresis / Search					Off	ms
Hysteresis Rate					Off	ppm

T   Temporary programmed value

7 Feb 2007 9:49

Mode

The presence of atrial and ventricular spikes indicates that this is a dual-chamber strip.

Rate

This strip is much more challenging than it looks at first glance! Although the printout states that the pacing rate is 60 ppm, there are no pacing intervals available on the strip to confirm that. However, there is a roundabout way to assess proper base rate pacing. The pacemaker reports that the paced AV delay interval is 150 ms. If we knew the VA interval (VP-AP) we could add that to the paced AV delay and get the pacing interval. There is actually one such interval on the strip (between the third and fourth complexes or AP-VP) and the VA interval measures about 850 ms with calipers. This confirms 60 ppm base rate pacing (1000 ms = 150 + 850).

Capture

Most of the atrial events on this strip are intrinsic. The third complex shows an atrial pacing spike, but it is not clear what happened. My interpretation is that this spike failed to capture the atrium, but it is

possible to view this event as pseudofusion or even appropriate capture. At the very least, we should be very suspicious about atrial capture.

On the other hand, there is a total loss of ventricular capture. Although ventricular pacing spikes appear on the strip, none of them captures the ventricle.

Sensing

Atrial sensing appears to be appropriate. Intrinsic atrial events inhibit the atrial output pulse; the intrinsic atrial event launches the sensed AV delay, which times out in about 150 ms to deliver a ventricular pacing spike.

There are five intrinsic ventricular events on this strip; the pacemaker senses the first, third, and fifth of them as indicated by the annotations and the fact that the ventricular event inhibited the ventricular spike and reset device timing.

The second and fourth intrinsic ventricular events are not sensed as evidenced by the fact that they have no effect on device timing and are not annotated. Whenever an event is not sensed, the next logical question has to be this: Should it have been sensed? In the case of these two non-sensed intrinsic ventricular events, the answer has to be no. This is functional non-sensing. The intrinsic event occurs within about 200 ms of the ventricular pacing spike, that is likely within the ventricular refractory period. Actually, ventricular sensing in this strip is appropriate.

Underlying rhythm

This patient has sinus node dysfunction and slow AV conduction.

What to do next

The most important first step for this patient is to restore capture. Begin with atrial capture (although some might argue there is appropriate atrial capture – I disagree and, at most, there is only one example of it on the whole strip).

Next ventricular capture should be restored. Test the pacing threshold and reprogram the output settings (pulse amplitude and pulse width).

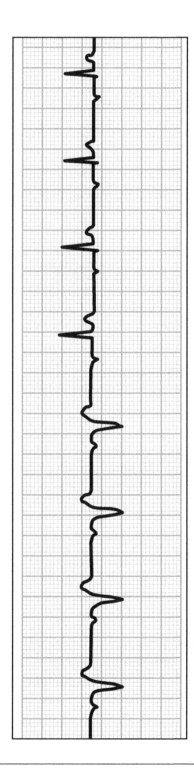

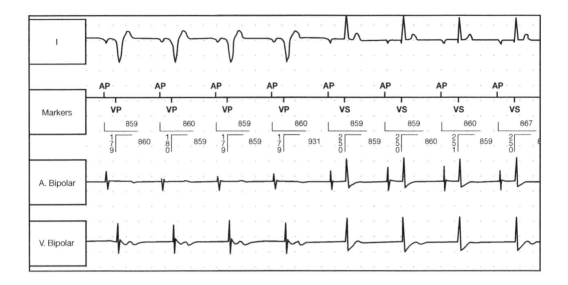

Mode

This is a programmer screen showing one surface ECG (top tracing) and two intracardiac electrograms (atrial and ventricular) from a dual-chamber pacemaker. Even from just the tracing, the presence of two types of ventricular events in close relationship to intrinsic atrial activity reveals that this is a dual-chamber device. The annotations confirm this.

Rate

The atrial pacing interval (AP-AP) is the best way to measure rate on a dual-chamber strip. This atrial pacing interval is 860 ms (70 ppm), an appropriate rate. Notice how this strip transitions from AP-VP pacing to AP-VS pacing. The paced AV delay (AP-VP) measures about 180 ms but when the strip transitions to AP-VS events, the AV interval is 250 ms. The paced AV delay interval setting of 180 ms should have been imposed. This kind of unusual behavior is not random; it occurs consistently. That strongly suggests some sort of special pacing algorithm is going into effect.

This is an example of AutoIntrinsic Conduction Search™ or Ventricular Intrinsic Preference™ technology or some other type of algorithm designed to encourage intrinsic ventricular activity by automatically prolonging the AV delay interval.

Capture

Atrial capture is appropriate.

Ventricular capture is also appropriate; note the distinct paced ventricular morphology.

Sensing

Atrial sensing cannot be evaluated from this paced ECG, since all atrial events shown are paced. When an atrial electrogram is available, it is always a good idea to compare what it shows versus what is on the surface ECG. Notice the atrial EGM shows four examples (right side) of far-field R-wave sensing which align with intrinsic ventricular events. The pacemaker did not respond to these events because they occurred during the ventricular blanking period. While this is far-field sensing, it did not affect the appropriate atrial sensing behavior of the pacemaker.

Ventricular sensing appears to be appropriate in that intrinsic ventricular events inhibit the ventricular output and reset device timing. The ventricular events on the surface ECG align well with what is shown on the ventricular EGM.

Underlying rhythm

This patient has sinus node dysfunction and slow AV conduction.

The nuts and bolts of paced ECG interpretation: variations in the AV delay interval

Ever since the DAVID clinical trial, many pacemaker specialists have been very concerned about pacing the right ventricle (the conventional way ventricular pacing is conducted with a pacemaker). As a general rule in medicine, the less intervention required for a patient, the better. That's true for pacing as well as other medical procedures. As much as possible, the patient's intrinsic rhythm should be given ample opportunity to emerge, providing it can support the patient's normal activities.

Recently, all major manufacturers of cardiac rhythm management devices have introduced specialty algorithms designed to encourage intrinsic ventricular activity. Most of them are based on some method of automatically extending the AV delay interval. This often allows intrinsic ventricular activity to occur without compromising rate support. Clinicians will likely be seeing more and more of such algorithms in action as new devices help pacing physicians attempt to minimize unnecessary pacing.

What to do next

Atrial sensing should be evaluated. The presence of far-field signals on the atrial intracardiac electrogram is not necessarily a cause for alarm, particularly since the device functioned appropriately and "blanked them out." Nevertheless, atrial sensing has to be checked and making the device less sensitive on the atrial channel would help, providing it could be done without compromising patient safety.

Otherwise, this is a great example of how an algorithm can successfully encourage ventricular activity. (While all algorithms work a bit differently, most of them are set up to automatically extend the AV delay during periods of ventricular pacing in order to "search" for intrinsic activity. Should intrinsic activity occur, as it did in this strip, the prolonged AV delay remains in effect until ventricular pacing is necessary again and resumes.)

SCRAMBLE TRACING #13

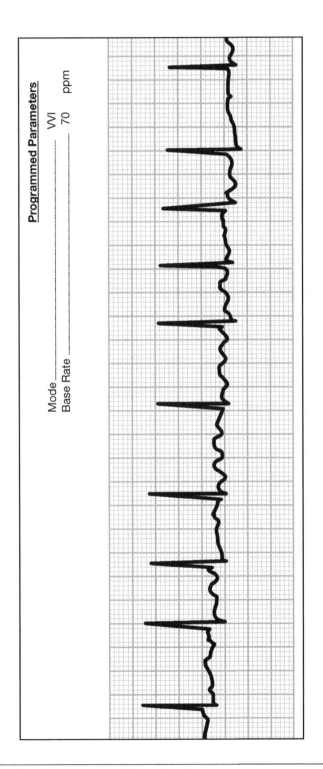

Programmed Parameters

Mode _____ VVI

Base Rate _____ 70 ppm

The Nuts and Bolts of Paced ECG Interpretation, 1st edition. By Tom Kenny.
Published 2009 by Blackwell Publishing, ISBN: 978-1-4501-8404-5.

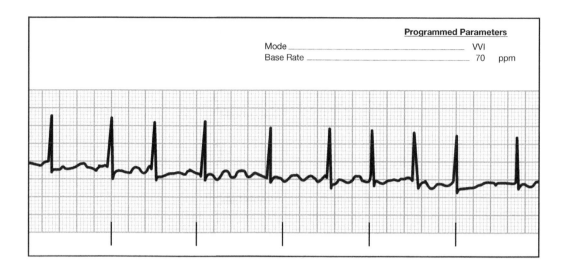

Mode

Looks can be deceiving! If somebody handed you this strip with no explanation at all, you would most likely assume that this patient does not have a pacemaker. After all, there's no evidence on this strip of pacing. However, from the printout, we know that this is actually an ECG from a VVI pacemaker patient.

Rate

There is no paced ventricular activity to measure since there is no pacing at all in this strip. The printout states a programmed base rate of 70 ppm. The ventricular activity on this strip is so erratic that it is hard to determine the ventricular rate. We can measure intervals between intrinsic ventricular events but every one is different.

One way to calculate the intrinsic ventricular rate in a strip like this is to mark off 6 seconds of time and multiply the number of ventricular events that occur in six seconds and multiply it by ten to arrive at how many ventricular events occur in 1 minute (6 sec × 10 = 60 sec = 1 min). Using the grid paper, you can count off five large boxes (5 × 200 ms = 1000 ms = 1 sec) to mark off 1 second (see tic marks above). This particular strip gives us exactly 6 seconds of "data." There are 10 intrinsic ventricular events that occur in these 6 seconds. Multiply that by 10 to get the beats per minute and this translates to an intrinsic ventricular rate of around 100 bpm (10 events

in 6 sec × 10 = 100 events in 60 sec = 100 events per min). Thus, the patient's ventricular intervals are erratic but his ventricular rate is around 100 bpm.

Capture

Ventricular capture cannot be evaluated from this strip.

Sensing

Ventricular sensing is appropriate in that the patient's intrinsic ventricular event inhibits the output pulse and resets device timing. No intervals on this strip are long enough to cause pacing to occur, that is, they are all less than 857 ms (the interval that corresponds to 70 ppm).

Underlying rhythm

This patient has atrial fibrillation (AF). This is evident primarily from two things: the rapid intrinsic atrial activity and the resulting erratic but rapid ventricular response. The latter – an irregular ventricular rate – is the giveaway that this is AF. The patient has some degree of intrinsic conduction in that some of the atrial activity seems to conduct down over the AV node to the ventricles to cause a native depolarization. Although the native ventricular rhythm is erratic, it is fast enough to inhibit the pacemaker.

What to do next

Based on our systematic analysis, ventricular capture has to be evaluated.

But the overriding concern at the moment is addressing this patient's AF. Device diagnostics may reveal how frequently the patient experiences these arrhythmias and the patient chart may show what has been done (if anything) to treat the AF. AF can occur suddenly, even in patients with no previous history, so it is quite possible that the AF has not been treated. The first line of defense against AF is drug therapy, which goes beyond the scope of this book. A good example of a drug used against AF is the beta-blocker. Some pacemakers offer overdrive algorithms or other features to help manage high intrinsic atrial rates, including the AF Suppression™ algorithm to suppress AF before it can start. Not all patients are candidates for such special features, but they do work well in some patients. Some patients may even be candidates for radio frequency ablation of AF or surgical ablation, but that is considered a more drastic step.

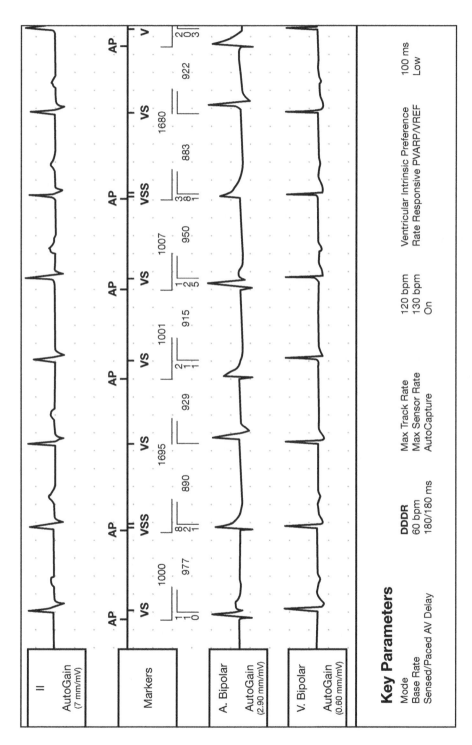

Key Parameters

Mode	**DDDR**	Max Track Rate	120 bpm	Ventricular Intrinsic Preference	100 ms
Base Rate	60 bpm	Max Sensor Rate	130 bpm	Rate Responsive PVARP/VREF	Low
Sensed/Paced AV Delay	180/180 ms	AutoCapture	On		

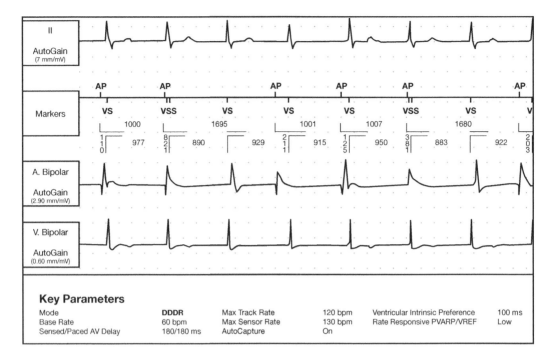

Mode

This comes from a programmer and demonstrates the value of going beyond the paced ECG for interpreting some particularly unusual pacemaker scenarios. Looking at just the ECG (top tracing), there is clearly ventricular activity on the strip but nothing is going on at all in the atrium. Moving down to the annotations, it is clear that this is a dual-chamber device and the AP annotations show the pacemaker is sending output pulses to the atrium. The parameters displayed on the bottom confirm this is a DDDR device.

Moving down to the atrial electrogram (next to last tracing), there is consistent activity. But look where these events align. The first three events on the atrial EGM align with ventricular activity – the atrial EGM was simply picking up ventricular events. The fourth event on the atrial EGM is an actual atrial event. As we evaluate this strip, we need to account for the inconsistencies across these tracings and annotations.

Rate

Using the annotations and intervals on the screen, the atrial pacing interval is 1000 ms (60 ppm),

which is appropriate for the device and matches the programmed settings. However, there are no atrial events at all on the paced ECG. The pacemaker "thinks" it's pacing the atrium at 60 ppm, but the paced ECG shows that the patient is being supported entirely by a native ventricular rhythm slightly above the base rate.

Capture

Atrial capture is not appropriate. The many annotations on the strip indicate that the pacemaker delivered atrial output pulses but the atria did not depolarize.

Before we get down to ventricular capture, it is important to evaluate the two annotated events called VSS. This stands for "ventricular safety standby." Twice, the patient is paced using the VSS feature. Ventricular safety standby occurs when an intrinsic ventricular event "falls into" the crosstalk detection window (part of the refractory period). The pacemaker responds to an intrinsic ventricular event during the crosstalk detection window by pacing the ventricle. This assures that even if the pacemaker should fail to see the intrinsic ventricular event, the patient still receives ventricular rate support. The double lines near the VSS annotation are meant to indicate the intrinsic event and the triggered pace-maker output. However, look at the paced ECG. The only event present is the intrinsic ventricular event. The ventricular output pulse fails to capture.

One way to confirm failure to capture in a situation like this is to study the QRS morphology as well as the T-wave morphology of the intrinsic beats and compare them to any event that might be paced. Both VSS events have QRS and T-wave morphologies that are similar to intrinsic activity. Furthermore, the intracardiac ventricular electrogram shows one intrinsic event at each of the VSS markers, not an intrinsic and a paced event. Thus, ventricular capture is not appropriate, either.

Sensing

Atrial sensing cannot be evaluated from this strip.

Ventricular sensing appears to be functioning appropriately. Intrinsic ventricular events inhibit the ventricular output pulse and reset device timing.

Underlying rhythm

This patient has sinus node dysfunction and slow AV conduction. He also is experiencing crosstalk, a phenomenon that occurs when the ventricular sensing circuits "overhears" what is going on in the atrium (in this case, atrial pacing) and inappropriately thinks it is an intrinsic ventricular event. The two crosstalk events on this strip are the ones associated with the VSS annotation.

What to do next

Both atrial and ventricular capture must be restored. Pacing threshold tests should be conducted and appropriate output parameters (pulse amplitude and pulse width) should be programmed. While it would be great to verify appropriate atrial sensing, it may not be possible in this patient since we have no evidence here of any intrinsic atrial activity.

The fact that atrial and ventricular events are not working in sync together is likely a function of the loss of capture in both chambers. Right now, the atrial event (not captured) occurs almost on top of the intrinsic ventricular event. When capture is restored, the appropriate AV delay interval (set to 180 ms in this example) will come into force and provide AV synchrony for the patient.

Crosstalk is being handled appropriately by the pacemaker's crosstalk detection window algorithm, but steps may be taken to minimize it. It could be minimized by extending the blanking period, reducing atrial output (if it can be done safely – which is likely not the case here), or making the ventricular channel less sensitive. Only initiate these actions if they can be programmed safely. If they cannot, crosstalk is still being managed for this patient through the VSS algorithm.

SCRAMBLE TRACING #15

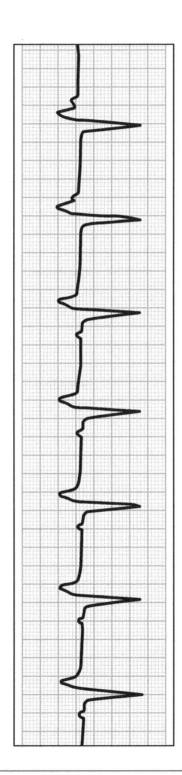

The Nuts and Bolts of Paced ECG Interpretation, 1st edition. By Tom Kenny.
Published 2009 by Blackwell Publishing, ISBN: 978-1-4501-8404-5.

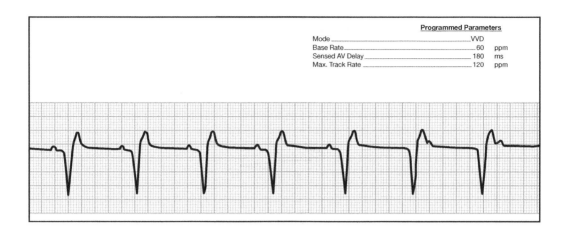

Programmed Parameters		
Mode	VVD	
Base Rate	60	ppm
Sensed AV Delay	180	ms
Max. Track Rate	120	ppm

Mode

The first several complexes on this strip look like atrial tracking – intrinsic atrial activity followed by ventricular paced events. That suggests the pacemaker is a dual-chamber system. The last two complexes on the strip tell a different story. There is neither sensed nor paced atrial activity present. These two complexes look like typical VVI pacing. A dual-chamber pacemaker would deliver an atrial pacing output in the absence of atrial intrinsic activity! This suggests the pacemaker is a single-chamber ventricular device. For a moment, you might be tempted to think the first five complexes on the strip were VVI pacing that just happened to be preceded by an intrinsic atrial event. Using calipers, you can see that a consistent AV delay of 180 ms is maintained. Five back-to-back events with a split-second perfect AV delay interval would be just too great a coincidence! These first five complexes are true atrial tracking. There is only one mode that can track the atrium but is unable to pace there: VDD.

VDD pacing is used mainly for testing today but there are dedicated VDD devices that will occasionally show up at the clinic. VDD is rare enough that it is not my first assumption when I see a strip like this; however, these devices have been and continue to be implanted, and this is classic VDD-style pacing.

Rate

The ventricular pacing interval (VP-VP) is 1000 ms (60 ppm), an appropriate rate. It can only be mea-

sured from the last two complexes, since the other events are tracked.

Capture

Atrial capture is not applicable to VDD pacing. Ventricular capture looks appropriate. Note that the ventricular events in this tracing all have the same "typically paced" morphology.

Sensing

Atrial sensing is functioning appropriately because the first five intrinsic atrial events launch the sensed AV delay which times out to a ventricular output pulse.

Ventricular sensing cannot be evaluated from this strip because all ventricular events are paced.

Underlying rhythm

The patient has slow AV conduction. In the first portion of the strip, sinus node function looks good, but it suddenly stops in the last two complexes. The patient has some form of sinus node dysfunction.

What to do next

Ventricular sensing should be evaluated, if possible. For dual-chamber systems, it is always preferable to encourage intrinsic ventricular activity by extending the AV delay. That is unlikely to work in a VDD patient, because the "typical VDD" patient has poor AV conduction to begin with. It could be attempted by extending the sensed AV delay (a VDD device has no "paced AV delay" because it does not pace the atrium) to 300 ms or more.

Probably the more effective way to allow intrinsic ventricular activity to appear on the strip is to temporarily program the pacemaker to VVI mode and then lower the base rate in 10-ppm increments until native ventricular events occur. Monitor the patient to be sure he tolerates such low rates. Even if the patient is doing fine and no intrinsic ventricular events occur, do not drop the base rate below 30 or 40 ppm.

SCRAMBLE TRACING #16

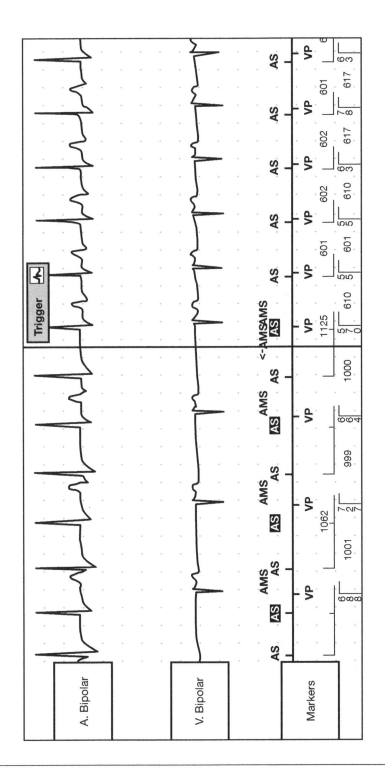

The Nuts and Bolts of Paced ECG Interpretation, 1st edition. By Tom Kenny.
Published 2009 by Blackwell Publishing, ISBN: 978-1-4501-8404-5.

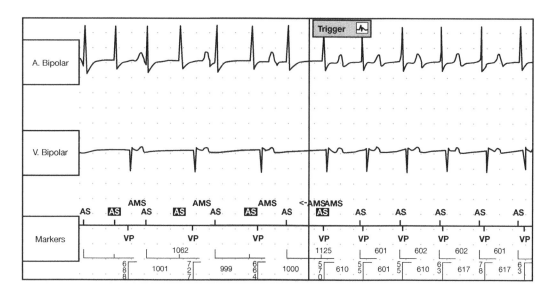

Mode

These are a pair (atrial and ventricular) of stored intracardiac electrograms from a programmer screen. The presence of an atrial and ventricular electrogram means that this is a dual-chamber system.

This electrogram was stored in the pacemaker's memory when the trigger event occurred (indicated at the top of the screen, near the middle). The annotations reveal that this pacemaker was operating in the AMS or auto mode switch algorithm until the trigger point was reached.

This is an automatically stored electrogram of the device exiting AMS and resuming normal operation. It is available from the pacemaker's memory so that the clinician can verify if AMS exit was appropriate. At first glance, it is a bit hard to tell if the AMS exit was appropriate, so let's examine it systematically.

Rate

The left side of the strip shows the device in AMS, so there is no atrial tracking going on. Thus, the rate would be assessed by measuring the ventricular pacing interval (VP-VP). It's consistent at 1000 ms or 60 ppm, an appropriate rate.

When the device exits mode switching (trigger), the ventricular pacing interval is much faster: it's about 600 ms or 100 ppm. The reason for this above-base-rate ventricular pacing is that as the

device leaves AMS, it resumes tracking the intrinsic atrial rate.

The patient has just experienced a rather abrupt increase in ventricular pacing rate. However, this is the expected and normal behavior of the device.

Capture

Atrial capture cannot be evaluated from this screen.

Based on the ventricular electrogram, capture seems appropriate. There is a response on the electrogram for every ventricular output (as annotated) and the presence of a resulting T-wave suggests depolarization.

Sensing

On the atrial electrogram, the taller, upward events are intrinsic atrial events while the smaller, slightly more rounded events are ventricular events that the atrial channel "overheard." The correlation of atrial annotations to atrial events on the electrogram suggests that atrial activity was properly sensed. Furthermore, the rather rapid intrinsic atrial rhythm inhibited atrial output pulses. When the device exits mode switching, atrial tracking occurs. All of this indicates proper atrial sensing.

Notice some atrial events are annotated AS, but others have the AS annotation in a little box. The box is a programmer convention and indicates that this particular atrial sensed event occurred during a refractory period. The pacemaker counted the event (for AMS purposes), but because it "fell into" the refractory period, there was no response to it.

Ventricular sensing cannot be evaluated here.

Underlying rhythm

This patient has intrinsic high-rate atrial activity and heart block.

What to do next

The big question is whether or not this exit from the AMS algorithm was appropriate. The intrinsic atrial rate slows down as you move across the strip from left to right. After the trigger line, the AS-AS interval is around 600 ms (100 ppm).

AMS exit is appropriate when the patient's intrinsic atrial rate drops below the programmed maximum tracking rate or MTR. MTR is typically programmed to around 100 or 120 ppm. Note that even though some atrial events occur in the refractory period (those in boxes), they are counted for determining AMS entry and exit. The atrial rate continues to slow down and by the far right section

of the strip it has already decreased to 100 bpm or 600 ms.

This is an appropriate AMS exit. However, it might be good to talk to the patient to determine if he experienced any symptoms or discomfort with the "rate bump" that occurred. The device went in a single beat from ventricular pacing at 60 ppm to ventricular pacing at around 100 ppm. In my experience, some patients find this unpleasant. To mitigate this abrupt rate transition, some devices allow you to program a "mode switch base rate." This rate – which is higher than the programmed base rate – is the interim base rate during the AMS algorithm. Had an interim mode switch base rate of say, 80 ppm, been used here, the patient would have experienced a much more subtle rate transition in and out of AMS.

In addition to possibly programming an interim AMS base rate, it would be useful to examine diagnostic reports to see how frequently this patient experiences AMS episodes. If AMS is a very frequent occurrence, the clinician ought to investigate ways of dealing with the atrial tachyarrhythmias since the patient is not getting full benefit of dual-chamber pacing during AMS episodes.

Furthermore, it is necessary to verify proper atrial capture and proper ventricular sensing.

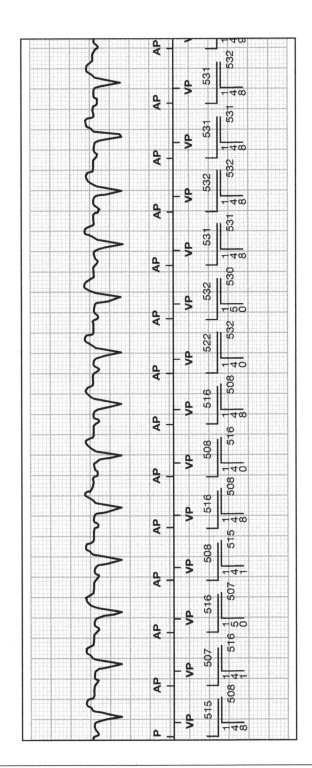

The Nuts and Bolts of Paced ECG Interpretation, 1st edition. By Tom Kenny.
Published 2009 by Blackwell Publishing, ISBN: 978-1-4501-8404-5.

459

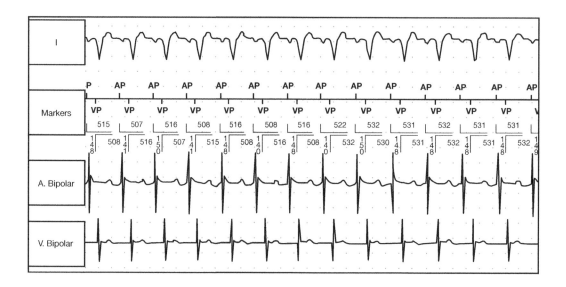

Mode

Using just the surface ECG, it might be difficult to determine the pacing mode since spikes are not clear. The annotations serve as spikes and show that this is a dual-chamber pacemaker. The full programmer screen provides a lot of other useful information – including an atrial and ventricular electrogram at the bottom. When evaluating so much information, we still use our systematic approach but we want to see alignment among the paced ECG (top), annotations and intervals, and electrograms (bottom). They should all be telling the same story!

Rate

The atrial pacing interval (AP-AP) drives the rate of a dual-chamber system, and here the atrial pacing interval is variable. It ranges from about 507 to 532 ms (113 to 118 ppm). This is of immediate concern since with consistent atrial pacing, one might expect the atrial pacing interval to be stable. Furthermore, this is a very high pacing rate, almost to the point of reaching the maximum tracking rate (MTR). Ventricular pacing is tracking the paced atrial rate to provide 1:1 AV synchrony. But the rate is much too high to be appropriate as a programmed base rate.

The most likely explanation for this higher-than-base-rate pacing is rate response. Rate-responsive pacemakers use a sensor of some sort to control the pacing rate in the presence of patient activity. When the sensor detects that the patient is active (and thus needs additional rate support), it elevates the pacing rate in accordance with the patient's activity level. Rate response is a very common feature in pacemakers today, so it is not at all unusual to see this kind of rhythm strip in the clinic. Confirm that the device is indeed rate responsive and under sensor control.

Capture

Atrial and ventricular capture both appear to be appropriate. Using the annotations as pacing spikes, it is evident that each pacing spike causes a depolarization on the surface ECG (top tracing). There is a one-to-one match of each annotation (AP or VP) and a waveform on the tracing. Notice that atrial and ventricular events appear on the intracardiac electrogram as well, but the tall narrow complexes indicate that the electrodes within the heart "saw" and recorded the pacemaker output pulse, not the cardiac depolarization. Thus, it is the surface ECG that helps confirm capture. All events on this strip are paced and the fact that they all have a similar morphology is further proof of proper capture.

Sensing

Neither atrial nor ventricular sensing can be evaluated from this strip.

Underlying rhythm

This patient has chronotropic incompetence, that is, his heart is unable to accelerate as needed to provide adequate rate support. The patient also has sinus node dysfunction and slow AV conduction.

What to do next

Atrial and ventricular sensing should be evaluated and sensitivity settings adjusted, if necessary. To verify sensing, intrinsic events have to occur. There is a different tactic to be used for encouraging atrial intrinsic events from encouraging ventricular intrinsic events.

Evaluate atrial sensing first by temporarily turning off rate response (you may be able to set it to PASSIVE for this test) and then lowering the base rate in small 10-ppm steps. Since the patient may feel this, tell him what you are doing and reduce the rate gradually. Even if he tolerates it well and even if no atrial intrinsic events occur, resist the urge to lower the rate below 30 or 40 ppm.

The best way to get ventricular intrinsic activity to occur in a dual-chamber system is to disable rate response temporarily and then extend the AV delay interval to 300 ms or higher. This can be done all at once; there is no need to proceed incrementally

like you do with a base rate change. This often results in ventricular intrinsic activity. If it fails, the other method is to temporarily program the device to VVI and reduce the base rate in the same manner as you did for the atrial sensing test. I do not recommend this method and use it only as a last resort because it evaluates sensing in an artificial environment, that is, it evaluates sensing as if the device were a VVI system. It's not; it's a dual-chamber device and dual-chamber pacemakers have many features where the atrial and ventricular channels interact. Thus sensing in VVI does not exactly provide a true picture of ventricular sensing in a DDDR pacemaker.

This patient has a rate-responsive pacemaker that functions appropriately. Diagnostic reports should be downloaded to find out how frequently and to what extent (how fast) rate response is used. Rate-responsive settings may require some adjustment.

For instance, this screen was captured during a particular event. If the patient had been exercising or exerting himself, this would be perfectly appropriate. However, if the pacemaker started doing this when the patient was sitting down quietly, then there is too much response from the rate response. This can be controlled by programming new rate response settings. The patient should be asked about his activities (for instance, how active or athletic he might be) and any symptoms.

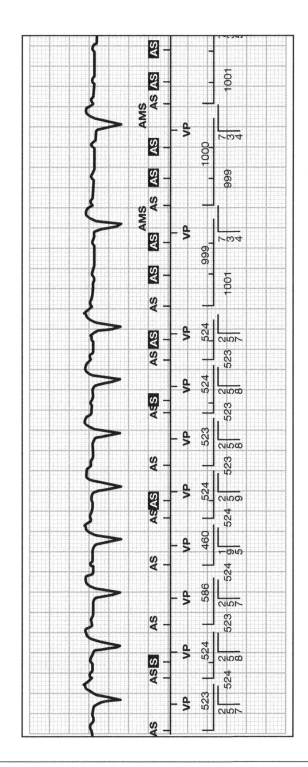

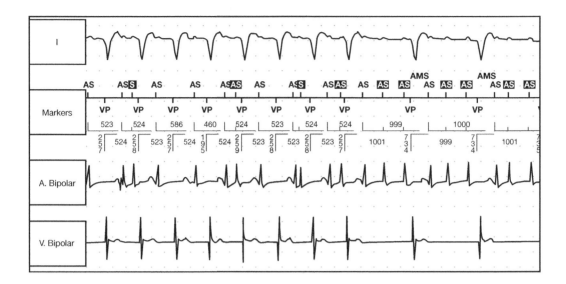

Mode

This comes from a dual-chamber device showing entry into AMS or mode switching. When AMS occurs, the clinician should always assess whether or not it was appropriate. For now, we know that the device is a dual-chamber system that is switching from an atrial-tracking to a non-atrial-tracking mode.

Rate

Up until the AMS letters appear, this pacemaker is tracking rapid and erratic atrial activity. Normally, the atrial pacing interval (AP-AP) would help ascertain the rate, but no such interval appears on this tracing. Since the pacemaker is tracking the atrium, the ventricular pacing interval (VP-VP) cannot verify the base rate. It can only say how fast the device is pacing right now in response to intrinsic atrial activity.

After entry into AMS, the ventricular pacing interval (VP-VP) is 1000 ms (60 ppm), an appropriate base rate. While atrial activity still occurs during AMS, the pacemaker ignores it.

Atrial events can be viewed in clearest detail from the atrial intracardiac electrogram (next-to-last tracing). The intrinsic atrial rate is fast, but it would be hard to measure in that it is so erratic no two intrinsic intervals (AS-AS) are alike!

Note that many of the intrinsic atrial events "fall into" the atrial refractory period and are annotated as AS events in a box. The AMS algorithm counts these events, but the pacemaker does not respond to them. AMS entry is appropriate.

Capture

Atrial capture cannot be evaluated here, but ventricular capture appears to be appropriate. Notice that all events on the surface ECG annotated as VP share the same morphology and have the same type of T-wave following the QRS complex. This further confirms appropriate ventricular capture.

Sensing

Atrial sensing appears to be appropriate. Every event on the atrial intracardiac electrogram can be found in the annotations. The atrial activity inhibits atrial pacing and, when atrial events fall in the alert period, reset device timing.

Ventricular sensing cannot be evaluated from this strip.

Underlying rhythm

This patient has some form of atrial tachyarrhythmia with very slow AV conduction. Since the ventricular response is erratic and the atrial events are quite rapid, I suspect this atrial rhythm disorder is atrial fibrillation (AF).

What to do next

AMS entry is appropriate.

Atrial capture should be evaluated, which requires atrial pacing to occur. This may or may not be possible in this patient. His atrial tachyarrhythmia might preclude it.

Ventricular sensing should be tested, and the atrial tachyarrhythmia could interfere with that as well. If possible extend the AV delay interval to 300 ms or higher. In cases like this, it may be necessary to program the pacemaker temporarily to VVI mode and lower the base rate in slow 10-ppm increments down to no lower than 30 or 40 ppm.

The larger issue is how to manage the atrial tachyarrhythmia. Diagnostic data should be retrieved to reveal how much intrinsic high-rate atrial activity is going on. If it is occasional, then AMS is a good solution. If it is very frequent or if the patient does not seem to tolerate it, other measures should be taken. The most likely next step in such cases is pharmacological therapy.

SCRAMBLE TRACING #19

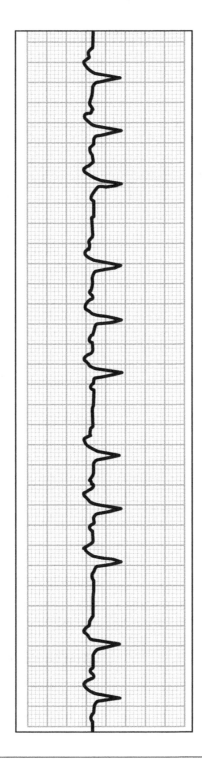

The Nuts and Bolts of Paced ECG Interpretation, 1st edition. By Tom Kenny.
Published 2009 by Blackwell Publishing, ISBN: 978-1-4501-8404-5.

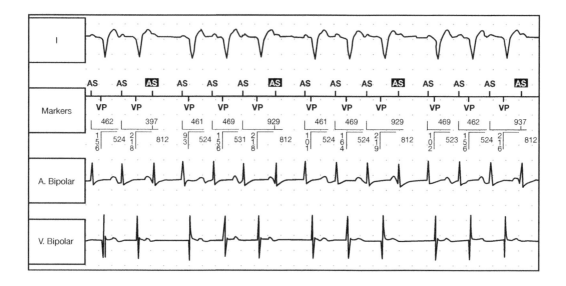

Mode

Even with just the surface ECG and no annotations, this has to be a dual-chamber pacemaker. The widened QRS morphologies indicate ventricular pacing and there is a close relationship of atrial activity to the ventricular pacing, indicating tracking. The programmer screen confirms that this is a dual-chamber device.

Rate

Rate cannot be evaluated here, because the pacemaker is tracking the atrium. The intrinsic atrial rate is stable but high (around 440 ms or 136 bpm).

However, the ventricular paced response shows an interesting pattern. This pattern appears on the surface ECG but it's even more striking in the annotations. For every run of four intrinsic atrial events, there are just three paced ventricular beats in response. Notice, too, that every fourth intrinsic atrial event appears in a box, meaning it occurs during the refractory period. This is 4:3 pacemaker Wenckebach behavior. The pacemaker tracks three atrial events but the fourth one occurs in the refractory period, and so the device will not respond to it, i.e., track it.

Capture

Atrial capture cannot be assessed from this infor-

mation, because all of the atrial activity shown here is intrinsic.

Ventricular capture is appropriate. It is difficult to discern the ventricular pacing spike in the surface ECG (top tracing) but using the VP annotations, it is apparent that every ventricular output corresponds to a ventricular depolarization. The paced ventricular events on the surface ECG all share the same widened morphology.

Sensing

Atrial sensing appears appropriate. Comparing the P-waves on the surface ECG to the annotations and the atrial electrogram, it appears that the pacemaker has "seen" and properly identified all intrinsic atrial events.

Ventricular sensing cannot be assessed from this strip.

Underlying rhythm

This patient has some kind of high-rate intrinsic atrial activity and slow AV conduction.

What to do next

First, atrial capture and ventricular sensing should be evaluated. Atrial capture testing may not be possible in that the pacemaker has to be able to pace the atrium (not desirable and sometimes not even possible during high-rate intrinsic atrial activity).

Ventricular sensing requires that intrinsic ventricular activity emerge. The best way to provoke this is to temporarily program an AV delay interval of 300 ms or higher.

The patient's high-rate atrial activity may be of some concern. Obtain diagnostic reports to see how frequently this occurs. If it is occasional, then probably so-called "upper rate behaviors" of the pacemaker (Pacemaker Wenckebach) may be sufficient to manage it. If it is frequent or causes symptoms, it may be necessary to find other ways to manage it. There are device-based options (mode switching,

the AF Suppression™ algorithm, and so on) to consider, but pharmacological therapy is the first-line treatment for treating symptomatic atrial tachyarrhythmias.

What about the 4:3 pacemaker Wenckebach? Pacemaker Wenckebach is the normal and expected behavior of the device in the presence of high-rate intrinsic atrial activity. This device appears to be programmed appropriately in that even in the presence of atrial rates around 136 bpm, the pacemaker avoids 2:1 block. This is a great example of how a pacemaker can help manage occasional high intrinsic atrial rates while continuing to deliver AV synchrony.

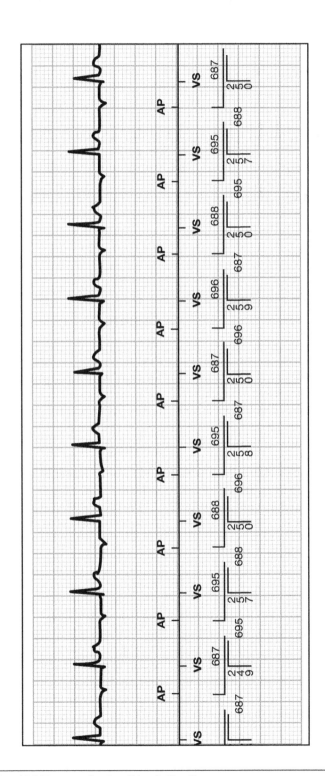

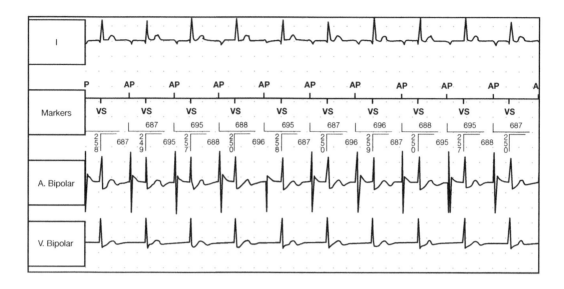

Mode

The surface ECG from the programmer does not exhibit prominent pacing spikes, but the annotations can serve that purpose. Even without annotations, there is a clear relationship between atrial and ventricular activity, suggesting dual-chamber pacing. Annotations point out that the rounded, downward atrial events are paced while the upward, pointed ventricular depolarizations are sensed events.

Use all of the information on the screen to get the big picture. The atrial pacing spikes (AP annotations) show up on the atrial electrograms as the largest spikes and they show up on the surface ECG as depolarizations. The intrinsic ventricular events appear appropriately on the ventricular electrogram but they also show up on the atrial electrogram. This is an example of far-field sensing.

Rate

The atrial pacing interval (AP-AP) is about 680 ms (90 ppm), which requires some kind of explanation. In the case of atrial tracking (AS-VP events), a rate of 90 ppm might be quite normal. But why would the pacemaker pace the atrium above the base rate? The most likely answer is that this device is rate responsive and that the sensor is in control of the pacemaker and has accelerated the pacing rate somewhat.

Capture

Atrial capture appears appropriate. The surface ECG (top tracing) reveals an atrial depolarization for every AP event annotated. All of these atrial events have the same morphology.

Ventricular capture cannot be evaluated here.

Sensing

Atrial sensing cannot be assessed from this information.

Ventricular sensing is a little bit more complicated. Ventricular events on the surface ECG are accurately reported on the annotations as VS events. These ventricular events inhibit the ventricular output and reset device timing. On the surface, it looks like appropriate ventricular sensing.

Looking at the ventricular intracardiac electrogram (bottom tracing), every ventricular event from the surface ECG appears here as well as with the resulting T-wave. This confirms appropriate sensing of the intrinsic ventricular activity and appropriate ventricular inhibition.

Moving up to the atrial intracardiac electrogram (next-to-last tracing), there is a lot more going on!

The largest events on this strip (very tall, narrow complexes) are the atrial output pulses. Since this electrogram is recorded from within the atrium, atrial events are going to be the most prominent events. These events do not confirm capture but they do indicate that the atrial electrogram picked up the atrial output pulses. But notice that there are events between the atrial output pulses that map onto the ventricular activity exactly. The ventricular events (QRS complexes) and the T-waves appear on the atrial electrogram as well!

This is a case of far-field sensing. The electrodes in the atrium are "eavesdropping" on what's going on in the ventricle. The reason far-field sensing occurs is that the ventricle is much larger and also "louder" in terms of signal size, so electrodes that are sensitive enough to pick up smaller atrial signals often also register ventricular signals.

The problem with far-field sensing is that the atrial channel cannot distinguish atrial activity from ventricular activity; all of these signals are "perceived" by the atrial channel as atrial events. This is the reason why far-field sensing often results in double-counting or other forms of oversensing. However, this is not occurring here. Except for the atrial intracardiac electrogram, one would never know that far-field sensing was even going on. So why is the atrial channel picking up far-field signals … and then ignoring them?

The reason is that these far-field signals are falling into the refractory period (the PVARP interval). This means they are overlooked by the pacemaker. By the way, this kind of far-field sensing is not unusual and as long as it does not affect proper pacemaker behavior should be no source of alarm.

Underlying rhythm

This patient has sinus node dysfunction with intact AV conduction. He also has some degree of chronotropic incompetence.

What to do next

Atrial sensing should be evaluated. To encourage intrinsic atrial activity, lower the programmed base rate in gradual 10-ppm steps down to no lower than 30 or 40 ppm. Be sure to tell the patient what is going on, since some patients find these rate decreases unpleasant. It may not be possible to evaluate atrial sensing in all patients.

Test ventricular capture by forcing the device to pace the ventricle. The easiest way to do this is to temporarily shorten the programmed AV delay interval to 130 ms or even shorter.

Since this patient uses rate response, it is good practice to check on rate-responsive settings. Diagnostic reports can reveal how frequently and to what extent rate response is used. Combined with a short patient interview about his activity level and symptoms, this information should be used to adjust rate-responsive parameter settings, if necessary.

Far-field sensing is occurring in this device but the pacemaker's own systems and timing cycles are managing it in such a way that it does not negatively influence device operation. While no adjustment is required here, it would be prudent to look at things that may help mitigate far-field sensing. For instance, it would be helpful if atrial sensitivity and the ventricular output could be reduced, but this should only be done if it in no way compromises patient safety.

Index

Printed and bound by CPI Group (UK) Ltd, Croydon, CR0 4YY

27/10/2024

14580203-0003

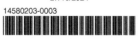